T0212114

Lecture Notes in Computer Science   11837

More information about this series at http://www.springer.com/series/7409

Hua Wang · Siuly Siuly ·
Rui Zhou · Fernando Martin-Sanchez ·
Yanchun Zhang · Zhisheng Huang (Eds.)

Health
Information Science

8th International Conference, HIS 2019
Xi'an, China, October 18–20, 2019
Proceedings

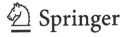 Springer

Editors
Hua Wang ⓘ
Victoria University
Footscray, VIC, Australia

Siuly Siuly ⓘ
Victoria University
Footscray, VIC, Australia

Rui Zhou ⓘ
Swinburne University of Technology
Hawthorn, VIC, Australia

Fernando Martin-Sanchez ⓘ
Instituto de Salud Carlos III
Madrid, Spain

Yanchun Zhang ⓘ
Victoria University
Footscray, VIC, Australia

Zhisheng Huang
Vrije University
Amsterdam, The Netherlands

ISSN 0302-9743   ISSN 1611-3349 (electronic)
Lecture Notes in Computer Science
ISBN 978-3-030-32961-7   ISBN 978-3-030-32962-4   (eBook)
https://doi.org/10.1007/978-3-030-32962-4

LNCS Sublibrary: SL3 – Information Systems and Applications, incl. Internet/Web, and HCI

This Springer imprint is published by the registered company Springer Nature Switzerland AG
The registered company address is: Gewerbestrasse 11, 6330 Cham, Switzerland

Preface

The International Conference Series on Health Information Science (HIS) provides a forum for disseminating and exchanging multidisciplinary research results in computer science/information technology and health science and services. It covers all aspects of health information sciences and systems that support health information management and health service delivery.

The 8th International Conference on Health Information Science (HIS 2019) was held in Xi'an, Shaanxi, China, during October 18–20, 2019. Founded in April 2012 as the International Conference on Health Information Science and Their Applications, the conference continues to grow to include an ever-broader scope of activities. The main goal of these events is to provide international scientific forums for researchers to exchange new ideas in a number of fields that interact in depth through discussions with their peers from around the world. The scope of the conference includes: (1) medical/health/biomedicine information resources, such as patient medical records, devices and equipments, software and tools to capture, store, retrieve, process, analyze, and optimize the use of information in the health domain; (2) data management, data mining, and knowledge discovery, all of which play a key role in decision-making, management of public health, examination of standards, privacy and security issues; (3) computer visualization and artificial intelligence for computer-aided diagnosis; and (4) development of new architectures and applications for health information systems.

The conference solicited and gathered technical research submissions related to all aspects of the conference scope. All the submitted papers in the proceeding were peer reviewed by at least three international experts drawn from the Program Committee. After the rigorous peer-review process, a total of 14 full papers and 14 short papers among 60 submissions were selected on the basis of originality, significance, and clarity and were accepted for publication in the proceedings. The authors were from Australia, Bangladesh, China, Finland, India, the Netherlands, the UK, and the USA. Some authors were invited to submit extended versions of their papers to a special issue of the *Health Information Science and System* journal and will be published by Springer.

The high quality of the program – guaranteed by the presence of an unparalleled number of internationally recognized top experts – is reflected in the content of the proceedings. The conference was therefore a unique event, where attendees were able to appreciate the latest results in their field of expertise, and to acquire additional knowledge in other fields. The program was structured to favor interactions among attendees coming from many different areas, scientifically and geographically, from academia and from industry.

Our thanks go to the host organizations, Shaanxi Normal University, China and Victoria University, Australia, as well as co-organizers/sponsors, Institute of Electronic and Information Engineering of UESTC in Guangdong, China and Guanzhou University, China. Finally, we acknowledge all those who contributed to the success of HIS 2019 but whose names are not listed here.

October 2019

Hua Wang
Siuly Siuly
Rui Zhou
Fernando Martin-Sanchez
Yanchun Zhang
Zhisheng Huang

Organization

General Co-chairs

Uwe Aickelin   The University of Melbourne, Australia
Chunxiao Xing   Tsinghua University, China
Yanchun Zhang   Victoria University, Australia and Guanzhou
                            University, China
Ruoxia Yao   Shaanxi Normal University, China

Program Co-chairs

Siuly Siuly   Victoria University, Australia
Zhisheng Huang   Vrije Universiteit Amsterdam, The Netherlands
Fernando Martin-Sanchez   Instituto de Salud Carlos III, Spain
Rui Zhang   Northwest University, China

Conference Organization Chairs

Hua Wang   Victoria University, Australia
Juanying Xie   Shaanxi Normal University, China

Publicity Co-chairs

Ji Zhang   University of Southern Queensland, Australia
Xiujuan Lei   Shaanxi Normal University, China

Industry Program Chairs

Chaoyi Pang   Zhejiang University, China
Jinli Cao   La Trobe University, Australia

Publication Chair

Rui Zhou   Swinburne University of Technology, Australia

Local Arrangements Chair

Xiaoming Wang   Shaanxi Normal University, China

Workshop Co-chairs

Zhu Wang   Northwestern Polytechnical University, China
Pinghui Wang   Xi'an Jiaotong University, China
Ickjai (Jai) Lee   James Cook University, Australia

Webmaster

Sarathkumar Rangarajan   Victoria University, Australia

Program Committee

Omer Faruk Alçin   Bingöl University, Turkey
Marcos-Gutierrez Alves   Zhejiang University Ningbo Institute of Technology,
                          China
Varun Bajaj   Indian Institute of Information, Technology Design
                          and Manufacturing, Jabalpur, India
Jiang Bian   University of Florida, USA
Genlang Chen   Zhejiang University, China
Soon Ae Chun   The City University of New York, USA
Licong Cui   The University of Texas Health Science Center
                          at Houston, USA
Yanhui Guo   University of Illinois Springfield, USA
Xiaolin Huang   Shanghai Jiao Tong University, China
Xia Jing   Ohio University, USA
Enamul Kabir   University of Southern Queensland, Australia
Rui Li   Xidian University, China
Jingwei Li   University Electronic Science and Technology
                          of China, China
Shaofu Lin   Beijing University of Technology, China
Gang Luo   University of Washington, USA
Saba Munawar   National University of Science and Technology,
                          Pakistan
Tao Qin   Xi'an Jiaotong University, China
Abdulkadir Sengur   Firat University, Turkey
Bo Shen   Donghua University, China
William Song   Dalarna University, Sweden
Le Sun   Nanjing University of Information Science
                          and Technology, China
Weiqing Sun   University of Toledo, USA
Xiaohui Tao   University of Southern Queensland, Australia
Ye Wang   Victoria University, Australia
Yimin Wen   Guilin University of Electronic Technology, China
Fangxiang Wu   University of Saskatchewan, Canada
Xiaofei Yang   Xi'an Jiaotong University, China

Xiaoran Yin	The Second Affiliate Hospital of Xian Jiaotong University, China
Peter Yum	Zhejiang Lab, China
Guo-Qiang Zhang	Case Western Reserve University, USA
Xiuzhen Zhang	RMIT University, Australia
Youwen Zhu	Nanjing University of Aeronautics and Astronautics, China

Additional Reviewers

Zhang, Ying
Chi, Shenqiang
Wang, Jing Jing
Ma, Jing
Xu, Yueshen
Li, Xiaojin
Zheng, Fengbo
Huang, Yan
Ahmed, Alshammari

Contents

EEG and ECG

Medical Image

Medical Information System and Platform

DocKG: A Knowledge Graph Framework for Health with Doctor-in-the-Loop

Ming Sheng[1], Jingwen Wang[2], Yong Zhang[1(✉)], Xin Li[3], Chao Li[1], Chunxiao Xing[1], Qiang Li[4], Yuyao Shao[2], and Han Zhang[5]

[1] RIIT&BNRCIST&DCST, Tsinghua University, Beijing 100084, China
{shengming,zhangyong05,li-chao,
xingcx}@tsinghua.edu.cn
[2] Beijing Foreign Studies University, Beijing 100089, China
{wjwen,shaoyuyao}@bfsu.edu.cn
[3] Beijing Tsinghua Changgung Hospital Medical Center,
Tsinghua University, Beijing, China
horsebackdancing@sina.com
[4] Center for Science and Technology Talents, MoST, Beijing 100045, China
liq@sttc.net.cn
[5] Beijing University of Posts and Telecommunications, Beijing 100876, China
zhanghan3281@bupt.edu.cn

Abstract. Knowledge graphs can support different types of services and are a valuable source. Automatic methods have been widely used in many domains to construct the knowledge graphs. However, it is more complex and difficult in the medical domain. There are three reasons: (1) the complex and obscure nature of medical concepts and relations, (2) inconsistent standards and (3) heterogeneous multi-source medical data with low quality like EMRs (Electronic Medical Records). Therefore, the quality of knowledge requires a lot of manual efforts from experts in the process. In this paper, we introduce an overall framework called DocKG that provides insights on where and when to import manual efforts in the process to construct a health knowledge graph. In DocKG, four tools are provided to facilitate the doctors' contribution, i.e. matching synonym, discovering and editing new concepts, annotating concepts and relations, together with establishing rule base. The application for cardiovascular diseases demonstrates that DocKG could improve the accuracy and efficiency of medical knowledge graph construction.

Keywords: Medical knowledge graph construction · Doctor-in-the-loop · EMR

1 Introduction

Knowledge graph serves as a repository that can integrate information from different sources together. There are concept knowledge graphs which contain only the concepts, and instance graphs which contains instance from the real world. In the medical domain, knowledge graph can support services like disease prediction, medication recommendation [1], etc. The quality of the services depends on the quality of the

© Springer Nature Switzerland AG 2019
H. Wang et al. (Eds.): HIS 2019, LNCS 11837, pp. 3–14, 2019.
https://doi.org/10.1007/978-3-030-32962-4_1

knowledge. Many attempts have been made to build the knowledge graphs completely automatically [2–4] from the data on the Internet [5]. When it comes to medical knowledge graphs, these fully automatic methods seem to be inadequate because of the following reasons:

1. The concepts and relations in medical domain are complex and obscure.
2. The data in medical domain follows inconsistent standards.
3. The data in medical domain is from different sources, heterogeneous and with poor quality.

Therefore, the general ways that have been used to construct knowledge graph automatically cannot be directly applied to the medical domain. On the one hand, it's very necessary to include some experts' experience in the process to improve the quality. On the other hand, if too many human activities are involved in the process, tremendous amount of expert time and effort will be needed and the efficiency of the whole construction progress will be too low [6]. What's worse, the whole system will be too brittle and unable to adapt to or expand to other new medical topics [7]. Therefore, an automatic method that involves an appropriate amount of expert effort is required. Therefore, the balance between the experts' effort and the knowledge graph construction is very delicate and needs to be carefully examined.

In this paper, we introduce DocKG, an overall framework that sheds light on when and where expert effort, also known as doctor-in-the-loop mechanism is needed to improve both the efficiency and quality of medical knowledge graph construction.

This paper is organized as follows. In Sect. 2, previous work related to DocKG will be introduced. In Sect. 3, the overall framework and workflow will be presented. In Sect. 4, when and where to involve doctors, i.e. doctor-in-the-loop will be explained in detail. Section 5 will summarize the paper and discuss possible improvements in the future.

2 Related Work

In this section, we will compare several mainstream knowledge graph building tools, and investigate human-in-the-loop mechanism.

2.1 Knowledge Graph Building Tools

Many automatic knowledge graph building tools have been proposed to process massive data and construct knowledge graphs without human involvement. Below is a summary of some typical knowledge graph building tools:

As Table 1 shows, the mainstream knowledge graph building tools include RDR, cTAKES, pMineR, I-KAT, etc. Among the six tools, less than half of them involve human activities in the construction process. None of them contain all of the four common functions in one single tool. Therefore, it's very inconvenient for the doctors and data engineers to build a high-quality medical knowledge graph with these tools.

Table 1. Comparison of functions between different building tools.

Name	Field	Data source	Entity recognition	Relation extraction	Entity alignment	ER/RDF mapping	Expert Involve
RDR [8]	Medical	–	×	×	×	×	√
cTAKES [9]	Medical	UMLS	√	√	√	×	×
pMineR [10]	Medical	EMR	×	×	×	×	×
I-KAT [11]	Medical	SNOMED-CT	×	×	×	√	√
myDIG [12]	General	csv, JSON	√	√	×	×	×
semTK [13]	General	csv...	×	×	×	√	×
DocKG	Medical	UMLS, EMR...	√	√	√	√	√

2.2 Human-in-the-Loop

In the medical domain, automatic methods based on machine learning have achieved promising results in many aspects like disease prediction and clinical notes classification. Despite that fact that automatic Machine Learning (aML) in medical domain has drawn many researchers' interest and have been growing rapidly, however, one disadvantage lies in their inexplicability [14] because the internal principles are beyond human's comprehension [15]. What's more, aML requires plenty of training sets to achieve promising results, but in the medical domain the researchers are sometimes faced with a small number of datasets or rare events. Therefore, it is necessary to develop algorithms that can interact with agents (like doctors) and can optimize their learning behavior. Through this interaction, training samples can be selected heuristically, and research time can be reduced dramatically. Algorithms that involves humans' interaction can be defined as "human-in-the-loop" [16]. Human-in-the loop has actually been applied to many aspects of artificial intelligence like named entity recognition [17] and rules learning [15] to improve the performance. However, in medical domain, few attempts have been made to incorporate human-in-the-loop mechanism to improve the performance, especially with regards of knowledge graph construction.

3 Framework and Data Flow

In this section, we are going to present the overall framework of the whole system. In order to explain the system in detail, the workflow of the whole construction process will also be presented. In order to store the information required and generated by DocKG, we used Apache Jena database.

3.1 Framework

In this part, the overall framework and workflow will be introduced based on an existing knowledge graph platform, HKGB.

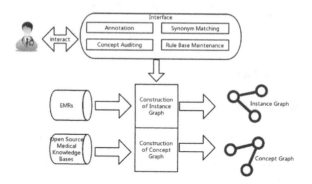

Fig. 1. Framework of medical knowledge graph construction with doctor-in-the-loop.

As Fig. 1 shows, a system that can construct disease-specific medical knowledge graph should include the following parts:

1. Doctors that focus on a particular field of disease.
2. A set of interfaces where the doctors can interact with the whole system.
3. Data sources.
4. Concept graph and instance graph constructors.

In the system, the doctors should be able to interact with the construction process through a set of interfaces. In this way, the doctors can influence the process by "injecting" their experience into the system. In the meantime, a set of automatic tools for constructing a medical knowledge graph is needed. Thus, by providing the interface we managed to combine the doctors' knowledge together with the automatic construction methods.

3.2   Workflow

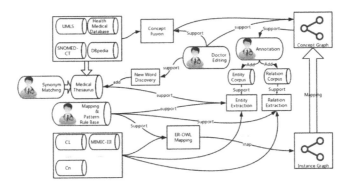

Fig. 2. Workflow of medical knowledge graph construction with doctor-in-the-loop

Figure 2 shows the workflow of the system in detail. In the system, there are four points in which the doctors should be involved.

1. Synonym matching in the fusion and alignment of concepts from different knowledge bases.
2. Doctor editing in the new word discovery and new concept selection.
3. Doctor annotation in the entity and relation extraction from EMRs.
4. Establishment of a rule base that contain both mapping rules and patterns for entity & relation extraction.

The four points will be explained in detail in Sect. 4.

4   Doctor-in-the-Loop in the Construction

In this section, we are mainly going to discuss the four points where the doctors should be involved in detail. Generally speaking, the doctors should provide their opinions on matching synonym, discovering and editing new concepts, annotating concepts and relations, together with establishing rule base to improve the quality of medical knowledge graph. In this section, we will use the construction of a health knowledge graph for cardiovascular diseases as example.

4.1   Synonym Matching Module

Existing medical knowledge bases are very important source of knowledge graph. In order for the information to be fully utilized, the different concepts and relations with the same meaning have to be properly aligned together. To improve the accuracy of the automatic matching methods and efficiency of manual alignment methods, we propose a synonym module that incorporate the results from doctors and matchers. There are two phases in this module: matching phase and aggregating phase (Fig. 3).

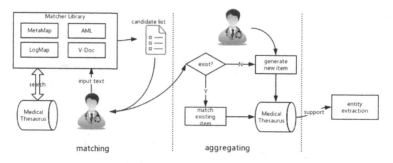

Fig. 3. Workflow of the synonym matching module

This module works on the corpus level and can operate across different data sources. The doctors can input new words or phrases into the module. Then the input text is passed onto the matcher library (a set of different matchers) to be processed. According to the matcher library, a list of candidates that are possible synonym to the input text is returned to the doctors. The list of candidates contains approximately 10 words or so, greatly narrowing down the doctors' search scope. The doctors can then decide by themselves whether the items in the list are synonyms to the input text or not. If there are items in the list that the doctors believe to be synonymous to the input text, then the doctor can align it to one of the existing items that they believe is the best match. If there are not, the doctors can create a new node to integrate the input text into the corpus. The words stored in the thesaurus can then support entity extraction.

The key part of this module is the organization the words and phrases with different spellings, different data sources but the same meaning. To address this problem, we introduce a hierarchical structure. We assign each different concept (words/phrases that have a unique meaning) with a unique concept identity (CID). A concept may have many expressions but only one expression is preferred. This preferred expression is the default representation for the concept. For the expressions that have the same meaning but different spellings or different data sources, we assign each of these expressions with a unique atom identity (AID). The AIDs are child nodes of the corresponding CID. In Fig. 4, we take "Amaurosis Fugax", a typical symptom for heart attack as an example to demonstrate the hierarchical structure.

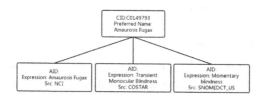

Fig. 4. Hierarchical structure of a concept

4.2   Concept Auditing Module

Unlike the synonym matching module that works on the corpus level, this module works beyond the corpus and on the concept level to provide the doctors with an interface to work directly with the concept graph. This concept auditing module provides two functions to the doctors: (1) concept selection & alignment and (2) new word discovery.

Concept Selection and Alignment

Due to the obscure nature of medical terms, the concepts in the medical thesaurus must be carefully inspected and selected before they can be added to concepts graphs. Figure 5 demonstrates the workflow of concept selection and alignment.

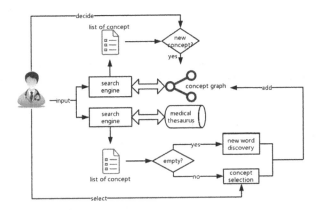

Fig. 5. Workflow of this function

If the doctors want to add a new concept to the concept graph, they can input the text, then the string will be passed onto the search engines on both the medical thesaurus and the conceptual graph. The search engine on the thesaurus will return a list of concepts corresponding to the input strings. The search engine on the conceptual graph will return a list of concepts from the graph that are similar to the concept corresponding to the input string. Instead of having to search manually through the large volume of concepts in the whole thesaurus, the doctors will only need to have a quick scan over the list of concepts provided by the search engines. The doctors can decide by themselves whether the concept corresponding to the input string is a new concept or not. If yes, the doctor can choose one from the list of concepts corresponding to the input string and add to the conceptual graph. However, if the search engine on the medical thesaurus returns no item corresponding to the input string, the doctors should use the new word discovery function described in the following section.

New Word Discovery

The new word discovery function provides the doctors with an interface to customize the terms and concepts that are not in the medical thesaurus. The new terms can be added through the following two methods:

Data-driven Method

This method aims to acquire information from the patients' EMRs. Some features of the EMRs that are not stored in the concept graph can be added.

Table 2. Part of a patient's EMR.

Item	Cardiac apex pulsation	Heart sound A2	Pericardial friction
Result	Accentuated	Split	Normal

Table 2 shows part of a patient's EMR in the cardiology department. Cardiac apex pulsation, heart sound A2 and pericardial friction are all important features for diagnoses on cardiac diseases. However, none of the three features can be aligned with concepts in the concept graph. Under this situation, the doctors can add new concepts to the graph through this module.

Demand-driven Method

The doctors can simply define some concepts and relations based on their own experience. Sometimes the information in the EMRs is simply too complicated and expands over many aspects. The features are too scattered while the doctors only want to narrow their attention down to a few more important features. In this need-driven method, the doctors can leave the EMRs behind and define concepts and relations on a higher level. Figure 6 shows an example of a graph defined by the doctors with a particular focus on the diagnoses of myocardial infarction.

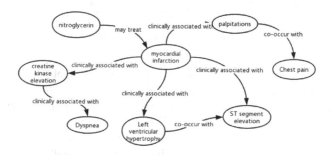

Fig. 6. A high-level graph defined by the doctors

4.3 Entity and Relation Annotation Module

In order to obtain information from the patients' EMRs, entity & relation extraction is needed. The quality of extraction is largely depended on the annotation. However, in the medical domain, there are plenty of entity classes that do not fit the traditionally defined four-class paradigm (PER, LOC, ORG, MISC). For example, in the clinical notes for cardiovascular diseases, there are chest pain location, onset period, etc. If these domain-specific labels are ignored, the quality of extraction based on deep learning methods will decline. Therefore, the annotation module provides the doctors with an interface to annotate the clinical notes in patients' EMRs.

As Fig. 7 shows, this interface is able to load in the patients EMRs and present the clinical notes to the doctors. On the left of the interface listed some pre-defined entity labels, including disease incentive, radiating location, medication name, etc. Apart from these pre-defined labels, the doctors can also customize their own labels. Then the doctors can select words or phrases and assign them with a proper label, or select pairs of entities from the EMR and assign a relation label (shown in Fig. 8) to the pair of entity. The results can then be added to entity & relation annotation respectively to support extraction. The data engineers should focus on using machine learning models, like CRF and CNN-LSTM for automatic extraction, while the doctors can focus on reviewing the results from the models and generating training materials for the models.

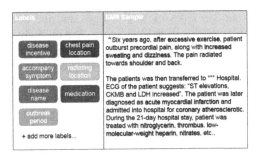

Fig. 7. Interface of entity annotation in detail

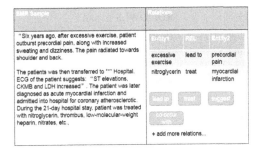

Fig. 8. Interface of relation annotation in detail

4.4   Rule Base Module

In order to support the construction process, there are two types of rules generated by the doctors that need to be stored. One type is mapping rules from ER model to RDF model, another type is extraction rules.

Mapping Rules

The instance graph is described in RDF/OWLS to better present the information in the form of graph. Data stored in ER models needs to be transformed into RDF/OWLS models.

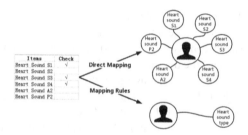

Fig. 9. Mapping process from ER to RDF

As Fig. 9 shows, on the left is an example of the checklist from one cardiovascular patient's EMR. There are six types of heart sounds and the doctors put a mark to suggest that the patient is positive of this symptom. The top right of Fig. 9 shows the direct mapping results: each type of heart sound is assigned to one attribute of the patient. Direct transformation of this ER model may cause the RDF/OWLS to be extremely complex and redundant. However, with the mapping rules (on the bottom right of Fig. 9) defined by doctors, the mapping result can become much simpler and more meaningful. All the six types of heart sound are assigned to one attribute called "heart sound type". With this attribute, the six types of heart sound actually become the values of this one attribute. Table 3 shows an example of mapping rules. The mapping rules will support the construction of instance graph.

Table 3. Example of mapping rules.

ER model	RDF/OWLS model
Heart Sound S1	Heart Sound Type CID:0008123
Heart Sound S2	
Heart Sound S3	
Heart Sound S4	
Heart Sound P2	
Heart Sound A2	
Transfusion of platelet	Blood Transfusion Type CID:0001023
Transfusion of RBC	
Transfusion of plasma	

Extraction Rules

There are two methods for entity extraction: one is based on sequence annotation method and the other is based on rules and patterns. Sequence annotation has been introduced in Sect. 4.3. Here we will focus on rules and patterns for extraction.

Extraction based on rules and patterns has shown some promising results because of its flexibility. This flexibility is especially important in the medical domain because the doctors' demands are frequently changing. By providing the doctors with an interface to customize the rules and patterns, more attention can be put to the more meaningful words that meet the doctors' needs.

First the doctors can define delimiters. Diagnosis of cardiovascular diseases requires extra attention on the patients' symptoms, so the doctors can customize regular expression like "showed symptoms of *". The * can match the words/phrases that suggest symptoms. Then industrial-level NLP tools like spaCy and Jieba with functions of matching and extracting can be applied on the clinical notes. Table 4 shows an example of extraction rules and the extraction result in cardiology. By incorporating the NLP tools, the doctors are freed of the labor to mark the entities manually and can focus more on the information that the text can provide.

Table 4. Example of extraction rules

Input:	
For further diagnosis and treatment, the patient is admitted to our department. The patient was diagnosed with "unstable angina" and "chest pain" in hospital. Since onset, the patient is conscious, he has been treated with nitroglycerin and heparin after admission.	
PATTERN 1:	PATTERN 2:
treated with + * + after admission	diagnosed with + * + in hospital
OUTPUT ENTITY:	OUTPUT ENTITY:
{nitroglycerin}	{unstable angina}
{heparin}	{chest pain}

5   Conclusion and Future Work

In the article, we introduce a knowledge graph framework for healthcare based on doctor-in-the-loop. The key point for the construction process is to combine the doctors' efforts with the automatic methods to achieve the balance between accuracy and efficiency. When and where to involve doctors in the loop is emphasized and there are four points in which the doctors' experience needs to be involved. The four points are: (1) synonym matching, (2) new concepts discovering and auditing, (3) concepts and relations annotation, (4) rule base establishment. Therefore, the quality for medical knowledge graph construction could be improved.

Acknowledgments. This work was supported by NSFC (91646202), National Key R&D Program of China (2018YFB1404400, 2018YFB1402700).

References

1. Wu, C., et al.: Prediction of fatty liver disease using machine learning algorithms. In: Computer Methods and Programs in Biomedicine, vol. 170, pp. 23–29 (2019)
2. Martínez Rodríguez, J.-L., López Arévalo, I., Rios Alvarado, A.B.: OpenIE-based approach for Knowledge Graph construction from text. Expert Syst. Appl. **113**, 339–355 (2018)
3. Wang, C., Ma, X., Chen, J., Chen, J.: Information extraction and knowledge graph construction from geoscience literature. Comput. Geosci. **112**, 112–120 (2018)

4. Qi, C., Song, Q., Zhang, P., Yuan, H.: Cn-MAKG: china meteorology and agriculture knowledge graph construction based on semi-structured data. In: ICIS: IEEE Computer Society, pp. 692–696 (2018)
5. Ye, M.: Text Mining for Building a Biomedical Knowledge Base on Diseases, Risk Factors, and Symptoms. Germany: Max-Planck-Institute for Informatics (2011)
6. Rotmensch, M., Halpern, Y., Tlimat, A., Horng, S., Sontag, D.: Learning a health knowledge graph from electronic medical records. Sci. Rep. 7(1), 5994 (2017)
7. Chen, P., Lu, Y., Zheng, V.W., Chen, X., Yang, B.: KnowEdu: a system to construct knowledge graph for education. IEEE Access 6, 31553–31563 (2018)
8. Hyeon, J., Oh, K., Kim, Y.J., Chung, H., Kang, B.H., Choi, H.-J.: Constructing an initial knowledge base for medical domain expert system using induct RDR. In: BigComp: IEEE Computer Society, pp. 408–410 (2016)
9. Savova, G.K., et al.: Mayo clinical text analysis and knowledge extraction system (cTAKES): architecture, component evaluation and applications. J. Am. Med. Inf. Assoc. 17, 507–513 (2010)
10. Gatta, R., et al.: Generating and Comparing Knowledge Graphs of Medical Processes Using pMineR. In: K-CAP: ACM, pp. 36:1–36:4 (2017)
11. Afzal, M., Hussain, M., Khan, W.A., Ali, T., Lee, S., Kang, B.H.: KnowledgeButton: an evidence adaptive tool for CDSS and clinical research. In: INISTA: IEEE, pp. 273–280 (2014)
12. Kejriwal, M., Szekely, P.: myDIG: personalized illicit domain-specific knowledge discovery with no programming. In: Future Internet, vol. 11, p. 59 (2019). https://doi.org/10.3390/fi11030059
13. semTK. http://semtk.research.ge.com/
14. Amaral, A.D., Angelova, G., Bontcheva, K., Mitkov, R.: Rule-based named entity extraction for ontology population. In: RANLP: RANLP Organising Committee/ACL, pp. 58–62 (2013)
15. Yang, Y., et al.: A study on interaction in human-in-the-loop machine learning for text analytics. In: IUI Workshops: CEUR-WS.org, (CEUR Workshop Proceedings), vol. 2327 (2019)
16. Holzinger, A.: Interactive machine learning for health informatics: when do we need the human-in-the-loop? Brain Inf. 3(2), 119–131 (2016)
17. da Silva, T.L.C., et al.: Improving named entity recognition using deep learning with human in the loop. In: EDBT: OpenProceedings.org., pp. 594–597 (2019)

At Home Genetic Testing Business Process Management Platform

Jitao Yang[(⊠)]

School of Information Science, Beijing Language and Culture University,
Beijing 100083, China
yangjitao@blcu.edu.cn

Abstract. At home genetic testing is currently accepted by a lot of people in many countries, and statistical data show that, currently, at home genetic testing has more than 26, 000, 000 customers all over the world. Generally, the business process for at home genetic testing is: after a user's order, a saliva collection kit will be sent to the user, the user should split saliva to a specific saliva collection tube and send the kit back to laboratory, then the laboratory will extract the DNA from the saliva, and sequence the DNA using next generation sequencing equipment or micro-array platform, the generated DNA sequencing data will be analyzed and genetically interpreted, finally, a genetic report will be sent to the user. To handle millions of samples in a year requires a scalable, robust, parallel, and easy to use business process management system to satisfy the external customer service and internal sample track and management requirement. In this paper, we first describe the detail business process of at home genetic testing, then based on our best practice, using spring cloud, spring boot, and microservices, we give the design and implementation of a business process management platform to support at home genetic testing business. The platform is flexible that supports both the business to business service as well as the business to customer service.

Keywords: Genomics · CRM · Genetic testing · Business process management

1 Introduction

At home genetic testing, also referred to as direct-to-consumer (DTC) genetic testing, is marketed directly to customers without the involvement of a clinical provider to get genetic testing of customers' DNA [3]. The testing generally requests the consumer to collect saliva, and send it to the genomics laboratory for DNA sequencing, analysis, and genetic interpretation. DTC genetic testing has many areas of application including nutrition genomics [4,5], sports genomics [1,2], skin care [6,8], ancestry [11], genetic health risk [9,10], and etc.

© Springer Nature Switzerland AG 2019
H. Wang et al. (Eds.): HIS 2019, LNCS 11837, pp. 15–22, 2019.
https://doi.org/10.1007/978-3-030-32962-4_2

A big at home genetic testing company needs to:

- process millions of samples in a year,
- track samples exactly,
- manage the sale, logistics, experiment efficiently,
- analyze DNA data in parallel,
- interpret DNA data accurately, and
- send genetic reports to customers friendly.

Therefore, it is necessary to design and develop an advanced management system to support the high complex DTC business.

The business management system should provide benefits not only for the customers but also company's internal employees from the departments of sales, marketing, product, laboratory, bio-informatics, genetics, after sale service, and finance; several main functions of the system are outlined below:

- sale, shopping cart, coupon, and the other online shopping functions,
- logistics management and statistics,
- accurate sample tracking and management,
- laboratory experimental steps quality control,
- communicate with laboratory equipment,
- integration with analysis pipelines,
- automated customer interpretation reports generation,
- reports audit,
- sample status sharing with customers and business partners,
- business process efficiency improvement,
- financial statistics,
- access control based on user roles,
- tens of thousands of samples processed in parallel,
- flexible to customize and provide new service for new business partners.

However, because at home genetic testing business is new and there are not many similar companies in the world, therefore, large ERP/CRM software providers such as SAP, Oracle, Microsoft and Salesforce do not have mature business process management software for at home genetic business. Since different business partners may require different experiment platforms (e.g. Next Generation Sequencing platform or micro-array platform) with different types of genetic reports (e.g. report format and testing items could be different), therefore, it is also very challenging for a platform to provide service for millions of customers directly as well as provide customization service for different business partners.

In this paper, we give the design and implementation of an at home genetic testing business management platform, which is a web-based platform that can help DTC genetic testing enterprises to track samples and experimental steps exactly, and bring accuracy, efficiency and flexibility to business workflows.

2 Business Process

Figure 1 demonstrates the business process of the at home genetic testing service. The management platform is composed by four systems: E-Market system, Customer Relation Management (CRM) system, Laboratory Information Management System (LIMS), and Interpretation & Report system.

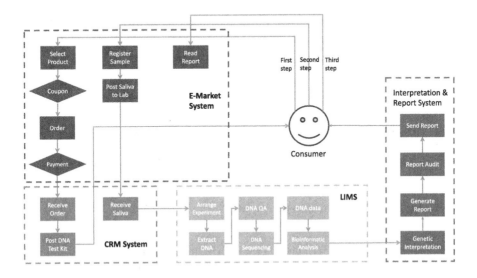

Fig. 1. The business process of at home genetic testing.

E-Market system, supports the customers to browse the genetic testing products online, add the product to cart, checkout the product with coupons, add shipping address, pay the product online. The E-Market system also has the function of providing order status and sample status to customers. The order status function helps customer to track the payment status and the logistics status. The sample status function will tell customer the sample status including sample registered, sample received by laboratory, sample processed in the laboratory, sample sequenced, sample under analysis and genetic interpretation, and genetic interpretation examined and verified.

Customer Relation Management system, will receive the order information from customers, then the staff will be notified to post DNS test kit (a box with instruction book and a saliva collection tube) to the customer. CRM needs to connect with logistics company to know the sample transportation status such as if the sample was posted, which city the sample was arrived in, and CRM will synchronize logistics information to the E-Market system, so that the customer can monitor the posting status of the products purchased.

After receiving the DNA test kit, the customer will first be asked to register the sample information by filling personal information (such as name, age, gender, contact information) together with the bar-code number on the saliva collection tube to the customer information module, which is embedded in the E-Market system. Please note that, the DNA test kit purchaser and the DNA test kit user could be different persons, therefore, the DNA test kit order information has no direct connection with sample registration information. Customer information will also be synchronized to customer relation management system for after sale service.

Laboratory Information Management System, tracks all the sample status and manages all the experimental operations in the laboratory. LIMS will first arrange the sample orders to be sequenced, the experimental procedures will include:

- cells extraction from saliva,
- DNA extraction from cells,
- DNA concentration evaluation,
- DNA amplification,
- DNA fragmentation,
- DNA precipitation,
- DNA resuspend,
- DNA and microarray hybridization,
- extension and dyeing of microarray, and
- microarray scan.

Then the sequencing data will be generated by sequencing equipment [7], and will be stored in persistent storage system. When the new generated sequenced data was detected, the SNP (Single Nucleotide Polymorphisms) [13] calling analysis pipeline [12] will be activated to analyze the sequenced DNA data. The data analysis pipeline can run in parallel to analyze thousands of samples at the same time.

Interpretation & Report system, will interpret the SNPs based on the SNP calling result, using the database (such as OMIM [14,15], and AutDB [16]), the published scientific papers such as Katherine A. et all [17], and the algorithms such as James J. Lee et all [10]. Different companies also have their own interpretation algorithms. The algorithms were encapsulated as an automatic interpretation engine that, the sequenced DNA data are input data, genetic report is the output data which is generated automatically in html or pdf format for customers. The system can generate multiple types of reports such as precision nutrition, precision sports, precision skin-care, etc. The genetic reports are in the format of HTML 5 web pages that can adjust to different web browsers (such as chrome, safari, firefox, and edge) and different electrical equipment (such as computer, iPad, and mobile phones). The system can also produce PDF genetic reports, which is convenient for customers to print their reports. The generated reports also need to be reviewed and verified by genetic experts, then the reports will be sent to customers through the E-market system. The customer will be notified through short messages to read the reports.

3 Platform Implementation

Generally, the business models of at home genetic testing companies are:

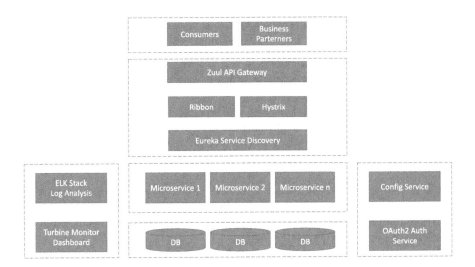

Fig. 2. Microservices with spring cloud.

- selling products to customers directly through their own websites, mobile apps, or the online e-commerce platform such as amazon.com, jd.com, and etc.;
- selling products to business partners, then the business partners sell the products to customers;

Therefore, apart from the support of direct selling of products to customer service, the business process management platform should also have the functions of collaborating with business partners that, the platform is required to provide business process and reports customization services for business partners. For different business partners, the platform will have different laboratory experiment process, different customer relationship management process and different report generation system.

Figure 2 describes the platform architecture, which is constructed using spring cloud [18] with microservices [26]. Each microservice can provide unique genetic reports customization service for one business partner, each business partner can have its own database structure. The microservices can share common data and common business functions.

We chose to use the microservice architecture is because:

- the service scaling is relatively convenient,
- the services are loosely coupled,
- the service could be small and focus on specific service or function,

- the services have well defined interfaces to provide services for external applications and communicate with each other,
- the services can be deployed independently and each service can be developed with different technologies.

In the platform:

- Zuul is the gateway service embedded in spring cloud, it is a server-side load balancer and router;
- Ribbon is a client-side load balancer which is used to control over the behavior of TCP and HTTP clients;
- Hystrix detects failures and uses the encapsulated logic to prevent failures from unexpected system difficulties and errors;
- Eureka is used for service discovery that, every microservice should be registered in Eureka server so that to be discovered and used through port and IP address;
- ELK (Elasticsearch, Logstash, and Kibana) stack is used to search, analyze, and visualize dynamic log data of system in a real time;
- Turbine monitor is used to aggregate hystrix stream to monitor and analyze the overall health of the platform;
- Config service provides a central place for server-side and client-side properties configuration across all the distributed computing environments;
- Oauth2 [21] uses token mechanism to enable external systems to obtain limited access time/authority to the platform.

The microservices in the platform were developed with Spring Boot [19], Spring Cloud, MyBatis [20], and MySQL. The user-interface was implemented with HTML5, CSS3, JQuery, Vue javascript framework [22], the user interface can adjust to different browsers (chrome, safari, firefox, internet explorer) and different screen sizes.

The E-Market mobile application was embedded in WeChat [25], which has more than one billion users. Through the web application service in WeChat, customers can browse the DTC products, place orders, pay the orders. The customers can also receive notifications from WeChat, when the genetic reports are ready, and the customers can read the reports in the web application of WeChat conveniently.

The API services of the platform were encapsulated as RESTful resources to communicate with external business partners.

The platform was deployed in Tencent Cloud [23], the microservices are scalable to be implemented to new docker environment, CDN (Content Delivery Network) [24] was used for high-performance caching files and images.

The platform has been delivered online, which can not only provide service to customers (to C) directly, but also can provide services to multiple business partners (to B). Meanwhile, the platform can accept samples from to C customers and to B customers, and process thousands of samples in parallel a day. Due to the space limitation we cannot show ER diagram of the database nor the interface of the platform in this paper.

Since different business partners have their own product customization requirement, therefore, the platform can support multiple customized business process pipelines and multiple customized reports for different business partners.

4 Conclusions

Currently, at home genetic testing has tens of millions of customers all over the world, and the DTC business is growing very fast in many countries. A big at home genetic testing company needs to process millions of samples in a year, which requires a powerful business process management system to: support scalable and parallel processing of samples, provide service to customers directly, collaborate with business partners, and communicate with multiple agents.

In this paper, we first introduce the at home genetic testing service, then describe the detail business process of at home genetic testing service. We give the design and implementation of a DTC business process management platform, which is composed by e-market system, customer relation management system, laboratory information management system, data analysis pipelines, genetic interpretation system, and report generation and verification system. The platform can process thousands of samples in parallel each day. The platform provides our best practice to at home genetic companies to use spring cloud, spring boot, and microservices to support the at home genetic testing business. The platform can provide service for millions of (to C) customers directly as well as provide customization service for different (to B) business partners.

Acknowledgment. This work was partially supported by the Science Foundation of Beijing Language and Culture University (supported by "the Fundamental Research Funds for the Central Universities") (19YJ040010, 17YJ0302, 15YJ030001, 18YJ030006)

References

1. Sawczuka, M., Maciejewska, A., Cieszczyk, P., Eider, J.: The role of genetic research in sport. Sci. Sports **26**(5), 251–258 (2011)
2. Guth, L.M., Roth, S.M.: Genetic influence on athletic performance. Curr Opin Pediatr. **25**(6), 653–658 (2013)
3. U.S. Food and Drug Administration (FDA): Direct-to-Consumer Tests. https://www.fda.gov/medical-devices/vitro-diagnostics/direct-consumer-tests. Accessed 11 June 2019
4. Simopoulos, A.P.: The impact of the bellagio report on healthy agriculture, healthy nutrition, healthy people: scientific and policy aspects and the international network of centers for genetics, nutrition and fitness for health. J. Nutrigenet Nutrige. **7**(4–6), 191–211 (2015)
5. Sales, N.M.R., Pelegrini, P.B., Goersch, M.C.: Nutrigenomics: definitions and advances of this new science. J. Nutr. Metab. **2014**, 202759 (2014)
6. Makrantonaki, E., Bekou, V., Zouboulis, C.C.: Genetics and skin aging. Dermatoendocrinol **4**(3), 280–284 (2012)

7. iScan System - Array scanner for extensive applications. https://www.illumina.com/systems/array-scanners/iscan.html. Accessed 11 June 2019

8. Gromadzka, G., et al.: Gene variants encoding proteins involved in antioxidant defense system and the clinical expression of Wilson disease. Liver Int. **35**(1), 215–222 (2015)

9. Sanchez-Roige, S., et al.: Genome-wide association studies of impulsive personality traits (BIS-11 and UPPS-P) and drug experimentation in up to 22,861 adult research participants identify loci in the CACNA1I and CADM2 genes. J. Neurosci. **39**(13), 2562–2572 (2019)

10. Lee, J.J., Wedow, R., Okbay, A., et al.: Gene discovery and polygenic prediction from a genome-wide association study of educational attainment in 1.1 million individuals. Nat. Genet. **50**, 1112–1121 (2018)

11. Alexander, D.H., Novembre, J., Lange, K.: Fast model-based estimation of ancestry in unrelated individuals. Genome Res. **19**(9), 1655–1664 (2009)

12. Nielsen, R., Paul, J.S., Albrechtsen, A., Song, Y.S.: Genotype and SNP calling from next-generation sequencing data. Nat. Rev. Genet. **12**(6), 443–451 (2011)

13. U.S. National Library of Health: What are single nucleotide polymorphisms (SNPs)? https://ghr.nlm.nih.gov/primer/genomicresearch/snp. Accessed 11 June 2019

14. Hamosh, A., Scott, A.F., Amberger, J.S., Bocchini, C.A., McKusick, V.A.: Online Mendelian Inheritance in Man (OMIM), a knowledgebase of human genes and genetic disorders. Nucleic Acids Res. **33**(Database issue), D514-7 (2005)

15. OMIM - Online Mendelian Inheritance in Man, an Online Catalog of Human Genes and Genetic Disorders. https://www.omim.org/. Accessed 11 June 2019

16. Pereanu, W., et al.: AutDB: a platform to decode the genetic architecture of autism. Nucleic Acids Res. **46**(D1), D1049–D1054 (2018)

17. Fawcett, K.A., Barroso, I.: The genetics of obesity: FTO leads the way. Trends Genet. **26**(6), 266–274 (2010)

18. Spring Cloud. https://spring.io/projects/spring-cloud. Accessed 11 June 2019

19. Spring Boot. https://spring.io/projects/spring-boot/. Accessed 11 June 2019

20. MyBatis. https://blog.mybatis.org/. Accessed 11 June 2019

21. The OAuth 2.0 Authorization Framework. https://tools.ietf.org/html/rfc6749. Accessed 11 June 2019

22. Vue - The Progressive JavaScript Framework. https://vuejs.org/. Accessed 11 June 2019

23. Tencent Cloud. https://intl.cloud.tencent.com/. Accessed 11 June 2019

24. Content Delivery Network. https://intl.cloud.tencent.com/product/cdn. Accessed 11 June 2019

25. WeChat. https://www.wechat.com/en/. Accessed 11 June 2019

26. Francesco, P.D., Malavolta. I., Lago, P.: Research on architecting microservices: trends, focus, and potential for industrial adoption. IEEE International Conference on Software Architecture (ICSA), Gothenburg, pp. 21–30 (2017)

A Smart Health-Oriented Traditional Chinese Medicine Pharmacy Intelligent Service Platform

Lei Hua[1], Yuntao Ma[3], Xiangyu Meng[2], Bin Xu[2], and Jin Qi[2(✉)]

[1] College of Telecommunications & Information Engineering,
Nanjing University of Posts and Telecommunications, Nanjing 210003, China
[2] School of Internet of Things, Nanjing University of Posts
and Telecommunications, Nanjing 210003, China
qijin@njupt.edu.cn
[3] Nanjing Pharmaceutical Company Limited, Nanjing 210012, China

Abstract. With the national emphasis on traditional Chinese medicine treatments and the development of the modern Internet, people are increasingly showing a strong interest in traditional Chinese medicine, leading to the transformation of traditional Chinese medicine enterprises. The optimisation and innovation of the traditional Chinese medicine pharmacy service has become a hot topic. Therefore, this study combines the advantages of traditional Chinese medicine with Internet technology to build a smart health-oriented traditional Chinese medicine pharmacy intelligent service platform. It integrates hospitals, pharmacies, drug decoction centres, distribution centres and other resources, and forms a traditional Chinese medicine decoction, distribution and traceability system. The system realises the informatisation, automation and standardisation of traditional Chinese medicine pharmacy services. In this study, the platform is implemented using the Internet of Things and the Internet in Nanjing Pharmaceutical Co., Ltd. to provide patients with standard modern drug decoction and distribution services, and to monitor and manage the decoction, distribution and traceability processes.

Keywords: Traditional Chinese medicine pharmacy service · Intelligent service platform · Smart health · Drug traceability

1 Introduction

With the rise of traditional Chinese medicine healthcare, the traditional Chinese medicine market has grown rapidly, becoming the second largest pharmaceutical market after the United States. People are increasingly seeking traditional Chinese medicine prevention and treatment. To benefit more patients, traditional Chinese medicine services have emerged as required [1]. The traditional Chinese medicine pharmacy service faces many problems, such as small workshops, lack of professional talent, poor decoction services, poor equipment maintenance, lax management, and untraceable logistics and distribution. To this end, President Xi announced the goal to

© Springer Nature Switzerland AG 2019
H. Wang et al. (Eds.): HIS 2019, LNCS 11837, pp. 23–34, 2019.
https://doi.org/10.1007/978-3-030-32962-4_3

'vigorously promote the revitalisation and development of traditional Chinese medicine'. On 9 February, 2017, the General Office of the State Council issued a report, 'Several Opinions on Further Reforming and Perfecting the Policy of Drug Production and Circulation Usage', striving to improve the small-scale and scattered state of the pharmaceutical industry [2]. Therefore, there is an urgent need to accelerate the development of the traditional Chinese medicine pharmacy service, improve management and policy systems, improve traditional Chinese medicine services, promote the optimisation and innovation of traditional Chinese medicine, accelerate the informatisation, automation and standardisation of traditional Chinese medicine, and halt the unbalanced development of the traditional Chinese medicine industry.

To this end, this study combines the advantages of traditional Chinese medicine and the Internet, integrating the decoction, distribution and traceability services of traditional Chinese medicine, to build a smart health-oriented traditional Chinese medicine pharmacy intelligent service platform to realise the informatisation, automation and standardisation of the traditional Chinese medicine pharmacy service.

The remainder of this paper is organised as follows: Sect. 2 presents related work and Sect. 3 describes the architecture of the proposed platform. Section 4 presents the processes involved in the proposed platform, including decoction, delivery and traceability services. Section 5 describes the implementation of the proposed platform. Finally, Sect. 6 presents the conclusions.

2 Related Work

The proposed platform involves three main aspects of the traditional Chinese medicine pharmacy services: decoction, distribution and traceability. In this section, we discuss related work along these three aspects.

Regarding the traditional Chinese medicine decoction service, previous studies [3] analysed the issues of the incomplete informatisation and inefficiency of the traditional Chinese medicine decoction business and developed a decoction information management system. Prior literature [4] explored how to successfully conduct traditional Chinese medicine decoction in grassroots hospitals along three dimensions: system, personnel and decoction machinery and provided the theoretical basis for clinical work. At present, most regions have started following the traditional Chinese medicine decoction method, saving patients' time and facilitating medicine consumption. However, decocting traditional Chinese medicine has some drawbacks in terms of efficacy, supervision and other issues, resulting in poor patient experience. To this end, this paper regulates the process of traditional Chinese medicine decoction, adopting the function control system of modern traditional Chinese medicine decocting centres, and uses modern automatic decocting and decoction packaging equipment to monitor the entire decoction process. The core personnel at each post have been professionally trained, and the operation process is necessarily scanned and recorded before each operation step, which helps to assign responsibility retroactively.

Regarding the traditional Chinese medicine distribution service, literature [5] states that human intervention has been reduced through strict control of the distribution process, improving work efficiency and protecting patient rights. Previous studies [6] have conducted the process reengineering of traditional distribution modes and the remote information monitoring of services through the construction of information platforms with traditional Chinese medicine characteristics. Currently, most distribution centres cooperate with third-party courier companies, the distribution equipment is relatively simple and the quality of traditional Chinese medicine cannot be fully guaranteed. To this end, this study utilises cold-chain vehicles for low-temperature distribution. To save costs and improve distribution efficiency, connection points are set at specific locations to achieve alternate delivery of feeder and cold-chain vehicles.

Regarding the traditional Chinese medicine traceability service, prior literature [7] put forward the concept of a two-dimensional code to represent traditional Chinese medicine quality, conceived the quality traceability system based on this two-dimensional code and proposed the online traditional Chinese medicine quality traceability cloud-platform conceptual model. In [8], the authors constructed a visual traceability system from planting and processing to circulation and drinking based on RFID technology and the circulation of Chinese herbal medicines. At present, research regarding the traceability of traditional Chinese medicine pharmacy services is still limited. The current study combines RFID, two-dimensional code and other sensing technologies to scan and trace each link in the traditional Chinese medicine decoction and distribution processes. Patients can utilise the WeChat Official Account, the Internet, public telephones, etc. to query the state of decoction and delivery and conduct real-time monitoring and traceability.

Most of the above literature only described a single aspect of traditional Chinese medicine services, either decoction, distribution, or traceability, and hence, these studies are incomplete and cannot help in providing efficient traditional Chinese medicine services. Therefore, this paper combines traditional Chinese medicine decoction, distribution and traceability services to propose a smart health-oriented traditional Chinese medicine pharmacy intelligent service platform, which is discussed in detail in Sect. 3.

3 Architecture of the Smart Health-Oriented Traditional Chinese Medicine Pharmacy Intelligent Service Platform

The proposed platform, whose architecture is shown in Fig. 1, is divided into five main modules: (1) data perception, (2) data management, (3) system support, (4) technical support and (5) core services.

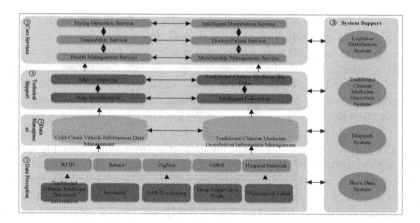

Fig. 1. Architecture of the smart health-oriented traditional Chinese medicine pharmacy intelligent service platform

The main functions of each module of the proposed platform's architecture are described below:

① Data Perception: It utilises RFID to collect decoction information, temperature and humidity sensors to collect environmental information and GPS to obtain vehicle information. Next, the acquired information is uploaded to a back-end database using 4G/5G, ZigBee, GPRS and other technologies for intelligent planning, real-time monitoring and abnormal operation alarms. Additionally, the prescription and delivery statuses are queried in real time by scanning the drug supervision code and related prescription labels.

② Data Management: This module mainly includes cold-chain vehicle information data management, which is required for intelligent route planning, real-time monitoring, abnormal alarms and full-process visualisation of the cold-chain distribution process, and traditional Chinese medicine distribution information management, which manages logistical and distribution-related information of the traditional Chinese medicine products.

③ System Support: This module comprises four parts: the basic data system, the dis-patch system, the traditional Chinese medicine decoction system and the logistics distribution system. The basic data system mainly includes the various types of traditional Chinese medicine data, prescription data, patient-related personal information and treatment information data. The dispatch system organises and analyses the data collected by the perception module, implements intelligent delivery route plans and dispatches the delivery vehicles. The traditional Chinese medicine decoction system standardises the decoction of traditional Chinese medicine. The logistics distribution system provides logistics distribution and cloud-query services for prescription status and logistics status.

④ Technical Support: This module includes related technologies such as traditional Chinese medicine big data, edge computing, intelligent perception and data visualisation. Edge computing enables real-time monitoring, positioning and optimisation of delivery paths. Intelligent perception technology, such as GPS, realises real-time dynamic collection, transportation, monitoring, alarming and visualisation of the entire distribution process, realises effective vehicle scheduling and ensures the quality of traditional Chinese medicine products. The data visualisation technology executes early warning and monitoring of the entire traditional Chinese medicine pharmacy service.

⑤ Core Services: This module comprises six services: frying operation service, intelligent distribution service, traceability service, doctor-patient service, health management service and membership management service. The frying operation service manages the traditional Chinese medicine decoction operation process; the intelligent distribution service provides traditional Chinese medicine quality information, vehicle position tracking and real-time query of prescription and delivery status in the traditional Chinese medicine cold-chain distribution process; the traceability service records the operation by scanning the drug supervision code for patient traceability query; the doctor-patient service provides periodic reports for hospitals and consultation services for patients; the health management service provides patients with health record services and manages personal health information; the member management service provides members with traditional Chinese medicine knowledge services and healthcare recommendations.

4 The Process of the Smart Health-Oriented Traditional Chinese Medicine Pharmacy Intelligence Service

The smart health-oriented traditional Chinese medicine pharmacy intelligent service platform includes processes such as patient visits, doctor prescriptions, decocting in decoction centres, distribution centre dispatch and patient tracking and forming the ordered chain of patient-hospital-decoction centre-distribution centre-patient. The specific processes involved in the traditional Chinese medicine pharmacy intelligent service is as follows: the patient goes to hospital for medical treatment, the doctor creates and uploads the prescription and the patient pays the fee at the billing office. Next, the decoction centre first receives the electronic prescription, audits and dispenses the prescription; subsequently, the formula is reviewed, soaked and fried; finally, the drug is packed and labelled for distribution; lastly, the distribution centre reviews the received invoices and scans the drug supervision code of the traditional Chinese medicine, and delivers the products to the patient. The patient receives the traditional Chinese medicine and confirms receipt by scanning the label on the package [9]. Patients can scan the drug supervision code to accurately trace decoction and distribution links. The service flow chart is shown in Fig. 2.

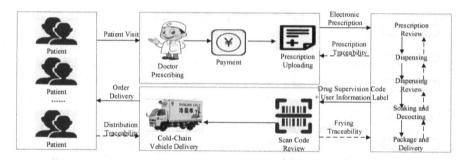

Fig. 2. Flow chart of the smart health-oriented traditional Chinese medicine pharmacy intelligent service

4.1 Traditional Chinese Medicine Pharmacy Decoction Service

The traditional Chinese medicine decoction service involves the following process flow: prescription review–drug formulation–prescription review–soaking–decoction–packaging [10]. The relevant flow chart is shown in Fig. 3.

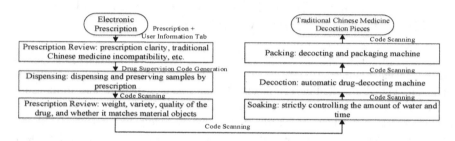

Fig. 3. Flow chart of traditional Chinese medicine pharmacy decoction service

The traditional Chinese medicine decoction centre receives the electronic prescription and the pharmacist reviews the user information label, the clarity of the prescription and contraindications of the Chinese medicine. The blending personnel dispense the medicine as per the prescription, weigh the prescription individually and leave the sample in the sample tray. The reviewer checks the weight of the drug and whether the drug is consistent with the physical sample. The soaking and invigorating personnel add water to soak the formula, strictly controlling the amount of water and time. Using the automatic drug-decocting machine, the decocting staff standardises the cooking of traditional Chinese medicine and strictly controls the heat and boiling time. The packaging personnel pack the medicine using the decoction packaging machine. Operators at each stage scan the drug supervision code for recording purposes, so that the patient can trace his/her query.

4.2   Traditional Chinese Medicine Pharmacy Delivery Service

Considering the drugs from different decoction centres and distribution centres, the traditional Chinese medicine delivery service utilises collaborative edge computing to achieve common distribution [11]. The distribution planning diagram based on collaborative edge computing is shown in Fig. 4.

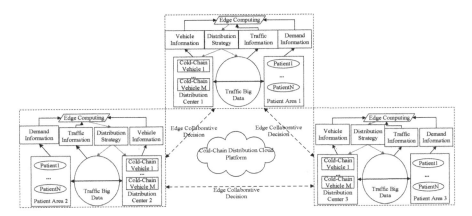

Fig. 4. Distribution planning diagram for edge collaborative decision

The distribution centre, the patient and the traffic big data platforms respectively provide feedback regarding vehicle, demand and road condition status to the edge platform, where it is analysed using edge computing to obtain the corresponding distribution strategy and feedback to the distribution centre's cold-chain vehicle and traffic data platforms for real-time traffic information management and command [12]. To improve distribution efficiency and reduce costs, we set up interchange station. The cold-chain vehicle can temporarily stop at the interchange station and transfer all or part of the traditional Chinese medicine products to one or more shuttle buses, which transport the products at low temperatures to alternate distribution between cold-chain vehicles and shuttle buses [13].

4.3   Traditional Chinese Medicine Pharmacy Traceability Service

The traditional Chinese medicine pharmacy traceability service provides patients with traditional Chinese medicine decoction and delivery services and monitors and records the whole process to facilitate accurate traceability by patients. The system of traditional Chinese medicine traceability service is presented in Fig. 5.

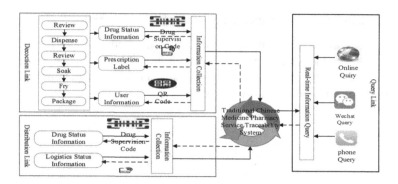

Fig. 5. The system of traditional Chinese medicine traceability service

During the decoction process, the auditing, provisioning, reviewing, soaking, decocting and packaging staff involved in each process is required to scan the drug supervision code to upload to the record, along with drug status information, prescription labels and user information. In the distribution process, drug and logistics status information must also be updated in real time using the scanning code. The key parameters of each link, information about responsible personnel and circulation information are collected and uploaded to the traceability system of the traditional Chinese medicine pharmacy intelligent service, which enables patients to trace and query the status of their product. Specific query methods include online query, WeChat query and telephone inquiry [14].

5   Implementation of the Smart Health-Oriented Traditional Chinese Medicine Pharmacy Intelligent Service Platform

The proposed platform was been implemented in Nanjing Pharmaceutical Co., Ltd. With the cooperation of medical institutions with decoction and logistics distribution centres, we provided patients with decoction, delivery and traceability services and implemented core business processes, such as system operation, traditional Chinese medicine decoction and distribution, user consumption and patient traceability. The implementation of the smart health-oriented traditional Chinese medicine pharmacy intelligent service platform is shown in Fig. 6.

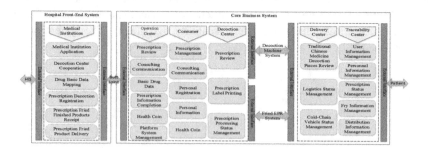

Fig. 6. Implementation of smart health-oriented traditional Chinese medicine pharmacy intelligent service platform

Nanjing Pharmaceutical Co., Ltd. utilises a standard modern decoction process, an automatic decocting machine and a decocting packaging machine produced by regular manufacturers. It has 64 decocting machines and 16 packaging machines in use and 48 decocting machines and 12 packaging machines ready to install. It is estimated that the daily prescription processing capacity can reach 5,000.

Nanjing Pharmaceutical Co., Ltd. builds the Nanjing Pharmaceutical Logistics Centre that implements unified storage management, unified logistics distribution, integrates drug storage and transportation resources, conducts upstream and downstream penetration, achieves multi-warehouse coordinated distribution and uses WMS/WCS, automated guided vehicle robots, automated warehouses, automatic picking points, barcodes/RFID, etc. to realise the informatisation, automation and intelligence of logistics operations. In the process of information transmission, the GS1 code and drug supervision code are uniformly shared and the basic data management platform is built, which leads to the gradual realisation of the traceability of the entire process of product replenishment, order, settlement and transportation. The scheduling decisions of the traditional Chinese medicine distribution centre are shown in Fig. 7.

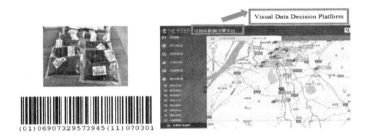

Fig. 7. The scheduling decision of the traditional Chinese medicine distribution center

Nanjing Pharmaceutical Co., Ltd. creates an Internet health service platform for patients to trace the company's activities. The patient generates a personal health file using the WeChat Official Account platform, which can query order information, such as processing and logistics status of the traditional Chinese medicine prescription as well as conduct online consultations and interactions with health assistant on the Internet health service platform. For each related process of frying and distribution, the WeChat platform can be utilised to check the relevant status. If an abnormal operation is detected, it can be traced back to the relevant person responsible, thereby enabling the whole process of monitoring and management. In addition, Nanjing Pharmaceutical Co., Ltd. also uses the supply chain collaboration platform to share data among hospitals, decoction centres, distribution centres and other systems, providing customers and hospital service systems, and understanding drug purchase, sales, storage and distribution information. Block chain technology is adopted to ensure the safety of medical institutions, and all prescriptions are using digital signature to ensure the authenticity of the pharmacist. The WeChat Official Account traceability service is shown in Fig. 8.

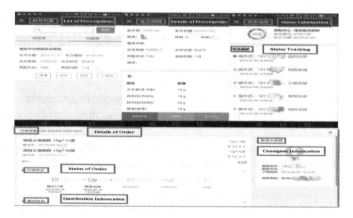

Fig. 8. The WeChat official account traceability service

The sales of the traditional Chinese medicine decoction service centre has grown from 12.38 million yuan/year in 2012 to 34.57 million yuan/year at the end of 2016, while the annual growth rate has remained above 35%. A total of 239,657 prescriptions were decocted and distributed in 2018. The number of traditional Chinese medicine pharmacy service monthly prescriptions in 2018 is shown in Fig. 9. The number of decoction and distribution prescriptions and the amount of sales from 2018 to 2020 are shown in Fig. 10. By the end of 2018, the number of users in the member management CRM system was about 1.5 million, 55 medical institutions were supported. About 5000 orders were processed daily, and the annual prescription was 1 million. The daily order was delivered by 12 noon the next day, and twice a day. The number of drug delivery was 25,000, accounting for 10% of the prescriptions, and the satisfaction of order service was as high as 95%.

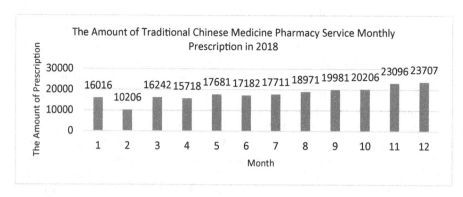

Fig. 9. The amount of traditional Chinese medicine pharmacy service monthly prescription in 2018

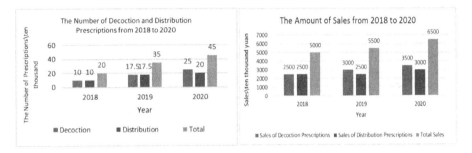

Fig. 10. The number of decoction and distribution prescriptions and the amount of sales from 2018 to 2020

6 Conclusion

In this study, combining the advantages of traditional Chinese medicine and the Internet, and integrating traditional Chinese medicine decoction, drug distribution and traceability services, we built a smart health-oriented traditional Chinese medicine pharmacy intelligent service platform, forming an order chain from patients to hospitals to decocting centres and then to distribution centres and finally to patients. Based on intelligent and automated decoction and logistics distribution facilities, the platform integrates technologies, such as edge computing and intelligent sensing, to better serve the public, reduce user waiting time and easing the pressure on hospitals. Additionally, through interactions with the Internet platform, it can effectively avoid the transmission of hard copy documents and materials, which has a certain degree of social and environmental benefits. Future plans involve extending the platform to grassroots community clinics, setting up regional decoction and delivery centres, establishing a library of Chinese medicine experts, attracting physicians to settle in community medical institutions, developing Chinese medicine clinics, building traditional Chinese medicine health and wellness malls, using 'cloud prescriptions' and 'health mall' platforms, expanding the sales of goods and realising the information management of the entire traditional Chinese medicine pharmacy service.

References

1. Xu, Y.F., Wang, L.X.: Discussion on the pharmacy service under the background of new medical reform. World Latest Med. Inf. **17**(29), 99–100 (2017)
2. Chang, F., Xia, Y.R., Lu, Y., et al.: Development and enlightenment of pharmaceutical service system in Taiwan. Health Econ. Res. **34**(10), 52–55 (2017)
3. Lv, Y.Q., Huang, Y.H., Liu, Y.K.: Design of traditional Chinese medicine decoction information management system. China Digital Med. **9**(06), 52–54 (2014)
4. Yu, K.B.: How to Improve the Quality of traditional Chinese medicine decoction of basic level hospital. China Health Ind. **16**(03), 20–22 (2019)

5. Luo, Y., Wang, X.Q., Chen, C., et al.: Application of traditional Chinese medicine decoction and distribution system based on internet of things. Electron. Technol. Software Eng. **8**(01), 254–255 (2019)

6. Yu, C., Liu, H.L.: Research and development of information platform based on distribution and quality control of traditional Chinese medicine decoction pieces. China Med. Educ. Technol. **30**(01), 98–100 (2016)

7. Cai, Y., Li, X.W., Ni, J.Y., et al.: Traditional Chinese medicine quality traceability system based on two-dimensional code. J. Chinese Med. Mater. **39**(2), 275 (2016)

8. Zhang, C.P., Li, S.X.: Design of traditional Chinese medicine material traceability system based on RFID. J. Sanming Univ. **32**(4), 65 (2015)

9. Wang, Z.M., Jing, S.Q., Gu, M.: Design and implementation of pharmaceutical service information platform. China Digit. Med. **9**(02), 5–7 (2014)

10. Wang, X.M., Shi, Y.: Discussion on the key issues of traditional Chinese medicine outsourcing and decoction in medical institutions. J. Tradit. Chinese Med. Manage. **24**(07), 3–5 (2016)

11. Wu, L.R., Lin, J., Liu, Y.Z., et al.: Regional collaborative distribution method based on vehicle delivery route. Comput. Eng. Appl. **54**(24), 7 (2018)

12. Tao, D.H., Liu, R., Lei, Y.J., et al.: Optimization of cold chain logistics distribution routing based on green supply chain. Industrial Eng. J. **22**(02), 89–95 (2019)

13. Yao, Y.G., He, S.Y.: Research on optimization of agricultural cold chain logistics distribution routing based on traffic big data. Manage. Rev. **31**(04), 240–253 (2019)

14. Wang, J.M., Zhou, Q.S., Jin, L.J., et al.: Reconstruction of traditional Chinese medicine pharmacy service based on WeChat official accounts. China Digit. Med. **11**(12), 92–94 (2016)

Research on a Blockchain-Based Medical Data Management Model

Xudong Cao[1], Huifen Xu[1], Yuntao Ma[3], Bin Xu[2], and Jin Qi[2(✉)]

[1] College of Telecommunications and Information Engineering, Nanjing University of Posts and Telecommunications, Nanjing 210003, China
[2] School of Internet of Things, Nanjing University of Posts and Telecommunications, Nanjing 210003, China
qijin@njupt.edu.cn
[3] Nanjing Pharmaceutical Company Limited, Nanjing 210012, China

Abstract. Medical data plays an important role in government regulation of resources, scientific research and precise treatment of medical staffs. Due to the different data management systems used by each hospital, it is difficult to exchange data among them, resulting in a waste of medical resources. In this paper, a medical data management model based on the blockchain is proposed, which takes advantage of the characteristics of the blockchain, such as decentralisation, tamper-proofing and realizability. A data-sharing reward mechanism was designed to maximise the benefits of both a medical data producer (MDP) and a medical data Miner (MDM) in the process of data sharing, while reducing the risk of leakage of a patient's private information. Finally, a reward mechanism was analysed through experiments, which proved the validity and reliability of the medical data management model based on blockchain.

Keywords: Blockchain · Medical data management · Reward mechanism · Privacy protection

1 Introduction

With the development of modern technology, a large amount of medical data is gathered in the hospital or regional data centre, and it is still growing at an explosive rate. Therefore, the load on the data centre will increase sharply as the amount of data continues to increase, and its security needs require an urgent upgrade, as well. Medical health data is a foundation for public health, academic researchers, pharmaceutical companies, and relevant government agencies for conducting disease prevention, medical research, and drug development through big data mining [1, 2]. However, patients' health data are not sufficiently shared among institutions because different hospitals or clinics have their own independent databases, often leading to repeated medical examinations when the patient transfers from one hospital to another. This not only increases the financial burden on patients, but also heavily wastes medical resources [3]. In addition, medical institutions have absolute control over patients' electronic health records and other data under the traditional mode, so hospitals can

© Springer Nature Switzerland AG 2019
H. Wang et al. (Eds.): HIS 2019, LNCS 11837, pp. 35–44, 2019.
https://doi.org/10.1007/978-3-030-32962-4_4

modify patients' information and health records arbitrarily, or even delete contents, which is unfair to patients [4].

In the medical industry, traditional data storage and processing mostly adopt a centralised strategy. However, the centralised management model cannot meet the growing data demand, and it cannot effectively guarantee security [5]. Blockchain technology has a special technical framework, having the characteristics of decentralisation, high reliability and low cost. Aiming at the problems existing in the traditional centralised management model of medical data, this paper proposes a novel medical data management model based on blockchain technology, and proposes a reward mechanism based on this model, which effectively realises the balance between patient privacy protection and economic interests. The main contributions of this paper are as follows:

- Aiming at the shortcomings of the traditional medical data management model, a new medical data management model based on blockchain technology is proposed.
- A reward mechanism is designed for the medical data management model based on blockchain technology, which can ensure maximum benefits of MDP and MDM.
- A large number of simulations were carried out to simulate the real medical data transaction scenario under realistic conditions, which proved the reliability and practicability of the designed reward mechanism.

The remainder of this paper is organised as follows. Section 2 outlines the related work in this area of research. Section 3 is a medical data management model proposal based on the blockchain. Section 4 discusses the reward mechanism in the data transaction model of this paper. Section 5 presents analyses of the experimental results. The last part summarises the work.

2 Related Work

In the medical industry, data storage and sharing are of great significance to the development of smart healthcare and academic research activities. Traditional medical data are generally adopting centralised data management, which means all medical data are maintained and stored by a large central service system. Centralised data management has the advantages of easy backup, easy implementation, low-cost, high-capacity and strong processing. Its model has been favoured by academia and the engineering fields.

Thilakanathan et al. [6] proposed a centralised cloud platform, which allows doctors to monitor, access and share patient medical data. The work in [7] considered using a large cloud platform to collect, store and process medical data through a unified standard that recognises the platform as a fully trusted central authority for all network entities. Li et al. [8] focused on a semi-trusted cloud computing environment, through attribute-based encryption technology to achieve fine-grained data access control and avoid exposing users' private information to unauthorised parties. The work in [9], a rural medical information system based on cloud computing, was proposed to provide lowest cost medical data management services for rural people. These tasks are to store user information in the cloud platform, through which authorised medical practitioners or patients can access information. However, the above traditional centralised data management cannot adapt to the growing volume of medical data, and its security is also difficult to guarantee.

In view of the problems existing in the centralised medical data management scheme, the use of blockchain technology to provide secure distributed medical data management services [10] have attracted extensive attention. An enhanced, trusted patient medical data-sharing model was proposed in [11], which had highly secure data encryption and decryption technology that encrypts patient information before sending it through the blockchain network. Doctors need to obtain the permission of the blockchain network to allow sharing of patient health information. Azaria et al. [12] designed a blockchain-based system called MedRec for electronic medical record management. In the MedRec, medical stakeholders such as medical scientist and public health authorities are involved as miners. The work in [13] adopted the distributed scheme of cloud computing and mobile computing to realise information sharing. The distributed virtual terminal was used to complete the communication and mining process, and the blockchain-based client server calculation ensured data integrity and traceability. The work in [14] used blockchain technology to share medical data through cloud computing. In this system, the author used intelligent contract and authentication permission to access data from different platforms.

A distributed medical data-sharing model based on blockchain technology has been studied, but most of the existing work has explored innovation in the medical data management model or new infrastructure. This paper proposes a medical data management model based on the blockchain, and on this basis, a new data-sharing reward mechanism and pricing calculation scheme, designed to ensure that both patients and medical data miners can achieve their best interests in data transactions, and further strengthen the protection of patients' privacy.

3   Blockchain-Based Medical Data Management Model

In order to further explore the medical data management based on the blockchain, a new blockchain-based medical data management model is proposed in this paper. There are three types of nodes in this model, namely, medical data producer (MDP), regulatory department and medical data miner (MDM), as shown in Fig. 1.

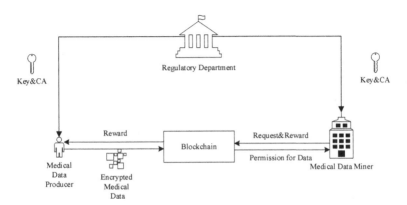

Fig. 1. Medical data management model based on blockchain

Medical Data Producer. MDP includes patient and medical staff group who produce a large amount of prescription information and electronic medical record data, which are usually stored in the hospital information system. First, the doctor checks the information with the patient and obtains the patient's consent. After obtaining permission, the data is packaged, encrypted and uploaded to the public blockchain in the form of a block. In addition, intelligent medical devices in patients' daily life can also generate a large amount of health data, which is packaged and encrypted by patients and uploaded to the public blockchain in the same way. Finally, all patients' medical data will be uploaded to the public blockchain for storage, laying the foundation for breaking the information barrier between medical institutions and data management departments.

Regulatory Department. Regulators are regarded as absolutely credible institutions in this framework, and this role is usually played by the relevant government departments. The main task of the regulatory department is responsibility for distribution and backup of the keys. At the same time, the users in the architecture are authenticated to ensure that the identity information is authentic and reliable, and digital certificates are issued for them. In order to ensure that the certificate cannot be tampered with, the regulatory department performs a hash calculation on the digital certificate, then digitally signs the generated digital digest with its own private key and puts this into the digital certificate.

Medical Data Miner. MDM refers to the users who need large-scale medical data mining and statistical learning, usually including pharmaceutical manufacturers, insurance companies, pharmaceutical distribution companies, scientific research personnel and so on. In the proposed model, MDM broadcasts data requirements to each node through the blockchain platform, and issues the required data amount, data type, reward for each data record and other parameters. Some users who are satisfied with the relevant conditions of their release, will separately trade with consumers through a series of smart contracts; then, consumers will get the right to use the corresponding data. At the same time, data owners will be rewarded.

4   Data-Sharing Reward Mechanism Oriented to the Blockchain

Medical data contains huge volumes of patients' private information. Using the blockchain as the carrier of stored medical data can ensure patients' privacy. In this paper, patient data (including medical records, personal health data generated by intelligent terminals, prescription information, medical record information, etc.) are confirmed by doctors and encrypted by patients, aiming to ensure the correctness of data by doctors and the safety of data by patients.

Medical data D_i generated by MDP_i and intelligent terminals are confirmed by the family or community doctor. Other medical data generated by medical records are confirmed by the doctor to ensure the correctness of the data, and personal ID D_{id_k} of doctor K is added to D_i [15]. Data digest A_i is generated by hash algorithm, and data digest and timestamp are encrypted by public key E_{PK_i} of MDP_i. Rcd_i is the medical data record to be uploaded. T_i is the timestamp when each data record is uploaded,

$hash(x)$ is a hash function, meaning that the variables in the function are mapped to the corresponding hash value, i.e. the summary of medical data is generated.

$$A_i = hash(D_i \&\& D_{id_k}) \tag{1}$$

$$Rcd_i = E_{PK_i}(A_i \&\& T_i) \tag{2}$$

In order to share medical information with MDM without harming the interests of MDP, it is necessary to choose a reasonable reward mechanism. This paper proposes an effective reward mechanism for medical data sharing to encourage patients to share data. In this data transaction model, MDM is the reward provider, while MDP is the reward recipient. We propose respective benefit functions for both parties, so that both parties can make the best decision under our proposed sharing reward mechanism.

For MDP, its comprehensive benefits are related to actual economic benefits and privacy costs. We suppose that MDP_i has the data in which MDM_j is interested. When MDM_j sends transaction requests to MDP_i, MDP_i chooses the number of data records n_i^j contributed to MDM_j according to its own interests, in order to achieve the highest comprehensive benefit H_i^j of MDP_i.

$$H_i^j = p_i^j n_i^j - e^{\alpha n_i^j} + 1 \tag{3}$$

Here, p_i^j means that MDM_j gives MDP_i a reward for each medical data record, and $p_i^j n_i^j$ represents the actual economic benefits of MDP_i. $e^{\alpha n_i^j} - 1$ denotes the patient's privacy cost, and α denotes the risk coefficient. The larger α is, the greater the risks of user privacy disclosure and the higher the privacy cost. In this paper, we use $e^{\alpha n_i^j}$ to describe the cost of user privacy, because the more data records shared by MDP, the more relevant information MDM has, and the more likely it is to infer the patient's privacy information, so that the risk will increase exponentially [16].

Formula (3) shows that the more data MDP_i chooses to share with data miner j, i.e., the larger n_i^j, the greater the economic benefits gained by MDP_i; the greater the n_i^j, the higher the risk of privacy disclosure MDP_i will assume. So, MDP_i needs to choose the shared data record volume n_i^j to maximise its overall benefits. In order to prove that formula (3) has a maximum value, the first and second partial derivatives of formula (3) are calculated as follows:

$$\frac{\partial H_i^j}{\partial n_i^j} = p_i^j - \alpha e^{\alpha n_i^j} \tag{4}$$

$$\frac{\partial^2 H_i^j}{\partial n_i^{j2}} = -\alpha^2 e^{\alpha n_i^j} < 0 \tag{5}$$

The second partial derivative is ≤ 0, meaning that the function H_i^j has a maximum value in its domain, so that MDP_i can choose the optimal shared data records quantity n_i^{j*} to maximise H_i^j. Where n_i^{j*} is the extreme point, i.e., the value of n_i^j when the first-order partial derivative is 0,

$$n_i^{j*} = \frac{\ln\left(\frac{p_i^j}{\alpha}\right)}{\alpha} \qquad (6)$$

Given the p_i^j of each data record, n_i^{j*} is the optimal number of shared data records. Considering that the number of shared data records cannot exceed the total number of data records N_i owned by MDP_i, there are the following restrictions:

$$n_i^{j*} = \begin{cases} \frac{\ln\left(\frac{p_i^j}{\alpha}\right)}{\alpha} & n_i^{j*} < N_i \\ N_i n_i^{j*} \geq N_i \end{cases} \qquad (7)$$

For MDM, its economic benefits are related to the capability of MDM to transform data values to economic assets after performing the data mining task and factoring in the market price and actual cost of each medical data record. We assume that MDM_j is interested in the data of N MDPs. Each MDP_i adjusts the shared data amount n_i^j according to the price p_i^j given by MDM_j. In turn, each MDM_j adjusts the pricing p_i^j according to the optimal shared data amount n_i^{j*} of MDP_i, so that the economic benefit function E_j of MDM_j reaches its maximum [17].

$$E_j = C_j \cdot m_j \sum_i n_i^j - \sum_i p_i^j n_i^j \qquad (8)$$

Here, $C_j \cdot m_j \sum_i n_i^j$ denotes the total economic benefits of MDM_j after data mining, $\sum_i p_i^j n_i^j$ denotes the cost incurred by MDM_j in obtaining data, C_j denotes the ability of MDM_j to convert collected data into the real economy, and m_j denotes the market price of each data record.

There are also corresponding constraints for MDM. First, MDM_j has an upper limit of l_{imax}^j for acquiring MDP_i data records to prevent the complete disclosure of MDP_i's data and protect his privacy interests; secondly, MDM has the minimum total data record demand L_{jmin} according to its actual needs [17]:

$$\max E_j \text{ when } n_i^j = \frac{\ln\left(\frac{p_i^j}{\alpha}\right)}{\alpha} \qquad (9)$$

$$\text{s.t.} 0 \leq n_i^j \leq \min\left(N_i, l_{imax}^j\right) \qquad (10)$$

$$\sum_i n_i^j \geq L_{jmin} \qquad (11)$$

Finally, in order to maximise the comprehensive interests of MDP, the reward mechanism adjusts the price of each data record to maximise the actual economic interests of data mining workers and maximises the interests of both sides when both sides make the optimal strategy.

Through the above analysis, the reward mechanism can iterate through the changing strategies of both sides, and finally converge to a certain optimal solution. This means that in the actual medical data sharing scenario, both MDP and MDM can maximise the interests of both sides, and realise the safe sharing and management of medical data.

5 Results and Analysis

Under the consideration that there are few researches on medical data management based on blockchain at home and abroad, especially the maximization of benefits of both parties in medical data transaction driven by incentive mechanism, it is difficult to conduct comprehensive analysis of this model and compare it with other researches. In order to realise the sustainable implementation of the incentive mechanism mentioned above under the proposed medical data-sharing model, we conducted multiple iterations in this experiment to simulate a real-life medical data trading scenario. First, MDM sent data requests to MDP to access relevant medical data records. Then MDM gave the price p_i^j of each medical data record, which led MDP to change the transaction volume n_i^j of data records correspondingly in order to achieve its maximum comprehensive benefits. Then MDM changed the price p_i^j to achieve its maximum economic benefits. When MDM_j achieved its maximum economic benefit, the price p_i^j changed again, which led to the change in the best data record transaction volume of MDP. We therefore iterated repeatedly until the benefits of both converged to a certain value. We could then get the best pricing and corresponding best data record transaction volume.

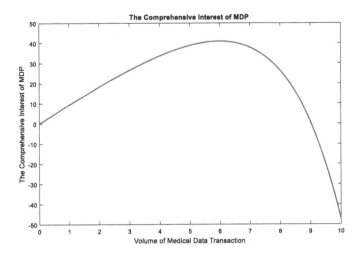

Fig. 2. Comprehensive interest curve of MDP

For MDP, we dynamically select the shared data n_i^j to maximise its benefits. The benefit function of MDP is shown in Fig. 2. It can be seen that as long as the appropriate data transaction volume is selected, its benefits can be maximised.

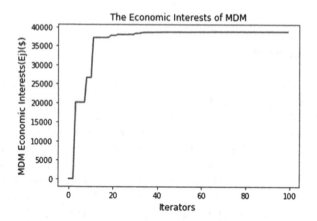

Fig. 3. Economic interest curve of MDM

For MDM, we assumed that there were 500 MDPs in the experiment. The ability of MDM_j to convert data into economic benefits was $C_j = 2.6$. The market price was one dollar for every thousand medical data records, that is, $m_j = 1 (\$/kilo)$, and the number of iterations was set to 100. Figure 3 shows that the best real economic benefits of MDM had stabilised around 50 iterations.

At the same time, we analysed the effects of different parameters on the interests of MDM in the experiment. First, we analysed the impact of MDM_j's ability to translate data into economic benefits C_j on the results. In Fig. 4, we show the impact of different average transaction volumes on MDM.

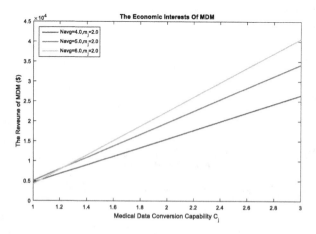

Fig. 4. Effect of parameter C_j on MDM's benefits

As shown in Fig. 4, with the same level of transformation capability C_j, the larger the average transaction volume, the greater the benefits MDM got; when the average transaction volume was the same, the stronger the transformation capability, the greater the benefits MDM got.

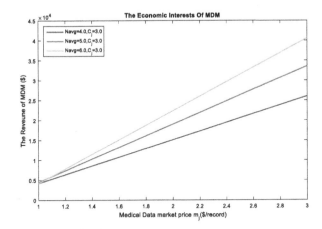

Fig. 5. Effect of parameter m_j on MDM's benefits

Finally, we analysed the impact of market price m_j on the interests of MDM. In Fig. 5, we can see that given the same average transaction volume of data record, E_j and m_j were linearly dependent, and the higher the market price m_j was, the higher the revenue of MDM would be; when given the same parameter m_j, the larger the average transaction volume of the data record was, the greater the revenue of MDM would be.

The experimental results showed that the reward mechanism could well support the blockchain-based medical data management model proposed in this paper and ensure the security of patients' privacy data while guaranteeing the best interests of both parties in the data transaction process.

6 Conclusion

In this paper, a blockchain-based medical data management model is proposed to encourage patients to upload and trade data, which helps to break through the barrier of different medical data management systems and improve the utilisation of medical data. In the proposed model, the regulatory department acts as a fully-trusted authority, responsible for the distribution and management of personnel keys and digital certificates. Patients have sole ownership and sharing rights of their medical data, and the rewards provided by MDM can be used for patients' medical expenditure. Moreover, we propose a data upload chain encryption method to achieve data security uploads. Finally, a reward mechanism was designed between MDP and MDM, which proved the feasibility of the reward mechanism and the reliability of the model through experimental analysis. Next, we will implement the blockchain-based medical data management system on the basis of the above model and the reward mechanism, at the same time fully combined with the actual situation of China's medical and health undertakings, and introduce the diversified technology, to realize the security of medical data sharing, lay a foundation for the development of China's medical and health undertakings, eventually improve the overall health level in our country.

References

1. Hunter, P.: The big health data sale: as the trade of personal health and medical data expands it becomes necessary to improve legal frameworks for protecting patient anonymity handling consent and ensuring the quality of data. EMBO Rep, p. e201642917 (2016)
2. Alkureishi, M.A., et al.: Impact of electronic medical record use on the patient-doctor relationship and communication: a systematic review. J. Gen. Internal Med. **31**, 548–560 (2016)
3. Abbas, A., et al.: A review on the state-of-the-art privacy-preserving approaches in the e-health clouds. IEEE J. Biomed. Health Inf. **18**(4), 1431–1441 (2014)
4. Kupwade Patil, H., et al.: Big data security and privacy issues in healthcare. In: 2014 IEEE International Congress on Big Data, pp. 762–765, Anchorage, AK (2014)
5. Tawalbeh, L.A., et al.: Mobile cloud computing model and big data analysis for healthcare applications. IEEE Access **4**, 6171–6180 (2016)
6. Thilakanathan, D., et al.: A platform for secure monitoring and sharing of generic health data in the cloud. Future Gener. Comput. Syst. **35**, 102–113 (2014)
7. Zhang, Y., et al.: Health CPS: healthcare cyber-physical system assisted by cloud and big data. IEEE Syst. J. **11**(1), 88–95 (2017)
8. Li, M., et al.: Scalable and secure sharing of personal health records in cloud computing using attribute-based encryption. IEEE Trans. Parallel Distrib. Syst. **24**(1), 131–143 (2013)
9. Padhy, R.P., et al.: Design and implementation of a cloud based rural healthcare information system model. Univ. J. Appl. Comput. Sci. Technol. **2**(1), 149–157 (2012)
10. Esposito, C., et al.: Blockchain: a panacea for healthcare cloud-based data security and privacy. IEEE Cloud Comput. **5**(1), 31–37 (2018)
11. Kim, K.J., et al.: A trusted sharing model for patient records based on permissioned Blockchain. J. Int. Comput. Serv. (JICS) **6**, 75–84 (2017)
12. Azaria, A., et al.: Medrec: using blockchain for medical data access and permission management. In: Proceedings 2nd International Conference on Open Big Data, pp. 25–30 (2016)
13. Yik Him, H., et al.: Mobile inter cloud system with blockchain. In: Proceedings of the International Multi Conference of Engineers and Computer Scientists, vol. 1 (2018)
14. Sharma, P.K., et al.: A distributed blockchain based vehicular network architecture in smart City. J. Inf. Proc. Syst. **13**(1), 84 (2017)
15. Manogaran, G., Thota, C., Lopez, D., Sundarasekar, R.: Big data security intelligence for healthcare industry 4.0. In: Thames, L., Schaefer, D. (eds.) Cybersecurity for Industry 4.0. SSAM, pp. 103–126. Springer, Cham (2017). https://doi.org/10.1007/978-3-319-50660-9_5
16. Romanosky, S., et al.: Privacy costs and personal data protection: economic and legal perspectives. Berkeley Technol. Law J **24**(1), 1061 (2009)
17. Li, X., et al.: EdgeCare: leveraging edge computing for collaborative data management in mobile healthcare systems. IEEE Access **7**, 22011–22025 (2019)

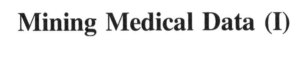

Mining Medical Data (I)

Identifying Candidates for Medical Coding Audits: Demonstration of a Data Driven Approach to Improve Medicare Severity Diagnosis-Related Group Coding Compliance

Yunyi Feng[1], Simon Lin[2], En-Ju Lin[2,3], Lesley Farley[2], Yungui Huang[2], and Chang Liu[1(✉)]

[1] School of Electrical Engineering and Computer Science,
Ohio University, Athens, OH, USA
liuc@ohio.edu
[2] The Research Institute, Nationwide Children's Hospital, Columbus, OH, USA
[3] Department of Biomedical Informatics, The Ohio State University,
Columbus, OH, USA

Abstract. Correct code assignment of Medicare Severity Diagnosis-Related Group (MS-DRG) is critical for healthcare. However, there is a gap currently on automatically identifying all potentially miscoded cases and prioritizing manual reviews over these cases. This paper reports a new process using a data-driven machine learning approach to flag potentially misclassified cases for manual review. We investigated using a stack of regularized logistic/softmax regression, random forest, and support vector machine to suggest potential cases for manual review by care providers, provided details addressing the data imbalance, and explored using features from various source including diagnosis and procedure codes, length of stay and the access log data from the electronic health record system. This potentially improves the efficiency of the coding review by care providers, providing another line of defense against miscoding to enhance coding compliance, and reduce the negative effects of upcoding and downcoding. We tested the new method with four common pediatric conditions and demonstrated its feasibility.

Keywords: Medical coding audit · MS-DRG

1 Introduction

Diagnosis-Related Group (DRG) is a system to classify inpatient stays into groups of similar illness, severity, prognosis, treatment difficulty, and resource utilization [1]. Since complications and comorbidities (CC) can increase medical complexity and increase resource utilization, the Medicare Severity DRG (MS-DRG) system further splits the DRG codes based on the presence or absence of CC or major CC (MCC). For example, *Simple pneumonia and pleurisy without CC/MCC (MS195)*, *Simple pneumonia and pleurisy with CC (MS194)*, and *Simple pneumonia and pleurisy with MCC*

H. Wang et al. (Eds.): HIS 2019, LNCS 11837, pp. 47–57, 2019.
https://doi.org/10.1007/978-3-030-32962-4_5

(MS193) reflects increased levels of medical severity. In this paper, we focus on MS-DRG coding and thus abbreviate MS-DRG to DRG from here on.

Proper coding is important for care providers in a number of ways [1]. First, accurate DRG ensures that the hospital is properly reimbursed by the Centers for Medicare and Medicaid Services (CMS) for the service delivered for their Medicare/Medicaid patients [2]. Secondly, DRG is used to calculate the Case Mix index of a hospital, which reflects the clinical complexity of the patient population a hospital cares for. CMS uses Case Mix index to adjust reimbursement, compensating hospitals caring for a more complicated patient mix, thus it directly affects cost recovery for the hospital. Moreover, an accurate Case Mix index allows a hospital to do appropriate quality comparison against other hospitals or benchmark measures for equivalent patient severity.

Beyond the financial impact to the providers, accurate DRG coding has significant impact on the whole healthcare system. In US, the healthcare cost is rising every year representing a significant portion of US's gross domestic product (17.7% by $3.3 trillion in 2016) [3]. Inaccurate coding, along with other reasons such as insufficient documentation and medical necessity, contributed to the $36.21 billion in gross improper payments by the CMS [4]. The high cost for recovery audit means more taxpayer dollars going towards administrative overheads rather than actual healthcare. Some of the high healthcare cost is transferred to patients as deductibles. In addition, there is intense interest in developing data-driven approach for healthcare applications such as readmission prediction, utilization prediction and resource allocation. Many clinical research studies also use these medical data to identify study cohorts. Thus, correct DRG coding ensures the validity of these secondary data analyses. Most hospitals use vendor software to assign a DRG after a patient is discharged. To ensure correct assignment, medical coders would select a subset of the records for manual review [5]. CMS conducts yearly audits through the Comprehensive Error Rate Testing (CERT) program to determine improper payments, which include both overpayments and underpayments. While overpayments are primarily due to insufficient clinical documentation, underpayments are more likely a result of assigning a lower-level DRG code [6]. Notably, both overcoding (or upcoding) and undercoding (downcoding) are considered coding errors and constitute noncompliance by the CMS. Overcoding, or upcoding, is the reporting of a higher-level service or a more complex diagnosis, than is supported by medical necessity or the provider's documentation. In contrast, undercoding, or downcoding, is when the code billed does not adequately represent the full extent of medical complexity of a patient and the service performed by the physician. One of the more effective ways to prevent coding errors and repercussions from noncompliance is to perform internal audits to address potential miscoding.

Here we propose an automated, data-driven method that can identify claims with the highest risk of falling into a different DRG severity code. This method comprises two modules: building a mapping between correct DRG coding and inpatient stays using historical audited data and using this built model to rate new cases based on the risk of miscoding. Our approach prioritizes the ambiguous cases for manual review by the care providers, ensures that the effort by the auditing staff makes the largest impact, and potentially provides another line of defense against miscoding before reaching CMS's auditing. It can catch both overcoding and undercoding errors.

2 Methods

2.1 Study Design and Data Source

To demonstrate the feasibility of our new method, we used clinical and billing records for inpatient visits at Nationwide Children's Hospital (NCH; Columbus, Ohio) from 2009 to 2016. Specifically, the DRG codes assigned for an inpatient stay, the International Classification of Diseases (ICD) diagnosis codes, Current Procedural Terminology (CPT) codes associated with the encounter and length of stay (LOS) were retrieved from the NCH electronic data warehouse. All ICD and CPT codes encountered in those historical visits in the dataset were used. The number of ICD codes varied from hundreds to over a thousand among the four different sets. The number of CPT codes are in the hundreds among the sets. In addition, electronic health record (EHR) access log variables extracted for this study include number of users, processes and sessions associated with the records of the hospital stay. In accordance with the Common Rule (45 CFR 46.102[f]) and the policies of Nationwide Children's Institutional Review Board, this study using a de-identified data set was not considered human participants research. For this reason, it was not subject to Institutional Review Board approval, and consent was not obtained from the patients.

We selected four base DRGs along with their subdivisions on level of severities (i.e. major CC, CC and non-CC categorization). The four base DRGs are bronchitis & asthma (2 levels), seizures (2 levels), simple pneumonia and pleurisy (3 levels), and premature birth (6 levels). They were chosen as they were the most frequent base codes in the hospital's data and the numbers of cases at each level of severities were relatively balanced. Our selection also encompasses the different types of DRG categorization in terms of their complexity: 2 levels includes with/without CC/MCC, or with/without MCC; 3 levels include with MCC, with CC, without CC/MCC; neonate/newborn code is unique in that the 6 codes picked are all related to newborn but of different medical complexity and resource needs. The DRGs selected for the study along with the number of cases for each code are shown in Table 1.

Table 1. Selected DRG codes for the study.

DRG	DRG Name	Number of cases
202	*Bronchitis & asthma with CC/MCC*	2836
203	*Bronchitis & asthma w/o CC/MCC*	5763
100	*Seizures with MCC*	578
101	*Seizures w/o MCC*	2874
193	*Simple pneumonia & pleurisy with MCC*	411
194	*Simple pneumonia & pleurisy with CC*	1211
195	*Simple pneumonia & pleurisy w/o CC/MCC*	1024
790	*Extreme immaturity or respiratory distress syndrome, neonate*	2356
791	*Prematurity with major problems*	1241
792	*Prematurity w/o major problems*	1596
793	*Full term neonate with major problems*	2421
794	*Neonate with other significant problems*	1947
795	*Normal newborn*	492

For each DRG set (i.e. MS202-203; MS100-101; MS193-195; MS790-795), 15% of cases were randomly selected and reserved for subsequent fine tuning of system parameters, and another random 15% were reserved as the test dataset. All other cases were used as the training dataset for the model.

2.2 Module 1: Learning from Historical Data

We hypothesized that ICD codes, CPT codes, LOS, and the access log features contribute to the determination of DRG codes of the hospitalization. The EHR access log features include the number of users, processes and sessions associated with the access to the EHR of an inpatient stay. The codes of each hospital stay were encoded as high dimension vector (determined by the total number of codes of relevant ICD and CPT in each base cases), and other variables were encoded together as a vector and normalized.

We used three heterogeneous classifiers and the ensemble of them on the aforementioned features to learn DRG coding on hospital stays. The three classifiers are (1) random forest, (2) support vector machine (SVM) with polynomial kernel and (3) regularized logistic regression (for two-level DRGs: Bronchitis & asthma and Seizures) or softmax regression (for multi-level DRGs: Simple pneumonia & pleurisy and Premature birth). Formally, we denote an example corresponding to a stay with (x, t) where x is a multi-dimensional feature vector, and t is the known coded DRG level. For the binary sets, we have $t \in \{0, 1\}$ where $t = 1$ denotes the DRG code of the higher severity; for multi-level sets, we have $t \in \{1, 2, 3, \ldots, K\}$ where K is the number of possible codes in a set, representing MS195, MS194, and MS193 respectively for the pneumonia set, and MS790, MS791, MS792, MS793, MS794 and MS795 for the newborn case (in that order). Then we can view the goal of the task as to predict $P(t|x)$: given x, the features of a stay, model the probability of the outcome t. In the case where regularized logistic regression classifier is used, $P(t|x)$ is modeled by:

$$P(t = 1) = \frac{1}{1 + e^{-w^T x}}, \tag{1}$$

And $P(t = 0) = 1 - P(t = 1)$. The parameter of the model w is what we will need to learn from the data. In the multi-level cases, $P(t|x)$ is modeled by softmax regression:

$$P(t = k) = \frac{e^{-w_k^T x}}{\sum_{k=1}^{K} e^{-w_k^T x}} \tag{2}$$

where w_k is the parameter to be learned from the data.

The parameters of logistic regression and softmax regression were estimated using gradient-based optimization of the objective function. The objective function for the binary cases is weighted cross entropy with L1 regularization:

$$J = - \sum_{n=1}^{N} \{ ut_n ln\, y_n + (1 - t_n) ln\, (1 - y_n) \} + \alpha \parallel w \parallel, \qquad (3)$$

for multi-level cases:

$$J = - \sum_{n=1}^{N} \sum_{k=1}^{K} u_k \delta_k(t_n)\, \ln y_n + \alpha \parallel w \parallel, \qquad (4)$$

where u and u_k are hyper-parameters, the class weights to tune in order to handle the unbalanced data, t_n is the DRG code for the n-th example in the training set containing N examples. y_n denotes the prediction by the model for the n-th example, using Formula (1) and (2) respectively for (3) and (4). The Delta function $\delta_k(t_n)$ evaluates to be 1 if n-th example has the DRG code denoted by k, or to be 0 otherwise. α is the weight decay, a hyper-parameter. The ensemble classifier is a logistic regression or a softmax regression over the estimation given by the three classifiers, using the same objective. To avoid confusion, from now on, logistic regression or a softmax regression will only be used to refer the classifier among the three and the ensemble classifier will be used to refer the ensemble classifier. The contributions of different feature variables were tested too and the result was shown in the evaluation result section. The hyper-parameters were fine-tuned by: (1) predefine search spaces for the hyper-parameters; (2) randomly select from the search spaces and train models using them; (3) run evaluation on the development set and select the best performing model by the F_2 score. For various combinations of the input features, the fine-tuning was performed separately.

Implementation Details. All the scripts for the experiments were written in Python along with scikit-learn and Tensorflow. The optimization of the objective functions were done using Adam algorithm [7]. The pre-defined search space for hyper-parameters for the *bronchitis & asthma* set (binary) are: {2, **5**, 10, 50} for the weighted cross entropy weight u, {0, 2, **5**} for the weight decay α of the logistic regression, {100, **500**} for the number of epochs over the training data, {**20**, 50, 100} for the number of trees in the forest, {5:1, 8:1, **12:1**} for the class weights in the random forest, {4, **5**, 6} for the degree of polynomial in the kernel SVM, {2, 3, **6**, 8} for the coefficient term of the polynomial kernel, {5, 10, **12**} for the weighted cross entropy weight u of the ensemble classifier, and {50, **100**, 500} for the epochs during training of the ensemble classifier. The optimal setting among the tested combinations varied when including different features (see the section "Selection of variables and model settings" below). For model using the variables we chose after the experiments, the hyper-parameters are highlighted in bold above.

For the *pneumonia & pleurisy* set (multi-class), we started fine-tuning similarly and found that the ensemble of the three classifiers did no better than SVM with polynomial kernel along. Thus, we selected SVM with polynomial kernel alone and fine-tuned the hyper-parameters for that. The degree of the polynomial kernel of SVM was chosen from {4, **5**, 6}. Moreover, the coefficient of the kernel was selected from {4, 8, 12}. In addition, the weights of the three classes was z : 1.5 : 1 (MS193:MS194:MS195) with z selected from {**8**, 10, 15}. The chosen hyper-parameters are highlighted in bold above.

For the *seizures* set (binary), the search spaces are {5:1, 10:1, 12:1} for the class weights in the random forest, and is {2, 4, 6, 8} for the coefficient term of the polynomial kernel. The search spaces for other hyper-parameters are the same as in the *bronchitis & asthma* set. For the model using the variables we chose after the experiments, we set α to be 0, number of epochs to be 100, u to be 10, number of trees to be 100, the class weights in the random forest to be 10:1, polynomial degree to be 4, and the coefficient of the polynomial to be 4.

For the newborn set (multi-class), we carried out hyper-parameter fine-tuning in the same manner but found that the ensemble classifier did no better than the regularized softmax regression, thus later we chose to use only regularized softmax regression and fine-tuned the hyper-parameters for that, including weight decay from {0, **2**, 5, 10}, number of epochs from {50, 100, **500**}, learning rate from {0.1, 0.01, **0.001**}, and batch size from {100, 120, 150}. For model using the variables we chose after the experiments, the chosen hyper-parameters are highlighted in bold shown above.

2.3 Module 2: Prioritizing Cases with Potential Errors

After obtaining a well-trained model, the system works by making a prediction of the DRG code of a given case with a confidence score using the trained model from Module 1. The confidence score is given by the estimated probability $P(t|x)$. Then we compare them with the assigned codes from other source (such as human assignment and rule-based coding tools), and prioritize those cases that do not aligned based on the confidence score. These cases are potential targets for manual review. In other words, the difference in coding assigned by the trained model based on historical audited data and those by the simple rule based system is used to make suggestions of cases to be reviewed. Figure 1 shows an overview of the workflow for the data-driven code auditing method.

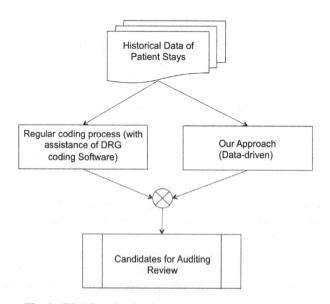

Fig. 1. Workflow for the data-driven code auditing method

2.4   Evaluation Metrics

To evaluate the performance of the models, we compared the DRG codes assigned to the test cases that were not used in the model training, against the actual codes assigned to them by (using the coding logic). For the binary sets, we rounded $P(t|x)$ into zero or one (0.5 was rounded to zero) and take t as the prediction if $P(t|x)$ rounds to 1. For multi-level cases, the predicted DRG level is the t that yields the maximum $P(t|x)$. Here we outline the evaluation metrics: recall, precision and F_2 score. To provide a clear view, Table 2 is used to show the definition of them in this scenario. In multi-level cases, macro average of F_2 is calculated.

$$accuracy = \frac{a+d}{a+b+c+d}$$

$$recall = \frac{a}{a+c}$$

$$precision = \frac{a}{a+b}$$

$$F_2 = (1+\beta)^2 \cdot \frac{precision \cdot recall}{\beta^2 \cdot precision + recall}, \beta = 2$$

Table 2. Possible outcome of the model comparing to the DRG from historical data

Number of cases		DRG from historical data	
		With CC/MCC	W/O CC/MCC
Model-assigned DRG	With CC/MCC	a	b
	Without CC/MCC	c	d

3   Model Evaluation

3.1   Evaluation on Test Dataset

The evaluation result along with the used model (algorithm) and features for the four sets are shown in Table 3.

Selection of Variables and Model Settings. The algorithms used for each set (shown in Table 3) were selected after comparing the performance of the four models (regularized logistic/softmax regression, SVM, random forest or the ensemble of them) using validation data. To determine if including LOS, CPT codes, and access log variables can improve the performance, we evaluated the model performance on the validation data using different combinations of the variables as shown in Table 4.

We added the analytical variables from the EHR access log with the hypothesis that a more medically complex patient may require more care and attention from the clinical staff. As a result, certain access log variables may reflect the level of a patient's medical severity. To the best of our knowledge, this is the first attempt to employ EHR analytical data on medical code auditing. The experiment shows that the increase of F_2 score when using the access log features is marginal. However, this does not reject the hypothesis, because the experiment was limited by the incomplete EHR access log data at hand. Due to the fact that the access log of EHR was recently implemented, and that the three variables were enabled in the access log on various date, only a small portion of the examples have all three access log features: Bronchitis & Asthma (2659, 31%); Pneumonia & Pleurisy (860, 32.5%); Premature Birth (3528, 35%); Seizures (1392, 38.5%). It would be interesting to see if the EHR analytical log data can be used to improve medical coding and auditing practices when sufficient high quality data available.

We also investigated using a medical code grouper to combine similar ICD into major groups but the preliminary result did not show its benefits. Therefore, we proceed with the ICD codes in its granular level.

Table 3. Model evaluation result on four common disease sets

Disease set	Model	Features	F_2 scores	Accuracy
Bronchitis & Asthma	ensemble	all ICD codes and all three EHR access log variables	95.03%	97.08%
Seizures	ensemble	ICD codes and the number of unique access log users	88.54%	96.75%
Simple pneumonia & pleurisy	SVM	ICD codes and the number of unique access log users	88.90%	89.85%
Premature Birth	regularized softmax regression	ICD codes and all access log variables	95.82%	96.18%

Table 4. Model performance (F2 score) with different variables and settings

Variables	Bronchitis & Asthma	Seizures	Pneumonia & Pleurisy	Premature Birth
ICD	95.18%	90.36%	89.30%	96.25%
ICD + # EHR access log processes	95.16%	90.95%	89.09%	96.34%
ICD + # EHR access log users	95.15%	91.43%	89.14%	96.27%
ICD + # EHR access log sessions	95.27%	90.35%	89.15%	96.20%
ICD + all access log variables	95.39%	91.07%	89.22%	96.27%
ICD + all access log variables + LOS + CPT	94.19%	86.86%	86.29%	93.42%

3.2 Manual Review Validation

A utilization review specialist (L.F.) reviewed the medical records for a small subset of patients from the bronchitis & asthma DRG set (n = 21). Utilization review specialists are trained to determine whether a patient's medical needs justify the medical care provided (e.g. inpatient stay, length of stay). Manual review showed that of the cases where our model scored a higher severity code (MS202) but the billing DRG was MS203 (without CC/MCC), over half (5 out of 7) were deemed medically complex by the UR specialist. This suggests that these cases may be good candidates for manual review by coding specialists.

4 Discussion and Conclusions

Using statistical modeling and machine learning methods to help address healthcare issues have been proven to be valuable and deserves more attention from both the healthcare and engineering domains, especially when large amount of health data are accumulated as a result of the adoption of EHR systems, while medicine was still heavily based one randomized controlled trails that are done in a limited and selected group of subjects and have its own limitations [8]. In recent years, there are increasing studies focusing on this topic and they demonstrate the effectiveness of data-driven methods in multiple applications, such as risk management [9–13], acceleration of bundled payment schemes [14], and treatment recommendation [15, 16].

Detecting and correcting coding error can be challenging. The traditional audit through a random sample can estimate the error rate, but it is impossible to identify many potentially problematic cases to review. Previous studies on miscoding detection are limited and focused only on upcoding detection [17]. Rosenberg et al. were the first trying to build a predictive model (hierarchical logistic Bayesian model) to detect miscoding and was based on an outdated coding system (UB82) [18]. Luo and Gallagher presented an unsupervised learning method to detect hospital level upcoding by comparing the different distributions of DRG codes in multiple hospitals [19].

To the best of our knowledge, here we have specified and demonstrated the first feasibility study of a data-driven approach to prioritize cases for manual review by care providers. Using our approach, the coding/auditing team can carry out automated batch run for the inpatient visits ready for DRG assignment on a daily base. The DRG classifier can run in parallel with the existing DRG grouper software used by the hospital. The cases whose DRG assignments differ between the two approaches will be tagged for manual review by a coding specialist. This algorithm leverages the fact that the different assignments of DRG level is potentially useful for coding specialist to identify miscoded cases, as the existing DRG coding software uses rule-based assignments based on limited information, whereas the DRG classifier learns from historical audited data using broader information.

By inspecting the classifiers, we found ICD codes are the most important feature. We also tested the potential of using EHR access measures as an indicator for medical resource utilization and medical complexity. The rationale is that more medically complicated patients require more attention by medical staff and the increased monitoring and procedures will be reflected by their EHR access. Our results show that EHR access log variables could improve the model slightly (less than 1% F_2 score on validation set) for some DRGs. For other sets, the additional EHR access log features made little contributions. This could be due to the nature of the medical condition and the clinical workflow of the specialty treating these patients. Notably, a limitation in this study is that access log was launched not long ago, and the collected variables are only available for the most recent years, thereby limiting the cases with these variables. As EHR access log data accumulate, the EHR access log variables may become a more reliable and accessible feature for medical analytics. Our study provides the first demonstration that EHR access log variables can be useful additional features for DRG auditing and other tasks that need to distinguish the levels of resources utilization and medical complexity.

There are a few limitations to this approach. First, the performance of the model is dependent on the number of cases available, making it difficult to model less frequent conditions. In addition, given that the model was built using historical audited data, its result would also be affected by the accuracy of the previous DRG assignment. For example, if there is systemic downcoding, the model trained on such data will be biased towards that direction. In order to address these issues, it would be useful to obtain larger dataset likely from multiple hospitals with equivalent case-mix index. A major potential roadblock towards the technology acceptance is whether it fits well in the existing workflow. Its implementation requires periodically retraining and improving the model using new data and comparing with existing coding to identify outliers, which implies interfacing with existing software tools in the workflow. Many of the existing tools are enterprise software that may or may not be able to add data pipelines.

In summary, we specified and demonstrated the potential application of a data-driven approach to identify encounters with DRG coding for manual review. This would potentially improve coding compliance, accelerate the reimbursement process, and reduce health care expenditure by lower the burden by audits from the payer side. We investigated and evaluated tailored algorithms to handle data imbalance and explored using multi-source information, including EHR access log data for developing solutions to assist miscoding detection for care providers. We anticipate that the reported study would lead to solutions that improve medical coding accuracy and efficiency.

Acknowledgment. Richard Hoyt and Beth Burkhart of Nationwide Children's Hospital helped prepare the data. Steve Rust and the rest of the data science team assisted in the project.

References

1. Rimler, S.B., Gale, B.D., Reede, D.L.: Diagnosis-related groups and hospital inpatient federal reimbursement. Radiographics **35**(6), 1825–1834 (2015)
2. Verdon, D.R.: Report: medicare coding errors signal need for physician education. Med. Econ. **91**(13), 55 (2014)

3. National Health Expenditures 2016 Highlights. Centers for Medicare and Medicaid Services. https://www.cms.gov/Research-Statistics-Data-and-Systems/Statistics-Trends-and-Reports/NationalHealthExpendData/downloads/highlights.pdf
4. CMS financial report FY2017. Centers for Medicare and Medicaid Services. https://www.cms.gov/Research-Statistics-Data-and-Systems/Statistics-Trends-and-Reports/CFOReport/Downloads/2017_CMS_Financial_Report.pdf
5. Stavrakas-Souba, L.: Avoiding audits by benchmarking your E/M coding. J. Med. Pract. Manage. 21(1), 51–53 (2005)
6. Medicare Fee-For-Service 2016 Improper Payments Report. Centers for Medicare and Medicaid Services. https://www.cms.gov/Research-Statistics-Data-and-Systems/Monitoring-Programs/Medicare-FFS-Compliance-Programs/CERT/Downloads/MedicareFeeforService 2016ImproperPaymentsReport.pdf
7. Kingma, D., Ba, J.: Adam: a method for stochastic optimization. In: Proceedings of the ICLR (2015)
8. Van Poucke, S., Thomeer, M., Heath, J., Vukicevic, M.: Are randomized controlled trials the (g) old standard? From clinical intelligence to prescriptive analytics. J. Med. Internet Res. 18(7), e185 (2016)
9. Wu, J., Roy, J., Stewart, W.F.: Prediction modeling using EHR data: challenges, strategies, and a comparison of machine learning approaches. Med. Care 1, S106–S113 (2010)
10. Radovanovic, S., Vukicevic, M., Kovacevic, A., Stiglic, G., Obradovic, Z.: Domain knowledge based hierarchical feature selection for 30-day hospital readmission prediction. In: Holmes, John H., Bellazzi, R., Sacchi, L., Peek, N. (eds.) AIME 2015. LNCS (LNAI), vol. 9105, pp. 96–100. Springer, Cham (2015). https://doi.org/10.1007/978-3-319-19551-3_11
11. Caruana, R., Lou, Y., Gehrke, J., Koch, P., Sturm, M., Elhadad, N.: Intelligible models for healthcare: predicting pneumonia risk and hospital 30-day readmission. In: Proceedings of the 21th ACM SIGKDD International Conference on Knowledge Discovery and Data Mining, pp. 1721–1730. ACM, 10 August 2015
12. Jovanovic, M., Radovanovic, S., Vukicevic, M., Van Poucke, S., Delibasic, B.: Building interpretable predictive models for pediatric hospital readmission using Tree-Lasso logistic regression. Artif. Intell. Med. 1(72), 12–21 (2016)
13. Xu, Y., Biswal, S., Deshpande, S.R., Maher, K.O., Sun, J.: RAIM: recurrent attentive and intensive model of multimodal patient monitoring data. In Proceedings of the 24th ACM SIGKDD International Conference on Knowledge Discovery & Data Mining, pp. 2565–2573. ACM, 19 July 2018
14. Zhang, W., Bjarnadóttir, M.V., Proaño, R.A., Anderson, D., Konrad, R.: Accelerating the adoption of bundled payment reimbursement systems: a data-driven approach utilizing claims data. IISE Trans. Healthcare Syst. Eng. 8(1), 22–34 (2018)
15. Chekroud, A.M., et al.: Cross-trial prediction of treatment outcome in depression: a machine learning approach. Lancet Psychiatry 3(3), 243–250 (2016)
16. Hughes, M.C., et al.: Prediction-constrained topic models for antidepressant recommendation. In: Neural Information Processing Systems (NIPS) Workshop on Machine Learning for Healthcare (2017)
17. Bauder, R., Khoshgoftaar, T.M., Seliya, N.: A survey on the state of healthcare upcoding fraud analysis and detection. Health Serv. Outcomes Res. Meth. 17(1), 31–55 (2017)
18. Rosenberg, M.A., Fryback, D.G., Katz, D.A.: A statistical model to detect DRG upcoding. Health Serv. Outcomes Res. Meth. 1(3–4), 233–252 (2000)
19. Luo, W., Gallagher, M.: Unsupervised DRG upcoding detection in healthcare databases. In: 2010 IEEE International Conference on Data Mining Workshops (ICDMW), pp. 600–605. Sydney, NSW, Australia; IEEE 2010, 13 December 2010

Classification of Skin Pigmented Lesions Based on Deep Residual Network

Yunfei Qi[1]([⊠]), Shaofu Lin[1,2], and Zhisheng Huang[3]

[1] College of Software, Faculty of Information Technology,
Beijing University of Technology, Beijing, China
qiyf@emails.bjut.edu.cn, linshaofu@bjut.edu.cn
[2] Beijing Institute of Smart City, Beijing University of Technology,
Beijing, China
[3] Vrije Universiteit Amsterdam, Amsterdam, The Netherlands
huang@cs.vu.nl

Abstract. There are various of skin pigmented lesions with high risk. Melanoma is one of the most dangerous forms of skin cancer. It is one of the important research directions of medical artificial intelligence to carry out classification research of skin pigmented lesions based on deep learning. It can assist doctors to make clinical diagnosis and make patients receive treatment as soon as possible to improve survival rate. Aiming at the similar and imbalanced dermoscopic image data of pigmented lesions, this paper proposes a deep residual network improved by Squeeze-and-Excitation module, and dynamic update class-weight, in batches, with model ensemble adjustment strategies to change the attention of imbalanced data. The results show that the above method can increase the average precision by 9.1%, the average recall by 15.3%, and the average F1-score by 12.2%, compared with the multi-class classification using the deep residual network. Thus, the above method is a better classification model and weight adjustment strategy.

Keywords: Deep learning · Residual network · Skin lesions ·
Multi-classification · Imbalanced data · Model ensemble

1 Introduction

Skin pigmented lesions are various and dangerous. For example, compared with stage I melanoma patients treated within 30 days of being biopsied, those treated 30 to 59 days after clinical have a 5% higher risk of dying from the disease, and those treated more than 119 days after clinical have a 41% higher risk [1]. In America, across all therapeutic stages of melanoma, the average five-year survival rate is 9%. The five-year survival rate of patients with early detection of melanoma is estimated to be 98%. The survival rate falls to 64% when the disease reaches the lymph nodes and 23% when the disease metastasizes to distant organs [2]. Therefore, timely detection and treatment is one of the effective means to deal with skin pigmentated lesions and improve the survival rate of patients.

© Springer Nature Switzerland AG 2019
H. Wang et al. (Eds.): HIS 2019, LNCS 11837, pp. 58–67, 2019.
https://doi.org/10.1007/978-3-030-32962-4_6

At present, the primary clinical diagnosis is dermoscopic image inspection, which relies on the experience of doctors and takes time and energy. Therefore, the research on the classification of skin pigmented lesions based on deep learning can relieve the pressure of doctors in the way of computer-assisted diagnosis and accelerate the diagnosis speed. It is valuable for doctors and patients.

There are similarities in skin pigmented lesions, and the data of skin pigmented lesions are imbalanced. Therefore, it is difficult in research that how to correctly distinguish the image of similar lesions and solve the imbalance of data. In this paper, SEResNeXt model [3] was used for feature extraction, and its Squeeze-and-Excitation module could increase the effect of feature channel and improve the recognition ability of similar lesions. The model ensemble is used to solve the problem of extremely imbalanced data.

The rest of this paper is organized as follows. Section 2 describes the related work. Section 3 introduces data and methods. Section 4 explains the experimental procedure. Section 5 shows the results and analysis. The last section includes conclusions and future work.

2   Related Work

Esteva et al. [4] proved that convolutional neural network (CNN) is an effective method to solve the classification of skin lesions through a large number of researches and experiments. It even surpasses the accuracy of human recognition in some image recognition categories and is comparable to the level of experienced doctors.

Most of the datasets of skin lesions are very small, and the number of images contained by the lesions is extremely imbalanced. Vasconcelos et al. [5] used Deep Convolutional Neural Networks (DCNN) to classify and achieved good results in the imbalanced dataset. Ge et al. [6] considered global features and local features equally in the algorithm, processed global information on a deep residual network and classified local information on SVM after processing with bilinear pooling technology of VGG. And they obtained the result of average accuracy of 0.625 in the test set. Yu et al. [7] proposed to use ResNet-50 to segment the lesion area and then use ResNet to classify the lesions, which pre-process data, by reducing background noise, to improve the model performance. Li et al. [8] used softmax loss function as class-weight to solved the multi-classification problem of imbalanced data, and also achieved good results. Today, some researchers classify lesions by using different CNN models, such as Inception, ResNet, DenseNet, etc. The accuracy of classification of similar lesions has been improved by the method of stacking network layer number, multi-model feature extraction or reclassification of lesions after segmentation. Some researchers, according to the number of data types, set class-weight or use weighted softmax Loss to deal with imbalanced data. But these methods depend on the experience of the experimenters and increase the time cost of training. However, there are still large errors in the results, and too many network layers increase the cost of experimental equipment as well.

In the experiment, we used SEResNeXt model to train the classifier, and without increasing the number of network-layers too much, we put forward an improved

Boosting model ensemble [9] through class-weight calculation method. We trained weak classifier by dynamically adjusting class-weight according to the data proportion of the training set, and then combined results of weak classifiers together. This method can deal with the imbalanced data by changing the model attention each lesion.

3   Dataset and Method

3.1   Dataset

The dataset from the HAM10000. More than 50% of lesions have been confirmed by pathology. And the ground truth for the rest of the lesions was either confirmed by follow-up, expert consensus or in-vivo confocal microscopy [10, 11]. The Images were manually cropped the scanned images with the lesion centered, and applied manual histogram corrections to enhance visual contrast and color reproduction. The dataset contains 7 types of skin pigmented lesions: melanoma, melanocytic nevus, basal cell carcinoma, actinic keratosis/Bowen's disease (intraepithelial carcinoma), benign keratosis (solar lentigo/seborrheic keratosis/lichen planus-like keratosis), dermatofibroma, vascular lesion. In addition, it also includes patients' age, gender, limb parts of image collection and classification confirmation method. Therefore, we focus on the research of image-based classification, so we do not consider the reference to classification by other factors (age, gender, etc.). The specific distribution of pigmented lesions in the dataset is as follows (Table 1):

Table 1. Distribution of pigmented lesions in dataset

Disease	Abbreviation	Amount
Melanoma	Mel	1113
Melanocytic nevus	NV	6705
Basal cell carcinoma	BCC	514
Actinic keratosis/Bowen's disease (intraepithelial carcinoma)	AKIEC	327
Benign keratosis (solar lentigo/seborrheic keratosis/lichen planus-like keratosis)	BKL	1099
Dermatofibroma	DF	115
Vascular lesion	VASC	142

According to the distribution of image types in the dataset, there are 6705 images of melanocytic nevus (NV), only 115 images of dermatofibroma (DF) and 142 images of vascular lesion (VASC) in the categories, so the number of images in each category is extremely imbalanced. We will describe the impact of unbalanced data in the Sect. 4.3.

3.2   Model

With the deepening of depth, the performance of ordinary convolutional neural networks decreases. But, the deep residual network (ResNet) [12] introduces a deep residual learning framework. Instead of hoping each few stacked layers directly fit a desired underlying mapping, they explicitly let these layers fit a residual mapping. Formally, H(x) is the optimal solution mapping. Then, let the stacked nonlinear layers fit another mapping of

$$F(x) = H(x) - x. \tag{1}$$

And it can be realized by feedforward neural networks with "shortcut connections" to let the original mapping recast into

$$F(x) + x, \tag{2}$$

identity "shortcut connections" and add neither extra parameter nor computational complexity. And it is already proved that this method improves the performance of the network by deepening the network depth.

Then, we can build ResNet by stacking build blocks, and use split-transform-merge strategy to form ResNeXt [13]. In the experiment, ResNeXt-50 achieves almost the same accuracy as ResNet-101, with less computation and parameters. The comparison of the residual structures of ResNext and ResNet is shown in Fig. 1.

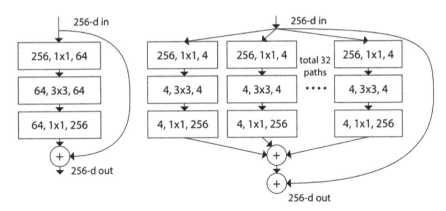

Fig. 1. Structure comparison between ResNet and ResNeXt. Left is ResNet and right is ResNeXt [13]

Finally, use the Squeeze-and-Excitation (SE) module to improve ResNeXt model performance. SE module structure consists of the squeeze and the excitation. The purpose is to improve model performance from feature channel by constructing SE module. In this paper, ResNeXt-50 model is used to add SE module to the residual branch. Then, reduce the dimension of input through some layers. After that, increase the dimension of result of the previous step through a ReLu and then get output. The channel outputs are weighted to the previous features by multiplication to complete the recalibration of the original features in the channel dimension. Through this method, the model can obtain the importance degree of each feature channel in training, and then, according to these importance degrees, promote the useful features in the task and suppress the features that have little effect [3].

3.3 Model Ensemble

In this paper, we improved Adboost, one of the boosting methods, to train multiple weak classifiers and finally form a strong classifier to solve the impact of imbalanced data. The traditional Adboost method uses exactly the same training class-weight to train the first weak classifier. According to the extremely imbalanced attributes of the dataset, the traditional class-weight adjustment scheme will undoubtedly reduce the training speed and the accuracy of the first weak classifier. Therefore, this paper proposes a dynamic class-weight adjustment method based on the input batch to train the first weak classifier. By adjusting the class-weight of different classes according to the results of this weak classifier, the attention of the classifier is changed to train the next weak classifier. We repeat the experiment, and finally take the average value of the predicted results of N weak classifier as the output result. The model ensemble structure is shown in Fig. 2.

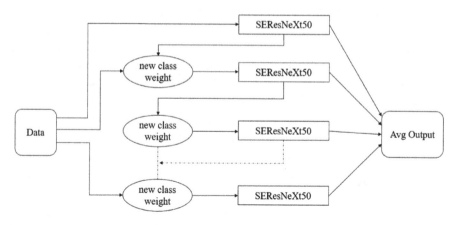

Fig. 2. Model ensemble structure

3.4 Transfer Learning

The purpose of transfer learning [14] is to use model pre-training parameters and network structure to speed up the training process of the experiment. As the amounts of training examples is insufficient for training a deep convolutional network from scratch, so we used the pre-trained imagenet model to initialize the network parameters and fine-tuned the last several layers.

4   Experimental Procedure

We wrote neural network code based on the advanced neural network API of keras [15], taken tensorflow [16] as the backend for computation, used cuda10 and cudnn7.3.0 for runtime environment, and divided picture labels into 0–6, a total of 7 categories for multi-classifier trained.

4.1   Data Preprocess

First, image name and image's disease classification label were read from CSV file. And redefined the labels as one-hot-encoding format. Second, loaded the images for numpy array and reshaped to (224, 224, 3). Then, fixed the array with random parameters. Last, we divided the dataset into 60% train set, 20% validation set and 20% test set. Under such split, it not only guarantees the richness of training set but also improved the training and testing of model generalization ability. Finally, test set has done not participate in training to ensure the effectiveness of test results.

4.2   Model Setting

In this paper, we used SEResNeXt-50 model for transfer learning with ImageNet data pre-training. In order to optimize the operational efficiency of the program and make the predicted results conformed to the expected results of the experiment, we modified the prediction layer of the model. Unlike the original ResNet fully connected layer, we used GlobalAveragePooling2D [17] instead of Flatten layer for dimensionality-reduction, so as to avoid the fully connected layers, we introduced a large number of parameters, and prevented this network to overfitting. It also increased stability and speed in transfer learning. Finally, there were two Dropout layers with drop factor 0.5, and a Dense layer with units 7 to predict the result.

4.3   Class-Weight

Imbalanced data can lead to serious errors in classifiers. The category of the maximum data volume leads to the over-attention of the classifier to this category, and it can also achieve high accuracy to judge the image as this category. However, this is not in line with the actual situation. Class-weight setting is added to the training process to make the classifier pay more attention to the types of lesions with fewer pictures in the training process. This method can change the punishment intensity of different kinds of judgment errors and improve the classification ability of classifiers. So we used this class-weight method to train different weak classifiers.

We used two methods to set up class-weight in training weak classifier, as follows:

1. According to the limitation of computer memory and graphics memory, input data only supports batch size of 16 for each epoch, which may lead to that batch processing do not contain smaller classified data. Therefore, the training of the first model is based on the image data of each input batch, and then the dynamic balance in the first training makes the model use the same degree of attention to the lesion types, so as to enhance the ability of the first weak classifier.

2. According to the test results of the weak classifier and the distribution of each disease in the train set, the class-weight is recalculated and adjusted for training the follow-up weak classifier. S is the number of lesion pictures and T is the target attention. The formula of class-weight calculation is as follows:

$$class\_weight = (1/S) \times T \tag{3}$$

5   Results and Analysis

5.1   Standard of Evaluation

The classification prediction results of the model are the diagnostic confidence representation of the multi-classification model, which represents the set of binary classifications, and the form is [0.0, 0.9, 0.03, ..., 0.01], which can be set as the type of predicted lesions when the confidence range exceeds 0.5.

P(precision), R(recall), and F(F1-score) are used as evaluation criteria in this experiment. The overall evaluation criteria are P, R and F of each single category. We calculate the average of all P, R and F to represent the performance of the classifier. They are defined as follows:

$$P = TP/(TP + FP), \tag{4}$$

$$R = TP/(TP + FN), \tag{5}$$

$$F = 2 \times (P \times R)/(P + R). \tag{6}$$

Where TP is true positive, FP is false positive, FN is false negative.

5.2   Experimental Results

We set learning rate of the model start from 0.01. If the value of loss in the validation set does not decrease, the learning rate will be adjusted to one tenth of the current value. Stop training when the loss of 10 epochs does not decrease. We listed the results of testing in the same test set with ResNet-50, SEResNeXt-50, and SEResNeXt-50 within model ensemble (Tables 2, 3 and 4).

Table 2. The result of ResNet-50

	Precision	Recall	F1-score	Support
MEL	0.65	0.58	0.61	214
NV	0.93	0.94	0.93	1323
BCC	0.81	0.81	0.81	103
AKIEC	0.77	0.50	0.61	66
BKL	0.72	0.80	0.76	241
DF	0.60	0.71	0.65	17
VASC	0.93	0.69	0.79	39
Avg	0.77	0.72	0.74	–

Table 3. The result of SEResNeXt-50

	Precision	Recall	F1-score	Support
MEL	0.67	0.68	0.67	214
NV	0.92	0.97	0.94	1323
BCC	0.88	0.81	0.84	103
AKIEC	0.93	0.42	0.58	66
BKL	0.83	0.74	0.78	241
DF	0.71	0.71	0.71	17
VASC	1.00	0.82	0.90	39
Avg	0.85	0.74	0.77	–

Table 4. The result of SEResNeXt-50 within model ensemble

	Precision	Recall	F1-score	Support
MEL	0.72	0.72	0.72	214
NV	0.95	0.96	0.95	1323
BCC	0.84	0.88	0.86	103
AKIEC	0.89	0.61	0.72	66
BKL	0.82	0.83	0.82	241
DF	0.67	0.94	0.78	17
VASC	1.00	0.87	0.93	39
Avg	0.84	0.83	0.83	–

Compared with ResNet-50, the test results of SEResNeXt-50 without model ensemble strategy, the average prediction increases by 10.3%, the average recall increases by 1.4%, and the average F1-score increases by 5.4%. Compared with the results of SEResNeXt-50 within model ensemble strategy, the average recall and F1-score of SEResNeXt-50 increase by 13% and 6% respectively.

From the results, we can conclude that the recognition rate of lesions with small amount of data has been successfully improved after weight adjustment, and the average performance of BCC, AKIEC, DF and VASC has been improved to some extent.

5.3   Comparison of Other Methods

We used auto class-weight to train different networks in keras, and the results are shown in Table 5.

Table 5. The result of SEResNeXt-50 within model ensemble

Table 5. The result of SEResNeXt-50 within model ensemble

Method	Validation score
PNASNet-5-Large	0.76
InceptionV3	0.67
DenseNet-201	0.77
ResNet-152	0.73
Ensemble of SEResNet-50	0.83

Table 5 shows that the average score of the method adopted in this paper is higher than that of the single model with class-weight balance in keras which class-weight is auto. Therefore, the method adopted in this paper can improve the performance of the model.

5.4 Conclusion and Future Work

Medical data are extremely imbalanced due to different rates of disease. These imbalances can lead to all lesions being considered benign and ignore malignant lesions in neural network training. The fusion model using class-weight adjustment strategy can adjust the model well to identify malignant lesions with low incidence rate, so weight adjustment and model fusion strategy are effective solutions to the imbalance of medical data.

Based on the low recall of some diseases in the experimental results, the future work should focus on the learning of lesion classification to improve the model performance, such as multi-scale model input, multi-CNN model input or model ensemble, so as to improve the generalization ability of the model. Secondly, the model only makes image prediction for 7 categories in the train set, but cannot identify abnormal classes. Therefore, the algorithm content or model method of relevant abnormal class detection is needed in the future work, so as to make the prediction results that the model have higher reference value.

Acknowledgments. This study was financially supported by program Research on Artificial Intelligence Innovation Technology for Mental Health Service, which is funded by the Beijing High-level Foreign Talents Subsidy Program 2019. The program number is Z201919. Our team continues to conduct research on artificial intelligence and big data analytics in the medical field, hoping to help human health with the power of data. And we are grateful to all study participants.

References

1. Conic, R.Z., Cabrera, C.I., Khorana, A.A., et al.: Determination of the impact of melanoma surgical timing on survival using the national cancer database. J. Am. Acad. Dermatol. **78**(1), 40–46 (2017)
2. Cancer Facts and Figures (2019). https://www.cancer.org. Last accessed 10 May 2019
3. Hu, J., Shen, L., Sun, G.: Squeeze-and-excitation networks. IEEE Transactions on Pattern Analysis and Machine Intelligence (2017)

4. Esteva, A., Kuprel, B., Novoa, R.A., et al.: Dermatologist-level classification of skin cancer with deep neural networks. Nature **542**(7639), 115–118 (2017)
5. Vasconcelos, C.N., Vasconcelos, B.N.: Experiments using deep learning for dermoscopy image analysis. Pattern Recognit. Lett. **16**(3), 68–77 (2017)
6. Ge, Z., Demyanov, S., Bozorgtabar, B., et al.: Exploiting local and generic features for accurate skin lesions classification using clinical and dermoscopy imaging. In: IEEE International Symposium on Biomedical Imaging (2017)
7. Yu, L., Chen, H., Dou, Q., et al.: Automated melanoma recognition in dermoscopy images via very deep residual networks. IEEE Trans. Med. Imag. **36**(4), 994–1004 (2017)
8. Li, Y., Shen, L.: Skin lesion analysis towards melanoma detection using deep learning network. Sensors **18**(2), 322 (2005)
9. Svetnik, V., Wang, T., Tong, C., et al.: Boosting: an ensemble learning tool for compound classification and QSAR modeling. J. Chem. Inf. Model. **45**(3), 786–799 (2005)
10. Tschandl, P., Rosendahl, C., Kittler, H.: The HAM10000 dataset, a large collection of multi-source dermatoscopic images of common pigmented skin lesions. Sci. Data 5, 180161 https://doi.org/10.1038/sdata.2018.161 (2018)
11. Codella, N., et al.: Skin Lesion Analysis Toward Melanoma Detection 2018: A Challenge Hosted by the International Skin Imaging Collaboration (ISIC). https://arx-iv.org/abs/1902.03368
12. He, K., Zhang, X., Ren, S., et al.: Deep residual learning for image recognition. Comput. Vis. Pattern Recogn. 770–778 (2016)
13. Xie, S., Girshick, R., Dollar, P., et al.: Aggregated residual transformations for deep neural networks. In: 2017 IEEE Conference on Computer Vision and Pattern Recognition (CVPR). IEEE Computer Society (2017)
14. Pan, S.J., Yang, Q.: A survey on transfer learning. IEEE Trans. Knowl. Data Eng. **22**(10), 1345–1359 (2010)
15. Keras. https://keras.io. Last accessed 10 May 2019
16. Tensorflow. https://tensorflow.google.cn. Last accessed 5 Apr 2019
17. Lin, M., Chen, Q., Yan, S.: Network in network (2013). https://arxiv.org/abs/1312.4400

Identifying lncRNA Based on Support Vector Machine

Yongmin Li[1], Yang Ou[1], Zhe Xu[2], and Lejun Gong[1(✉)]

[1] Jiangsu Key Laboratory of Big Data Security & Intelligent Processing,
Nanjing University of Posts and Telecommunications, Nanjing 210003, China
glj98226@163.com
[2] Nanjing Foreign Language School, Nanjing 210008, China

Abstract. With the development of high-throughput sequencing technology, it brings a large volume of data of transcriptome. Long non-protein-coding RNAs (lncRNAs) identification is pervasive in transcriptome studies in their important roles in biological process. This paper proposed a computational method for identifying lncRNAs based on machine learning. The method first selects feature using k-mer for traversing the transcript sequence to obtain a large class of features, integrated GC content and sequence length. Then it uses variance test to select three kinds of features by grid searching and reduce the data dimension and support vector machine pressure to establish a recognition model, the final model has a certain stability and robustness. The method obtain 95.7% accuracy, 0.99 AUC for test dataset. Therefore, it could be promising for identifying lncRNA.

Keywords: lncRNA · SVM · Feature selection · Classification · Grid searching

1 Introduction

In recent years, with the development of high-throughput sequencing technology, more and more sequencing data of genomes and transcripts of different species have been recognized. The mRNA content of proteins translated into mammalian genome is only 1%–2%. Most of the rest play only as RNA, and RNA molecules with a length greater than 200 nucleotides are long non-coding RNAs(lncRNA) [1, 2]. lncRNAs are a class of non-coding RNAs that play important roles in various developmental processes and stress responses. Studies have shown that lncRNA plays an important role in many life activities such as dose-compensation, epigenetic regulation, cell cycle regulation and cell differentiation regulation. lncRNA-related functions are also directly or indirectly related to many diseases, including Parkinson's disease, Alzheimer's disease, spinocerebellar ataxia, and Huntington's disease such as neurodegenerative diseases and cardiovascular diseases [3, 4]. It has been reported that lncRNA is closely related to nervous system related diseases [5], adding additional complex layers to brain function, which may be involved in unique brain function. lncRNA is also an indispensable molecular layer in the pathogenesis of heart failure [6], which is a kind potential signaling molecules. Moreover, lncRNA are stable and unique in plasma, could

H. Wang et al. (Eds.): HIS 2019, LNCS 11837, pp. 68–75, 2019.
https://doi.org/10.1007/978-3-030-32962-4_7

actively respond to stress and may have the potential to diagnose and treat heart failure. The lncRNA BACE1-AS is associated with the pathogenesis of Alzheimer's disease [7]. The lncRNA MALAT1 regulates the spread of cancer cells and the probability of disease progression [8]. At present, researchers have established a corresponding database lncRNADisease2.0 [9] related to lncRNA. The database contains multi-species test confirmation and predicted distribution results, and integrates 3878 literature data. Currently, 529 diseases have been included in the statistics. And continuous updating is important for further study of the biological mechanism of lncRNA. Since lncRNA is closely related to cell regulation and disease, it is important to study its biological mechanism and role. Therefore, accurately identifying and annotating lncRNAs is important to further understand long-chain non-coding RNA. There are that work could identify lncRNAs by experimental validation [10]. However, it is generally too expensive and time-consuming to perform experimental validation. This paper proposed a computational methods for identifying lncRNAs based on machine learning. The method uses the support vector machine as identified model with grid searching model's variance using k-mer feature integrated GC content and sequence length.

Aiming at the test dataset, the method obtain more performance than other method. More details are shown in the following sections.

2   Materials and Methods

The proposed method extracts features containing k-mer, GC content, and sequence length from lncRNA and mRNA transcripts respectively. Then it executes feature selection by variance, and puts in the support vector machine for classification model using grid searching technology. The proposed method's pipeline is shown in Fig. 1.

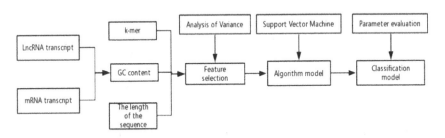

Fig. 1. The proposed method's pipeline

2.1   Feature Selection

The k-mer divides the reads into strings containing k bases [11], and the reads L can be divided into L-k + 1 sub-chains. The sub-sequence of length k in the RNA transcripts slides from the first base to the right according to the size of k like a sliding window as shown in Fig. 2 with k value of 3.

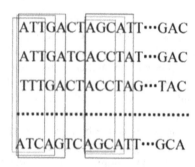

Fig. 2. k-mer with value of 3 sliding window

Since there are only four bases A, C, G and T at each position of the RNA, the number of features traversed by the k-mer can also be calculated. The number of subsequences with a length of k is 4 k which details. Assuming k is 5, the number of features extracted in this paper is 4^5 with 5-mer, 4^4 with 4-mer, 4^3 with 3-mer, 4^2 with 2-mer, 4 with 1-mer, totaling 1364 features. This paper considers all of these features.

The GC content is defined as the ratio of Guanine and Cytosine in the genome or specific DNA and RNA fragments [12]. The GC content is different in different species, and the human genome content is about 40%. This feature can be used to determine the preference of sequencing data and to determine whether the sequencing process meets random criteria. The GC content can also be used for related studies such as separation and measurement of DNA. In the study, we also extract GC contents as features. In addition to this, the length of sequence is also as features. Extracted above features are selected by analysis of variance (ANOVA).

2.2 Classified Model

The basic theory of the support vector machine (SVM) [13, 14] method is the VC dimensional theory and the structural risk minimization principle of statistical learning theory. It is able to obtain excellent classification results based on a small amount of sample data. At the time, it has strong adaptability.

The support vector machine method is inspired by the optimal classification plane in the case of linear separability. According to the case where the two-dimensional space is linearly separable as shown in Fig. 3, the black point and the white point represent two types of training samples respectively, and the optimal class classification surface is to find a line to accurately separate the two categories, and to maximize the classification interval. This classification idea is not only applicable to two-dimensional planes, but can be mapped to high-dimensional spaces for complex data to find the optimal classification hyperplane in high-dimensional space.

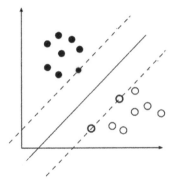

Fig. 3. The optimal hyperplane of the two-dimensional space

Generally, the kernel functions in SVM are linear kernel function, polynomial kernel function, radial basis kernel function, sigmoid kernel function. For different samples, the classification models obtained by different kernel function training are also different, so different kernel functions should be selected for different samples to classify. Experiments show that the radial basis kernel function has a high recognition score in different samples, which is optimal in performance. Thus, this study uses the radial basis nucleus function.

2.3   Grid Searching

In this study, the grid search method is to divide the required sample parameters into grids in a specific space, and then find the optimal parameters in the grid through continuous traversal. This traversal method can find the global optimal solution when the optimal interval is large enough and the step size is small enough. However, since the optimal parameters exist only in some small intervals, and many mesh parameter groups with low classification accuracy also need to be traversed. The grid search method [15] consumes a large amount of time in traversing all the parameter groups. It takes a lot of time to search for the optimal parameters in the grid, but the performance of the support vector machine is greatly improved, and the performance of recognition model is more than other machine learning algorithm such as decision tree and linear regression.

3   Results and Discussions

This study uses python programming language to implementation in Pycharm integrated development environment using anaconda 4.4.0 and biopython packages. The lncRNA and mRNA data were all sequenced in the GENCODE V29 database [16] with the human species. Among them, there are 29,273 non-coding RNA transcript sequences and 98,548 protein-encoding RNA transcript sequences, all of which are FASTA biological files as shown in Fig. 4. These FASTA files are preprocessed by perl script which facilitates the extraction of transcript sequences as shown Fig. 5. Using undersampling to process unbalanced raw data, it balances the number of lncRNA and mRNA transcripts by collections package.

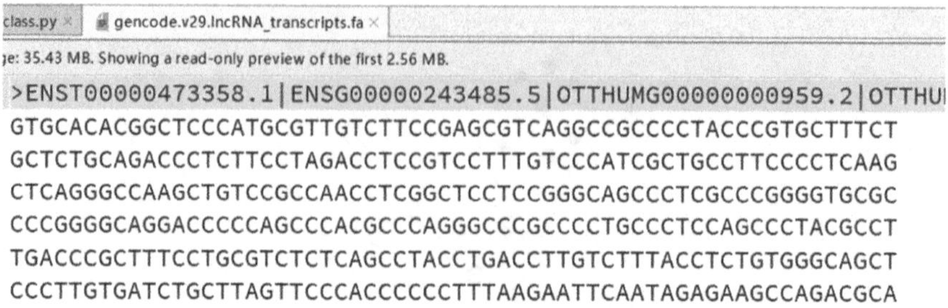

```
class.py ×    gencode.v29.lncRNA_transcripts.fa ×
je: 35.43 MB. Showing a read-only preview of the first 2.56 MB.
>ENST00000473358.1|ENSG00000243485.5|OTTHUMG00000000959.2|OTTHUl
GTGCACACGGCTCCCATGCGTTGTCTTCCGAGCGTCAGGCCGCCCCTACCCGTGCTTTCT
GCTCTGCAGACCCTCTTCCTAGACCTCCGTCCTTTGTCCCATCGCTGCCTTCCCCTCAAG
CTCAGGGCCAAGCTGTCCGCCAACCTCGGCTCCTCCGGGCAGCCCTCGCCCGGGGTGCGC
CCCGGGGCAGGACCCCCAGCCCACGCCCAGGGCCCGCCCCTGCCCTCCAGCCCTACGCCT
TGACCCGCTTTCCTGCGTCTCTCAGCCTACCTGACCTTGTCTTTACCTCTGTGGGCAGCT
CCCTTGTGATCTGCTTAGTTCCCACCCCCCTTTAAGAATTCAATAGAGAAGCCAGACGCA
```

Fig. 4. Raw fasta data

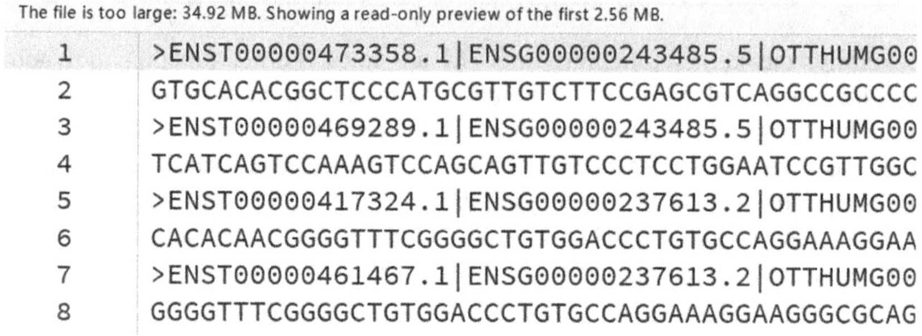

```
The file is too large: 34.92 MB. Showing a read-only preview of the first 2.56 MB.
 1    >ENST00000473358.1|ENSG00000243485.5|OTTHUMG00
 2    GTGCACACGGCTCCCATGCGTTGTCTTCCGAGCGTCAGGCCGCCCC
 3    >ENST00000469289.1|ENSG00000243485.5|OTTHUMG00
 4    TCATCAGTCCAAAGTCCAGCAGTTGTCCCTCCTGGAATCCGTTGGC
 5    >ENST00000417324.1|ENSG00000237613.2|OTTHUMG00
 6    CACACAACGGGGTTTCGGGGCTGTGGACCCTGTGCCAGGAAAGGAA
 7    >ENST00000461467.1|ENSG00000237613.2|OTTHUMG00
 8    GGGGTTTCGGGGCTGTGGACCCTGTGCCAGGAAAGGAAGGGCGCAG
```

Fig. 5. Preprocessed data by perl scrip

By solving the variance fitting of the feature matrix, two analytical parameters of F value and P value are obtained. The Table 1 show the features of top 20 F value of features with k value of 4. Figure 6 is the features' visualization.

Table 1. Features of top 20 F values of K-mer with value of 4.

No.	F value	P value	K-mer
1	729.4078	6.39E−121	CG
2	678.8432	1.75E−114	CGG
3	630.8785	3.40E−108	ACG
4	617.7548	1.92E−106	GC
5	588.1771	1.94E−102	CGGC
6	579.7021	2.81E−101	G
7	538.9209	1.34E−95	AAT
8	521.4722	4.01E−93	GCG
9	508.26	3.14E−91	CGA
10	491.1873	9.30E−89	GCGG

(*continued*)

Table 1. (*continued*)

No.	F value	P value	K-mer
11	473.0101	4.28E−86	GGCC
12	466.7324	3.63E−85	GGC
13	459.2299	4.71E−84	CCG
14	429.5591	1.37E−79	T
15	426.7886	3.61E−79	GACG
16	426.5942	3.86E−79	CGAG
17	426.0169	4.73E−79	TAA
18	418.8301	5.92E−78	GCCG
19	415.3607	2.02E−77	AAA
20	409.2284	1.77E−76	CGC

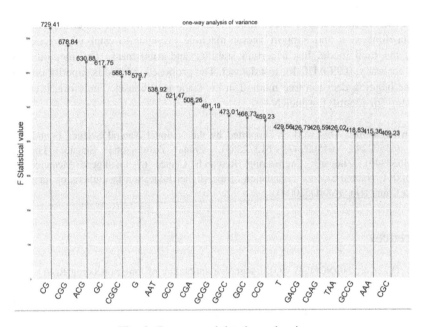

Fig. 6. Preprocessed data by perl scrip.

In order to compare the submitted methods, aiming at the same test dataset, we also use bagging decision tree [17] to classify for lncRNA which obtain 80% overall accuracy. This shows the proposed method is superior to the bagging decision tree method (Fig. 7).

```
GridSearchCV best score accuracy is 0.8912448979591836
-------------------------------------------------------
svm model para is SVC(C=1, cache_size=200, class_weight=None, coef0=0.0,
    decision_function_shape='ovr', degree=3, gamma=1, kernel='rbf',
    max_iter=-1, probability=True, random_state=1, shrinking=True, tol=0.001,
    verbose=False)
-------------------------------------------------------
best model fit all data, the accuracy is 0.9566532258064516
-------------------------------------------------------
```

Fig. 7. Grid searching parameters.

4 Conclusions

This paper proposed an identified method for lncRNA based on support vector machine. The method first selects feature using k-mer for traversing the transcript sequence to obtain a large class of features, integrated GC content and sequence length. Then it uses variance test to select three kinds of features by grid searching and reduce the data dimension and support vector machine pressure to establish a recognition model, the final model has a certain stability and robustness. The method obtains 95.7% accuracy, 0.99 AUC for test dataset. The proposed method is superior compared with the bagging decision tree method in the same test dataset. Therefore, it could be promising for identifying lncRNA.

Acknowledgments. This work is supported by the National Natural Science Foundation of China (61502243, 61502247, 61572263), China Postdoctoral Science Foundation (2018M632349), Zhejiang Engineering Research Center of Intelligent Medicine under 2016E10011, Natural Science Foundation of the Higher Education Institutions of Jiangsu Province in China (No. 16KJD520003).

References

1. Bu, D., et al.: NONCODE v3.0: integrative annotation of long noncoding RNAs. Nucleic Acids Res 40, D210–D215 (2012)
2. Derrien, T., et al.: The GENCODE v7 catalog of human long noncoding RNAs: analysis of their gene structure, evolution, and expression. Genome Res. **22**, 1775–1789 (2012)
3. Cheetham, S.W., Gruhl, F., Mattick, J.S., Dinger, M.E.: Long nonconding RNAs and the genetics of cancer. Br. J. Cancer **108**, 2419–2425 (2013)
4. Li, D., Chen, G., Yang, J., Fan, X., Gong, Y., Xu, G., et al.: Transcriptome analysis reveals disti-nct patterns of long nonconding RNAs in heart and plasma of mice with heart failure. PLoS ONE **8**, e77938 (2013)
5. Chen, L., Guo, X., Li, Z., He, Y.: Relationship between long non-coding RNAs and Alzheimer's disease: a systematic review. Pathol. Res. Pract. **215**(1), 12–20 (2019)
6. Li, D., Chen, G., Yang, J., et al.: Transcriptome analysis reveals distinct patterns of long noncoding RNAs in heart and plasma of mice with heart failure. PLoS ONE **8**(10), e77938 (2013)
7. Vucicevic, D., Schrewe, H., Orom, U.A., et al.: Molecular mechanisms of long ncRNAs in neurological disorders. Front. Genet. **4**, 48 (2014)

8. Gutschner, T., Hammerle, M., Eissmann, M., et al.: The noncoding RNA MALAT1 is a critical regulator of the metastasis phenotype of lung cancer cells. Cancer Res. **73**(3), 1180–1189 (2013)

9. Bao, Z., Yang, Z., Huang, Z., et al.: LncRNADisease 2.0: an updated database of long non-coding RNA-associated diseases. Nucleic Acids Res. **47**(D1), D1034 (2019)

10. Wang, H., Hu, H., Xiang, Z., Lu, C., Dai, F., Tong, X.: Identification and characterization of a new long noncoding RNA iab-1 in the Hox cluster of silkworm Bombyx mori identification of iab-1. J. Cell Biochem. **120**(10), 17283–17292 (2019)

11. Zhang, Y., Wang, X., Kang, L.: A k-mer scheme to predict piRNAs and characterize locust piRNAs. Bioinformatics **27**(6), 771–776 (2011)

12. Banerjee, T., Gupta, S., Ghosh, T.C.: Role of mutational bias and natural selection on genome-wide nucleotide bias in prokaryotic organisms. Biosystems **81**(1), 11–18 (2005)

13. Kong, L., Zhang, Y., Ye, Z.Q.: CPC: Assess the protein-coding potential of transcripts using sequence features and support vector machine. Nucleic Acids Res. **35**, W345–W349 (2007)

14. Zhou, Z.H.: Machine Learning. Tsinghua University Press, Beijing (2016)

15. Pang, H.-X., Dong, W.-X.: Novel linear search for support vector machine parameter selection. J. Zhejiang Univ. Sci. C **12**, 885 (2011)

16. Derrien, T.: The GENCODE v7 catalog of human long noncoding RNAs: analysis of their gene structure, evolution, and expression. Genome Res. **22**, 1775–1789 (2013)

17. Achawanantakun, R., Chen, J., Sun, Y., Zhang, Y.: LncRNA-ID: long non-coding RNA IDentification using balanced random forests. Bioinformatics **31**(24), 3897–3905 (2015)

Research on the Evaluation of Chinese Herbal Medicine Quality and Safety Credit Index Based on TOPSIS

Zhi-kang Wang and Hua Guan[✉]

College of Information Engineering, Hubei University of Chinese Medicine,
Wuhan, China
3018@hbtcm.edu.cn

Abstract. Quality and safety evaluation of Chinese herbal medicine has always been a difficult and key issue in the research and application of Chinese herbal medicine, which restricts the modernization and internationalization of Chinese herbal medicine. In this paper, we present a quality and safety credit evaluation index of Chinese herbal medicines production, and the numerical value was used to reflect the quality and safety credit status of Chinese herbal medicine enterprises. TOPSIS method is introduced into the field of quality and safety evaluation of CHM. Considering the multi-level characteristics of the evaluation index system, the weight of the index is calculated by analytic hierarchy process (AHP), and the ranking of quality and safety credit of CHM in the region is obtained. The quality and safety credit evaluation index of Chinese herbal medicine was constructed. It is an important basic application platform for establishing a sound quality supervision system for Chinese herbal medicine.

Keywords: Chinese herbal medicine · Quality and safety credit index ·
Technique for order preference by similarity to ideal solution (TOPSIS) ·
Analytic hierarchy process (AHP)

1 Introduction

Chinese Herbal Medicine(CHM), with its rich resources and unique curative effect, has attracted more and more attention from all countries in the world. The safety of CHM caused by environmental pollutants has been affected, and it has attracted more and more attention. In the international market, many of China's export products are blocked by so-called 'green barriers', such as heavy metals and pesticide residues. The safety of CHM has become a bottleneck restricting the development of Chinese medicine.

The method for designing the quality and safety credit index for Chinese herbal medicines(QSCI4CHM) is mainly based on the inspection and testing indicators of heavy metals and pesticide residues, we design the quality and safety evaluation indicators of CHM, and the numerical value was used to reflect the quality and safety credit status of Chinese herbal medicine enterprises. The Analytic Hierarchy Process (AHP) is used to calculate the index weights. The Technique for order of Preference by Similarity to Ideal Solution(TOPSIS) method was introduced into the field of regional

© Springer Nature Switzerland AG 2019
H. Wang et al. (Eds.): HIS 2019, LNCS 11837, pp. 76–85, 2019.
https://doi.org/10.1007/978-3-030-32962-4_8

Chinese herbal medicine quality and safety evaluation, and the CHM quality and safety credit evaluation index was constructed. The numerical value was used to reflect the quality and safety credit status of Chinese herbal medicine enterprises. Finally, the credit index of each Chinese herbal medicine enterprise is weighted and averaged to form the QSCI4CHM of industry and region.

2 Related Research

In 2005, the Japanese Chinese prescription Biopharmaceutical Preparation Association established the 'Industry Standard for Pesticide Residues in Chinese prescription and Biopharmaceutical Preparations', and a limited standard for organochlorine pesticides, organophosphorus pesticides and pyrethroids of several Chinese herbal medicines and proprietary Chinese medicines was prescribed. The German National Botanical Pharmacopoeia strictly limits the heavy metal content and pesticide residues of botanicals. The United States Pharmacopoeia [1] contains detection methods for 34 pesticide residues such as organochlorine, organophosphorus and pyrethroid, and specifies the limit standards and calculation formulas. China has also gradually improved the standard of harmful substances in traditional Chinese medicine, which is necessary for the safe use of Chinese medicine.

In terms of credit and safety evaluation, Aydogan [2] uses the rough set-based AHP to determine the index weight, and then combines the fuzzy TOPSIS method to conduct a multi-factor comprehensive evaluation of business performance. Wang [3] proposed a fuzzy TOPSIS method based on alpha level sets and presents a nonlinear programming (NLP) solution procedure. Rijia [4] constructed a comprehensive credit evaluation method for life insurance companies by using AHP and fuzzy comprehensive evaluation. Xiujin [5] tested and analyzed the pesticide residues and major heavy metals of 10 kinds of commercially available vegetables in 11 prefecture-level cities, and used AHP to calculate the comprehensive pollution index of vegetables of different varieties and different sub-regions. Based on the established meropenem drug utilization evaluation standard, Rong [6] used the weighted TOPSIS method to evaluate 147 cases of meropenem in a hospital in China from 2011 to 2012, and explored the establishment of meropenem drug evaluation method. Huanan [7] proposed the evaluation of the safety of livestock food based on the Fuzzy-AHP method.

3 The Design of QSCI4CHM

Figure 1 is the process of our method. Firstly based on guarantee of CHM safety factors and the process of agricultural from growth to flowing into the market, the evaluation indicator has been established.Secondly, the data related to the quality and safety of CHM collected through the Internet of Things, traceability platform, inspection and test data platform are put into the basic database, and then each indicator data is extracted in the database. Single factor or comprehensive index analysis is processed. Thirdly, considering the characteristic of multi-level index system,AHP method is used to calculate the weight assignment of each index, then, calculate QSCI4CHM of each product of each enterprise. Lastly,by TOPSIS method,the evaluation model was constructed to evaluate each product of each enterprise, and obtain the regional safety credit index of CHM. The evaluation results will be helpful to predicate the safety of CHM.

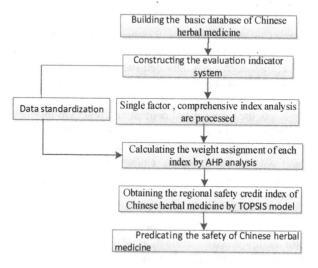

Fig. 1. The process of QSCI4CHM

4   Construction of Credit Index Evaluation System

4.1   Introduction to Credit Indicator Evaluation Index

The quality and safety credit evaluation index system is divided into three levels. The first-level indicator is the comprehensive evaluation of CHM quality and safety credit, which is indicated by A. The second-level indicators include three kinds of macro-qualification indicators. There are 9 individual indicators in the indicator layer, which are represented by C1–C9. The specific indicators are shown in Fig. 2.

The Chinese Pharmacopoeia [8] (2015 edition) stipulates the heavy metal limit requirement for CHM(Lead ≤ 10 mg/kg, cadmium ≤ 1 mg/kg, copper ≤ 20 mg/kg, arsenic limited range of 5 mg/kg, per person per day safe intake of 50–200 μg chromium, mercury ≤ 1 mg/kg).

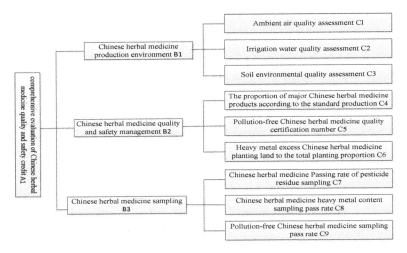

Fig. 2. The quality and safety evaluation index system of CHM

4.2   The Evaluation Method Based on Single Factor Index

The method for evaluating the pollution of heavy metals and pesticides in the soil of CHM planting adopts the single factor index method. Take the pollution of heavy metals as an example, the formula can be represented as following: $P_i = C_i/S_i$.

For a certain point, if there are many heavy metals in the soil, the single factor index method is used to calculate the maximum value of the index. That is: in $P_{max} = MAX\ Pi()$, P_{max} is the pollution index of various heavy metals in the soil; P_i is the pollution index of the type i heavy metal in the soil. The pollution level is shown in Table 1.

A certain soil has been tested to contain four heavy metals: arsenic, lead, cadmium and copper, and their contents are 0.04 mg/L, 0.03 mg/L, 0.005 mg/L, and 0.5 mg/L, respectively. The known standard contents are 0.05 mg/L, 0.05 mg/L, 0.01 mg/L, and 1.0 mg/L, respectively. The calculated $P_1 = 0.8$, $P_2 = 0.6$, $P_3 = 0.5$, and P4 = 0.5. At this time, $P_{max} = 0.8$, compared with the above table, the over-standard grade is I, which is the degree of cleanliness and meets the standard.

Table 1. The pollution of heavy metals in the soil

The degree of exceeding the limitation	Pi	P_{max}	The degree of pollution
I	$P_i <=1.0$	$P_{max} <=1.0$	Clean
II	$1.0 < P_i <=2.0$	$1.0 < P_{max} <=2.0$	Slight clean
III	$2.0 < P_i <=3.0$	$2.0 < P_{max} <=3.0$	Mild pollution
IV	$3.0 < P_i <=5.0$	$3.0 < P_{max} <=5.0$	Medium pollution
V	$P_i > 5.0$	$P_{max} > 5.0$	Heavy pollution

4.3   The Evaluation Method Based on Comprehensive Index

The comprehensive pollution index reflects the comprehensive pollution level of toxic elements such as heavy metals and pesticides measured in CHM. Take the pollution of heavy metals as an example. The formula for the comprehensive pollution index is:

$$P = \sqrt{\frac{\max\left(\frac{C_i}{S_i}\right)^2 + avg\left(\frac{C_i}{S_i}\right)^2}{2}}$$

The evaluation criteria are shown in Table 2:

Table 2. The grading criteria of comprehensive evaluation

Degree classification	P	Pollution degree	Pollution degree
1	P = 0.85	Non-pollution	Clean
2	0.85 < P = 1.71	Mild pollution	Polluted
3	1.71 < P = 2.56	Medium pollution	Exceed the limit
4	P > 2.56	Heavy pollution	Severely exceed the limit

The heavy metal content of a base has been tested, as shown in Table 3. According to the comprehensive evaluation formula, P = 0.45 < 0.85, which meets the standard and is not contaminated by heavy metals. When $Pi \leq 1$, it means that the CHM is not contaminated, and when $Pi > 1$, it means that the CHM is contaminated.

Table 3. The pollution in the soil

Area	Lead	Cadmium	Arsenic	HG	Chromium	HCH	DDT
I	0.11	0.10	0.23	0.04	0.39	0.02	0.02
II	0.13	0.12	0.23	0.04	0.59	0.02	0.02
III	0.10	0.08	0.23	0.04	0.42	0.02	0.02

4.4   Weight Determination and Index Design Based on AHP

Compared with the Chinese herbal medicine product quality safety degree A (target layer), the index of the criterion layer (B1, B2, B3), is compared in pairs, and the judgment matrix is obtained, then the basic steps of AHP are as following:

First, the structural model of AHP is established, and the '1–9 proportional method' is used in constructing the judgment matrix.

Then calculate the weight vector and perform the consistency test. When CR < 0.1, pass the consistency test. The RI indicators are shown in Table 4:

Table 4. The random consistency index RI

Order	1	2	3	4	5	6	7	8	9
RI	0	0	0.58	0.90	1.12	1.24	1.32	1.41	1.45

Finally the combined weight vector is calculated. Based on the above-mentioned Chinese herbal medicine quality and safety credit evaluation index system, and sorting the importance degree of each index in the system, the judgment matrix is as follows:

(1) The comprehensive evaluation of the quality and safety credits of the target layer of CHM is shown in Table 5.

Table 5. The judgment matrix of target layer A

A	B1	B2	B3
B1	1	1/3	1/4
B2	3	1	1/2
B3	4	2	1

It is calculated that W1 = (0.1220, 0.3196, 0.5584)T, λmax = 3.018, CI = (λmax-n)/(n-1) = 0.009147, because of the 3rd order matrix, RI = 0.58, at this time CR = CI/RI = 0.015771 < 0.1. Pass the consistency test.

(2) Guidelines layer weight analysis

The judgment matrix is constructed in turn for the criterion layers B1, B2, and B3, as shown in Table 6, 7 and 8.

Table 6. The judgment matrix of target layer A

B1//B2//B3	C1	C2	C3
C1	(1)//(1)//(1)	(1/3)//(1/4)//(2)	(1/5)//(3)//(1/2)
C2	(3)//(4)//(1/2)	(1)//(1)//(1)	(1/2)//(5)//(1/3)
C3	(5)//(1/3)//(2)	(2)//(1/5)//(3)	(1)//(1)//(1)

The calculated relative weights of B1, B2, and B3, λmax, CI, RI, and CR are shown in Table 7:

Table 7. The detailed parameters of criterion layer

Criterion layer	W	λmax	CI	RI	CR
B1	$(0.1095, 0.3090, 0.5816)^T$	3.004	0.0018	0.58	0.0032
B2	$(0.2255, 0.6738, 0.1007)^T$	3.0858	0.0429	0.58	0.0739
B3	$(0.2970, 0.1634, 0.5396)^T$	3.0092	0.0046	0.58	0.0079

It can be seen from the Table 7 that the values of CR are all less than 0.1, so the consistency test is passed. The data of a company's Chinese herbal medicine products are as follows:

Table 8. The detailed parameters of each Chinese herb medicine index

Product	C1	C2	C3	C4	C5	C6	C7	C8	C9
A	78.53	92.33	87.72	98.23	81	70.56	97.76	96.14	97.08
B	85.62	89.96	85.88	96.26	84	76.23	96.55	97.34	96.06
C	60.78	94.55	94.65	97.17	96	80.32	98.25	96.26	97.88
D	69.57	86.69	92.12	99.11	90	82.45	95.18	98.03	97.47

QSCI4CHM of each Chinese herb medicine product is calculated as follows:

Table 9. QSCI4CHM of each Chinese herb medicine

	A	B	C	D
Index	78	82	85	87

It can be seen from the Table 9 that the product D quality is the best and the A is the worst.

4.5 Comprehensive Evaluation of Chinese Herbal Medicine Products Based on TOPSIS

TOPSIS is a decision making method for solving problems with multiple criteria. The Basic principle of TOPSIS requires the chosen alternatives to have the shortest distance from the positive ideal choice and the farthest distance from the negative ideal solution.

① Building the original matrix, as shown in Table 10.

Table 10. The quality and safety of each regional Chinese herbal medicines

Region	A	B	C	D
1	78	82	85	87
2	83	84	86	77
3	90	82	88	83
4	79	89	84	86

② Making indicators have the same trend, absolute indicator using inverse method(1/X).For example, area 1 (A):After processing, value equals 0.012821.

③ Normalized. After normalizing, the parameters are as shown in Table 11.

Table 11. The credit index of each regional Chinese herbal medicines (after normalized)

Region	A	B	C	D
1	0.526381	0.512866	0.504189	0.476801
2	0.494672	0.500655	0.498326	0.538724
3	0.456197	0.512866	0.487001	0.499780
4	0.519718	0.472528	0.510191	0.482346

④ Determining the optimal value of the index and the worst quality constitute the optimal value vector Z^+ and the worst value vector Z^-

$$Z^+ = (Z_{max1}, Z_{max2}, Z_{max3}......Z_{maxn}) \quad Z^- = (Z_{min1}, Z_{min2}, Z_{min3}......Z_{minn})$$

The best scheme: 0.526381 0.512866 0.510191 538724
The worst scheme: 0.456197 0.472528 0.487001 0.476801

⑤ Calculate the distance between the index value of each evaluation unit and the optimal value and the worst value:

$$S_j^+ = \sqrt{\sum_{i=1}^{m} (f_{ij} - Z_i^+)^2} \quad S_j^- = \sqrt{\sum_{i=1}^{m} (f_{ij} - Z_i^-)^2}$$

The distance obtained by this example is as shown in Table 12:

Table 12. The distance of each regional schemes

Region	D+	D–
1	0.062212	0.082755
2	0.035992	0.078956
3	0.083548	0.046423
4	0.069642	0.067849

⑥ The merits of each evaluation unit are ranked according to the proximity degree. The larger C, the closer to the optimal level.

$$G_j = \frac{S_j^-}{S_j^+ + S_j^-}$$

The evaluation reference values are obtained by using the formula: Dbest/ (Dbest + Dwors). The smaller the reference value is, the higher the evaluation result is, that is, the scheme is optimal, and the region 1:0.429146, region 2:0.313115, region 3:0.642820, region 4: 0.506520. That is, Area 2 > Area 1 > Area 4 > Area 3.

5   Conclusion and Future Work

Based on the data management platform of Chinese herbal medicine quality and safety evaluation, we designs the QSCI4CHM, and establishes a safety evaluation method and technology which is suitable for the characteristics of traditional Chinese herb medicine.

The release of the 'quality and safety credit index of Chinese herbal medicine' has played a significant role in promoting Chinese herbal medicine enterprises to improve the quality and safety awareness of CHM. It is an important basic application platform for establishing a sound quality supervision system, accelerating the construction of a quality credit system, it helps to improve the public's knowledge and participation in pesticide management.

For the control of the quality and safety of Chinese herbal medicine, what we have done is only a little bit. There is still a long way to go before establishing a complete evaluation system for the quality and safety of CHM. We hope that the evaluation of the QSCI4CHM can be reflected in the quality and safety operation process of the entire Chinese herbal medicine supply chain, rather than an isolated evaluation of the safety control of a certain node enterprise, it should include suppliers, manufacturers, distributors, retailers, Carriers, etc. We also hope to send quality and safety warning information for Chinese herbal medicine products through the early-warning model.

Acknowledgment. This work has been supported by humanities and social science Research Program of Hubei province under Grant No. 17Y059.

References

1. United States Pharmacopoeia Commission. US Pharmacopoeia. 35 edition. Washington: United States Pharmacopoeia Commission, 1–1258 (2012)
2. Aydogan, E.K.: Performance measurement model for Turkish aviation firms using the rough-AHP and TOPSIS methods under fuzzy environment. Expert Syst. Appl. **38**(4), 3992–3998 (2011)
3. Wang, Y.M., Elhag, T.M.S.: Fuzzy TOPSIS method based on alpha level sets with an application to bridge risk assessment. Expert Systems with Application **31**, 309–319 (2006)
4. Ri-Jia, D., Hua-Ming, W., Chao, X.: Research on credit evaluation of china's life insurance companies based on ahp-fuzzy comprehensive evaluation. Coal Econ. Res. **23**(6), 1147–1156 (2008)
5. Xiu-jin, D., Xiao-li, W., Jia-hong, Z., Gui-xian, H.: Assessment on quality and safety of the vegetables in Zhejiang market based on AHP. Acta Agriculturae Zhefiangensis **23**(6), 1147–1156 (2011)

6. Xing, R., Zhu, Y.-L., Song, J.-W.: Evaluation on meropenem using based on weighted TOPSIS method. Chin. J. New Drugs Clin. Rem. **32**(5), 389–393 (2013)
7. Hua-Nan, L., Feng, X.: Meat food safety credit evaluation indicators and methods. Stat. Decis. **10**, 65–68 (2006)
8. National Pharmacopoeia Committee. Pharmacopoeia of People's Republic of China. Part 1. Beijing: China Medical Science Press (2015)

Mining Medical Data (II)

ICU Mortality Prediction Based on Key Risk Factors Identification

Rui Tan[1,2], Shuai Ding[1,2(✉)], Jinxin Pan[1,2], and Yan Qiu[1,2]

[1] School of Management, Hefei University of Technology, Hefei, China
2018110737@mail.hfut.edu.cn, dingshuai@hfut.edu.cn,
xiaoyu_pjx@163.com, qy2017110732@gmail.com
[2] Key Laboratory of Process Optimization and Intelligent Decision-Making
(Ministry of Education), Hefei University of Technology, Hefei, China

Abstract. Predicting ICU mortality and finding key risk factors make sense for both doctors and patients. Although there has been a number of research pertaining to ICU mortality prediction systems and algorithms, plenty of room still exists for improvement in practical prediction results and identification of important risk factors. In this study, we use C5 decision tree model to predict mortality of ICU patients and identify key risk factors. Totally 4367 records of ICU patients from a local grade-A tertiary hospital were selected for motality prediction, including 244 dead records with demographic information and physiological parameters. In order to solve the problem of inconsistent data sampling frequency, we extracted 96 statistical indicators based on the original records, such as the kurtosis value of red blood cells (HXB_kurt), the skewness coefficient of red blood cells (HXB_skew). Totally 41 indicators as the final input of the prediction model were extracted through feature extraction method. The experimental results show that C5 decision tree model outperform C&RT, CHDID, KNN, Logistic, SVM and Random Forest in five different performance indicators. Moreover, worst-case status and state of changes in respiratory, body temperature, care level, diastolic blood pressure and age were found to be the key risk factors.

Keywords: ICU · Mortality prediction · Risk factor C5 decision tree

1 Introduction

Intensive care unit (ICU) is a place in the hospital that provides medical services with high-efficiency and high-quality by concentrating manpower resource, strengthening equipment and facilities, and reducing deaths for critical patients [1, 2]. More than 5 million patients in the United States receive intensive care in the ICU every year, and the mortality rate is as high as 25%, partly because of the limitations of the availability of nursing staff and treatment equipment in the hospital [3, 4]. ICU nurses inevitably treat patients differently according to their condition [1, 5]. Meanwhile, ICU mortality has been proposed as an important indicator of the hospital medical quality [6]. Therefore, predicting ICU mortality and identifying risk factors have practical significance for effective allocation of ICU resources, reducing mortality and improving the quality of hospital medical service.

© Springer Nature Switzerland AG 2019
H. Wang et al. (Eds.): HIS 2019, LNCS 11837, pp. 89–97, 2019.
https://doi.org/10.1007/978-3-030-32962-4_9

With the wide application of information technology in the medical field [7, 8], hospitals have massive amount of clinical data through monitoring equipment and experimental testing, providing support for developing clinical prediction models for ICU. Among them, the study of mortality prediction is of paramount importance for ICU clinical treatment [9]. From scoring systems based on APACHE II [10] to advanced machine learning (ML) techniques [11, 12], many scholars have achieved good results in ICU mortality prediction. In the Physical Network ICU Mortality Challenge [13], the advantages of the state-of-the-art ML techniques are well presented in mortality prediction, such as Bayesian networks [14, 15], random forest models [16] and time series based dynamic prediction [17, 18]. Although the above algorithms may obtain accurate prediction results, it does not point out the relationship between the key factors and cannot effectively assist doctors to intervene in treatment.

In this study, the statistics of vital signs and experimental indicators of ICU patients are used to predict the mortality of ICU patients based on decision tree model. Compared with other methods, i.e., C&RT, CHDID, KNN, Logistic, SVM and Random Forest, our model yielded the best results in a comprehensive analysis of misdiagnosis rate, missed diagnosis rate, precision, F1 score and AUC. The main findings and contributions are as follows: (1) The C5 decision tree algorithm has great potential for mortality prediction for patients in ICU. (2) Using statistics like kurtosis coefficient, maximum value, mean value helps solve the data sparse problem, and we can describe the patient's health status by these statistics. (3) We identify key risk factors for ICU patients, such as the kurtosis value of breathing(huxi_kurt), the skewness coefficient of body temperature (TW_skew), which provides doctors with more convincing clinical decisions and helps reduce ICU mortality. (4) According to the results using the C5 decision tree, we can conclude that there is an evident relationship between the parent and child node variable.

The rest of the paper is organized as follows: Sect. 2 mainly reviews the ICU mortality prediction research works; Sect. 3 introduces the research method; Sect. 4 introduces the experiment setup; Sect. 5 presents the experimental results and discussion; the last section gives conclusion and the future direction for ICU mortality prediction.

2   Related Work

With the increase in ICU medical costs and mortality [9, 19], more and more scholars are engaged in the study of ICU mortality prediction.

Several methods have been proposed, which are based on the ICU baseline risk assessment systems (such as APACHE II, SAPS, etc.) that have been widely used in clinical practice. [20] and [21] conducted a prospective observational study of ICU patients to seek for factors influencing mortality prediction relying on patient-based SAPS-II and APACHEII scores, respectively; [22] improved the predictive performance of regression models by adding physiological variables to the existing scoring systems. But on the one hand, the models of these studies belong to logistic regression which may be affected by multicollinearity among variables; on the other hand, these experimental variables are derived from the scoring systems such as APACHEII, which has certain limitations.

In recent years, ML algorithms have been used more frequently in ICU mortality predictive research, which emerged after the 2012 ICU mortality prediction challenge initiated by PhysioNet. For example, [23] used the support vector machine (SVM) classifier to use patient's descriptive information and physiological data as model input features, and achieved higher scores in the PhysioNet mortality prediction challenge. [24] proposed a sequential contrast patterns classification framework to detect the critical events of patients in the ICU. This kind of algorithm can achieve more accurate prediction of death probability by mining and analyzing the physiological time serialization information of ICU patients.

However, the above learning and prediction processes belong to "black box" approaches for clinicians and patients. On the contrary, the C5 decision tree is easier to understand than many other models. More importantly, ICU patient data is constantly fluctuating over time, the sampling frequency of each indicator is inconsistent. The C5 decision tree is robust in the case of data omissions and excessive input fields.

3   Methodology

Clearly, it is crucial to extract the most relevant impact variables to predicting ICU mortality, and identifying the key factors is important for doctors' intervention and treatment. In this study, there are three steps to predict mortality of patients in ICU and identify the risk factors, as shown in Fig. 1.

3.1   Data Description and Preparation

The data used in this study is obtained from the case information of 4693 ICU patients from March 2017 to December 2018 in the First Affiliated Hospital of Anhui Province, PR. China. The data set mainly includes demographic information and time series characteristics of 4693 patients. For example, the demographic information of the patient includes age, gender, etc. The physiological parameters include fraction of inspiration, the number of red blood cells and white blood cells, etc.

In the data preprocessing stage, we solve the following problems: (1) eliminate cases with errors; (2) quantitative qualitative indicator; (3) for patients who have been admitted to the hospital multiple times, it is considered to be the corresponding number of patients. After data pre-screening, the final number of cases available is reduced to 4,367, of which 244 were deaths, accounting for 5.60% of the total patients.

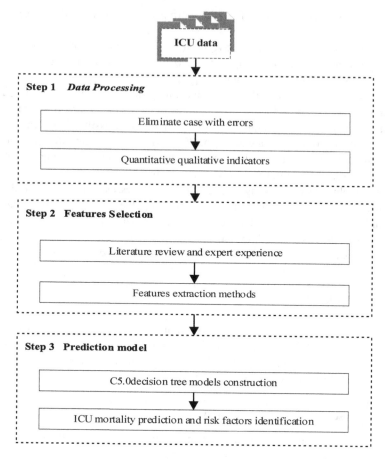

Fig. 1. Overall framework

3.2 Feature Selection

The selection of input characteristic variables in this study is mainly divided into two steps.

Firstly, we summarize 5 demographic factors and 13 physiological parameters, which are likely to have an impact on predicting ICU mortality. The 5 demographic factors include age, gender, weight, severity of illness (Idegree) and level of care (CareLevel). The 13 physiological parameters include fraction of inspiration(FiO2), red blood cells (HXB), white blood cells(BXB), breathing (huxi),heart rate(xinlv), body temperature (TW), potential of hydrogen (PH), potassium(K), sodium (Na), systolic blood pressure (SSY), diastolic blood pressure (SZY), creatinine (JG) and Glasgow Coma Scale(GCS).

ICU data sampling frequency is usually inconsistent and has uneven distribution characteristics. So, we use kurtosis coefficient, maximum value, mean value, median, minimum value, skewness coefficient and standard deviation of 13 physiological parameters to describe the overall distribution of the patient's various indicators. Then, the number of initial input variables is 96.

When using feature extraction methods to analyze ICU data, the variable with the importance greater than or equal to 0.90 is used as the final input variable of the prediction model according to the Pearson coefficient.

3.3 Prediction Model

In this study, we choose C5.0 decision tree to predict patients' mortality in ICU. The C5.0 algorithm is based on the information gain splitting method. The first split determines the sample subset and then splits again according to another filed. This process is repeated until the sample subset cannot be split. Meanwhile, this algorithm uses the rate of decline of information entropy, which is the variable that can bring the maximum information gain, as the basis for determining the optimal branching variable and the segmentation threshold. The decline in information entropy means that the uncertainty of information declines.

4 Experimental

4.1 Experimental Setup

The experimental environment of this study is comprised of SPSS Modeler and SPSS. Based on the real medical records of in-hospital ICU patients, we perform predicting the mortality of ICU patients using the C5.0 model and finding the most relevant influencing factors.

In the process of building the C5.0 model, in order to effectively prevent the over-fitting problem, we firstly check the validity of the predictor variables and remove the unrelated predictors. Then, in the model, the data set is divided into training set and test set by ratio of 7:3 using the Partition variable. Thirdly, we use boosting and tenfold cross validation to improve the accuracy of the model. The boosting is a special method used to improve the accuracy of C5.0 model. It works by building multiple models in a sequence, the first model is built in the usual way; when building the second model, the focus is on the records misclassified by first model, and so on. And we use a weighted voting method to combine the individual predictions into one total prediction.

4.2 Performance Evaluation

In order to assess the performance of our model more accurately, we selected the following commonly used medical indicators: misdiagnosis rate (Mr) and missed diagnosis rate (Mdr). And we expect Mr and Mdr to decrease. Meanwhile, we found that the alive and dead samples of our data set are seriously imbalanced. So, we also introduce precision (Pre), F1 score (F1) and AUC to evaluate our prediction model. The larger the values of Pre, F1, AUC, the better the performance of our model. Recall, specificity, precision, F1 score, misdiagnosis rate and the missed diagnosis rate are calculated as Table 1.

Table 1. Computational formula for evaluation indicators

Indicator	Computational formula
Misdiagnosis rate	$Mr = 1 - \frac{TP}{TP+FN}$
Missed diagnosis rate	$Mdr = 1 - \frac{TN}{TN+FP}$
Precision	$Pre = \frac{TP}{TP+FP}$
F1 score	$F1 = \frac{2TP}{2TP+FP+FN}$

where TP (Ture Positive) represents the number of cases that our model correctly identifies the surviving patients; TN (Ture Negative) represents the number of cases that our model correctly identifies the dead patients; FP (False Positive) indicates the number of cases that our model incorrectly identifies the dead patients as alive one; and FN (False Negative) indicates the number of cases that our model incorrectly identifies the surviving patients as death.

5 Results and Discussion

5.1 Results

Table 2 shows the 41 final input variables after feature selection, together with their importance. These variables are then used as input variables for the decision tree model. Table 3 shows the top ten key feature variables selected by the decision tree prediction model in the final input variables. This suggests that these ten variables play an important role in helping predict mortality in ICU patients. As shown in Table 4, it compares the performance of our C5 decision tree model with classification and regression tree(C&RT), chi-squared automatic interaction detection (CHAID), KNN, Logistic, Rand Forest and SVM in five different performance indicators. Obviously, according to the comprehensive analysis, the performance of the C5 decision tree is better than that of other models.

Table 2. 41 Final input variables.

Variable	Importance of variable	Variable	Importance of variable	Variable	Importance of variable
Weight	1.0	xinlv_std	1.0	huxi_min	1.0
huxi_kurt	1.0	huxi_skew	1.0	Age	1.0
SZY_min	1.0	xinlv_max	1.0	SSY_std	1.0
JG_max	1.0	JG_median	1.0	PH_kurt	1.0
xinlv_mean	0.999	JG_min	0.999	JG_std	0.999
FiO2_kurt	0.998	SSY_min	0.998	Level of care	0.998
FiO2_skew	0.997	Idegree	0.996	xinlv_median	0.996
K_skew	0.991	Gender	0.99	GCS_max	0.989
huxi_std	0.984	BXB_median	0.981	GCS_mean	0.974
GCS_min	0.964	huxi_max	0.964	GCS_median	0.962
TW_skew	0.962	BXB_mean	0.958	K_std	0.954
huxi_mean	0.951	HXB_min	0.948	HXB_std	0.943
JG_kurt	0.938	FiO2_max	0.929		

Table 3. Top ten key feature variables.

Variable	Importance of variable	Variable	Importance of variable	Variable	Importance of variable
huxi_mean	0.03	JG_mean	0.03	JG_std	0.03
TW_skew	0.03	xinlv_max	0.02	SSY_std	0.02
huxi_kurt_	0.02	K_skew	0.02	huxi_skew	0.02
JG_median	0.02				

Table 4. Comparison of experimental results.

Model	Mr	Mdr	Pre	F1	AUC
C5-Death	0.020	0.342	0.981	0.980	0.819
C&RT-Death	0.052	1.000	0.948	0.973	0.500
CHAID-Death	0.558	0.070	0.991	0.611	0.686
KNN-Death	0.000	0.988	0.948	0.973	0.506
Logistic-Death	0.001	1.000	0.948	0.973	0.504
Random Forest-Death	0.256	0.160	0.988	0.849	0.792
SVM-Death	0.019	0.465	0.974	0.978	0.758

5.2   Discussion

Firstly, as shown in Table 3, the worst-case status and state of changes in respiratory, body temperature, care level, diastolic blood pressure, potassium content, creatinine content, and oxygen saturation (especially respiratory value) of ICU patients during the first 48 h may reflect the severity of patient to some extent. The medical staff can set a threshold for the above-mentioned influential factors according to medically relevant regulations. Once the patient's vital signs exceed the threshold or the magnitude of the change is too large, the patient needs to be intensively treated and cared for.

Secondly, from the final result of the decision tree model, age is the basic premise for judging the life status of ICU patients. As is known to all, when a patient is older, the probability of death increases accordingly. In our decision tree prediction model, when the patient's age is greater than 88, it is more meaningful to pay attention to the magnitude of changes in creatinine content and the magnitude of change in breathing. If the changes in the values of these two indicators are too large, the patient's condition is deemed unstable and the probability of death will become greater. At this time, it is necessary to strengthen the treatment of patients. Conversely, when the patient's age is less than or equal to 88, the focus is on heart rate.

6   Conclusion and Future Work

This study uses the real data of hospital ICU patients to predict the mortality of ICU patients using C5 decision tree model, and helps doctors to accurately grasp the patient's overall condition and development through the patient's first 48 h of vital signs data. Moreover, most accurate risk factors can be found by this model to help doctors intervene at the earliest possible time, which has practical significance for ICU assisted diagnosis and treatment.

However, this study also has some limitations, mainly in: (1) the data of this study are from a specific hospital, which is relatively simple and not representative. So, the research results cannot be extended to other clinical environments. (2) Without considering the patient's complete time sequence data in the ICU, important feature may be lost. (3) In the experiment, only the possible influencing factors were found, but the relationships between the influencing factors were not identified.

The studies on ICU mortality prediction now are attempting to establish a global, averaged predictive model that may not be suitable for every patient. So, we consider developing an ICU mortality model that is more suitable for individual patient, enabling more accurate prediction for each ICU patient. This can help doctors intervene earlier in the treatment more effectively, reduce ICU mortality, and improve the quality of hospital's medical service.

Acknowledgments. This work is fully supported by the National Natural Science Foundation of China [Nos. 91846107, 71571058, and 71690235], Anhui Provincial Science and Technology Major Project [Nos. 17030801001, and 18030801137], and the Fundamental Research Funds for the Central Universities [No. PA2019GDQT0021].

References

1. Chan, C.W., Farias, V.F., Escobar, G.J.: The impact of delays on service times in the intensive care unit. Manag. Sci. **63**(7), 2049–2072 (2016)
2. Jing, L., Ming, D., Zhao, W.: Admissions optimisation and premature discharge decisions in intensive care units. Int. J. Prod. Res. **53**(24), 7329–7342 (2015)
3. Rouzbahman, M., Jovicic, A., Chignell, M.: Can cluster-boosted regression improve prediction of death and length of stay in the ICU? IEEE J. Biomed. Health Inform. **21**(3), 851–858 (2016)
4. Ghosh, Shameek, Feng, M., Nguyen, H., Li, J.: Hypotension risk prediction via sequential contrast patterns of ICU blood pressure. IEEE J. Biomed. Health Inform. **20**(5), 1416–1426 (2015)
5. Chan, C.W., Green, L.V., Lekwijit, S., Lu, L., Escobar, G.: Assessing the impact of service level when customer needs are uncertain: an empirical investigation of hospital step-down units. Manag. Sci. **65**(2), 751–775 (2018)
6. Armony, M., Chan, C.W., Zhu, B.: Critical care capacity management: Understanding the role of a step down unit. Prod. Oper. Manag. **27**(5), 859–883 (2018)
7. Luo, G.: PredicT-ML: a tool for automating machine learning model building with big clinical data. Health Inf. Sci. Syst. **4**(1), 5 (2016)
8. Thabtah, F., Abdelhamid, N., Peebles, D.: A machine learning autism classification based on logistic regression analysis. Health Inf. Sci. Syst. **7**(1), 12 (2019)
9. Hu, W., Chan, C.W., Zubizarreta, J.R., Escobar, G.J.: An examination of early transfers to the ICU based on a physiologic risk score. Manuf. Serv. Oper. Manag. **20**(3), 531–549 (2018)
10. Rudin, C., Ustun, B.: Optimized scoring systems: toward trust in machine learning for healthcare and criminal justice. Interfaces **48**(5), 449–466 (2018)

11. Gao, Y., Xu, A., Hu, P.J.-H., Cheng, T.-H.: Incorporating association rule networks in feature category-weighted naive Bayes model to support weaning decision making. Decis. Support Syst. **96**, 27–38 (2017)
12. Jagadeeswari, V., Subramaniyaswamy, V., Logesh, R., Vijayakumar, V.: A study on medical Internet of Things and big data in personalized healthcare system. Health Inf. Sci. Syst. **6**(1), 14 (2018)
13. Silva, I., Moody, G., Scott, D.J., Celi, L.A., Mark, R.G.: Predicting in-hospital mortality of icu patients: the physionet/computing in cardiology challenge 2012. In: 2012 Computing in Cardiology, pp. 245–248. IEEE (2012)
14. Abu-Samah, A., Razak, N.N.A., Suhaimi, F.M., Jamaludin, U.K., Chase, G.: Linking Bayesian network and intensive care units data: a glycemic control study. In: TENCON 2018-2018 IEEE Region 10 Conference, pp. 1988–1993. IEEE (2018)
15. Thanathornwong, B.: Bayesian-based decision support system for assessing the needs for orthodontic treatment. Healthcare Inform. Res. **24**(1), 22–28 (2018)
16. Lin, K., Hu, Y., Kong, G.: Predicting in-hospital mortality of patients with acute kidney injury in the ICU using random forest model. Int. J. Med. Inform. **125**, 55–61 (2019)
17. Ghasemi, P., Raoufy, M.R.: Prediction of mortality in patients with sepsis using detrended fluctuation analysis of heart rate variability. In: 2016 23rd Iranian Conference on Biomedical Engineering and 2016 1st International Iranian Conference on Biomedical Engineering (ICBME), pp. 150–154. IEEE (2016)
18. Li-wei, H.L., et al.: A physiological time series dynamics-based approach to patient monitoring and outcome prediction. IEEE J. Biomed. Health Inform. **19**(3), 1068–1076 (2014)
19. Wong, E.G., Parker, A.M., Leung, D.G., Brigham, E.P., Arbaje, A.I.: Association of severity of illness and intensive care unit readmission: a systematic review. Heart Lung: J. Acute Crit. Care **45**(1), 3–9 (2016)
20. Aminiahidashti, H., Bozorgi, F., Montazer, S.H., Baboli, M., Firouzian, A.: Comparison of APACHE II and SAPS II scoring systems in prediction of critically ill patients' outcome. Emergency **5**(1), 4 (2017)
21. Wang, X., et al.: A new method to predict hospital mortality in severe community acquired pneumonia. Eur. J. Intern. Med. **40**, 56–63 (2017)
22. Itani, R., Minami, Y., Haruki, S., Watanabe, E., Hagiwara, N.: Prognostic impact of disseminated intravascular coagulation score in acute heart failure patients referred to a cardiac intensive care unit: a retrospective cohort study. Heart Vessels **32**(7), 872–879 (2017)
23. Citi, L., Barbieri, R.: PhysioNet 2012 challenge: predicting mortality of ICU patients using a cascaded SVM-GLM paradigm. In: 2012 Computing in Cardiology, pp. 257–260. IEEE (2012)
24. Ghosh, S., Nguyen, H., Li, J.: B. T.-I. C. of the I. E. in M. & B. S.: Predicting short-term ICU outcomes using a sequential contrast motif based classification framework (2016)

Can Heart Rate Variability Parameters Be a Biomarker for Predicting Motor Function Prognosis in Patients with Chronic Stroke?

Xiaoyu Zhang[1], Xin Li[2(✉)], Haoyang Liu[3], Guigang Zhang[4], and Chunxiao Xing[5]

[1] Beijing Boai Hospital, China Rehabilitation Research Center,
Rehabilitation Medical College, Capital Medical University,
Beijing 100068, China
nmbrbd@hotmail.com
[2] Beijing Tsinghua Changgung Hospital Medical Center, Tsinghua University,
Beijing 100084, China
horsebackdancing@sina.com
[3] Beijing University of Posts and Telecommunications, Beijing 100876, China
[4] Institute of Automation, Chinese Academy of Sciences, Beijing 100190, China
[5] Research Institute of Information Technology, Tsinghua University,
Beijing 100084, China

Abstract. Stroke patients are often associated with lower levels of heart rate variability, suggesting that autonomic dysfunction is very common in stroke patients. Recent studies have shown that heart rate variability (HRV) is an early predictor of prognosis in patients with acute stroke, but the relationship between HRV and functional status in chronic rehabilitation patients is not clear. The purpose of this study was to investigate the clinical value of heart rate variability parameters in predicting motor function assessment in convalescent stroke patients. Methods: Sixty-four patients with strokes admitted to Beijing Bo'ai Hospital from October 2015 to October 2016 were enrolled. Dynamic electro-cardiogram was used to continuously record the data of 24-h monitoring and analyze the heart rate variability, including time domain parameters [standard deviation of all NN intervals (SDNN, where NN intervals refer to the RR intervals of sinus beats), standard deviation of the 5-mins average NN intervals (SDANN), percentage of successive NN intervals greater than 50 ms (PNN50), root mean square of differences between adjacent RR intervals (RMSSD)], frequency domain parameters [high frequency component (HF), low frequency component (LF), very low frequency component (VLF), ratio of low frequency to high frequency component (LF/HF)] and heart rate variability triangular index. And by using the Barthel Index for Activities of Daily Living (ADLs) and the Fugl-Meyer Motor Assessment (FMA) simultaneously, the patients' functional status was assessed. Results: The correlation analysis with related factors controlled showed that the HRV parameters were significantly correlated with the recovery of motor function [time domain indicators RR triangular index (r = 0.252; P = 0.05) and frequency domain indicator VLF (r = 0.302; P = 0.018)] and there was no relationship with HRV parameter and the improvement in activities of daily living of stroke patients in the chronic rehabilitation period. The monitoring of HRV-related parameters of stroke patients in their chronic rehabilitation period has a certain correlation with their motor function outcomes and daily living ability. Non-invasive monitoring of HRV may be an alternative method to judge the prognosis of stroke. In the future, further research is needed to verify the relevance of HRV to clinical outcomes.

Keywords: Heart rate variability · Stroke · Motor function · Prognostic

1 Introduction

Impaired autonomic function is a common disease in stroke patients and is associated with poor functional outcomes and higher mortality [1–3]. Heart Rate Variability (HRV) is a simple, non-invasive ECG-derived measurement method, which is used to monitor the control of cardiovascular activity by the autonomic nervous system (ANS) including the vagus nerve and sympathetic nerves [4, 5]. Given its accessibility and low invasiveness, HRV measurements are representative functional indicators of ANS activity. Non-invasive analysis of spontaneous heart rate variability (HRV) has been widely used in many studies to assess autonomic function [6, 7]. In addition, the reduction in HRV is considered to be a predictor of general mortality [8, 9] and cardiovascular risk factors (including hypertension and obesity) [10]. Heart rate variability is reported to be lower in patients with stroke or cardiovascular disease. In patients with severe ischemic stroke, autonomic dysfunction particularly inhibits parasympathetic tone [11–13]. The relationship between HRV and stroke provides information not only about the clinical status, but also about the prognosis of stroke. The study investigated the relationship between HRV analysis and post-stroke complications and/or functions such as patient mortality [14–16] and functions [17–19], severe stroke [20], post-stroke motor function [21, 22], as well as specific HRV changes (mainly in the time and frequency domain) [23], HRV SDNN and other parameters, and CMI; and the predictions with HRV succeeded in some cases. In particular, changes in frequency domain HRV parameters, mainly LF and HF, and time domain HRV parameters (including SDNN and RMSSD), and provide predictors of stroke function for stroke severity, stroke-related sports injuries [21, 22] Prognosis related. However, considering that there is little research on the influence of motor system impairment after stroke upon the autonomic nervous system, none of the parameters in HRV has been commonly accepted as a predictor of motor functional outcomes after stroke. The purpose of this study was to investigate the relationship between motor function in stroke patients during rehabilitation and HRV parameters reflecting autonomic dysfunction. The predictive biomarkers of HRV parameters reflecting the motor function of stroke patients were determined, which laid a theoretical foundation for strengthening the management of autonomic nervous function of stroke patients.

2 Patients

We collected data from some of the stroke patients during their convalescence at a time ranging from September 2015 to September 2016 at the Chinese Rehabilitation Research Center in Beijing Bo'ai Hospital. We chose patients meeting the following criteria: (I) aged 18–90 years; (II) 1–3 months after onset of stroke; (III) ischemic or hemorrhagic stroke confirmed by CT scan or magnetic resonance imaging; (iv) first onset, single lesion, and with unilateral exercise weakness. The exclusion criteria are: (I) major concomitant diseases, including heart failure with NYHA ≥ 3, chronic obstructive pulmonary disease, renal failure, malignancy and liver failure; (II) complicated with severe arrhythmia, such as Atrial fibrillation; (iv) stroke involving brainstem and cerebellum; (iv) previous myocardial infarction, coronary bypass grafting, carotid artery stenting, artificial pacemaker implantation. This study was approved by the Ethics Committee of Beijing Bo'ai Hospital. All participants signed an informed consent form.

3 Assessment

Data of patients in the rehabilitation department were collected with detailed demographic and clinical variables such as hypertension, diabetes, hyperlipidemia, and smoking and drinking history. 24-h holter monitoring was performed within one week after admission. Specifically, we monitored each patient with the 12-channel digital dynamic electrocardiograph (the MIC-12H 12-lead dynamic electrocardiogram developed by Beijing Jinco Medical Equipment Co., Ltd.) for more than 24 h. Thereby we obtained the following heart rate variability parameters: time domain parameters: standard deviation of all sinus beat RR intervals (referred to as NN interval)(SDNN), standard deviation of the average NN intervals (SDANN), percentage of successive NN intervals greater than 50 ms (PNN50), and the total number of all NN intervals divided by the height of the histogram of all NN intervals measured on a discrete scale (HRV triangular parameter); and time domain indicators: very low frequency components (VLF, Very low-frequency 0.003–0.04 Hz), low frequency components (LF, Low-frequency 0.04–0.15 Hz), high frequency components (HF, High-frequency 0.15–0.4 Hz), LF/HF ratio (LF/HF, Ratio of LF /HF). After admission (baseline, t0) and after 1-2 months of rehabilitation (t1), the following functional indicators were recorded: FMA and the Barthel Index scores were used to evaluate the patient's motor function and daily living ability. All participants received rehabilitation training for at least 3 h per day after admission.

4 Statistical Analysis

All statistical analyses were performed using SPSS version 25.0 (SPSS, Inc., Chicago, Illinois, USA). The distribution of continuous variables was determined by the Kolmogorov-Smirnov test. The mean and standard deviation of continuous variables, the median of non-normal distribution variables ((interquartile range, IQR)), and the frequency of classified variables were calculated. The categorical variables were expressed as a percentage of each group of patients. Correlation analysis was performed on each of the HRV parameters with the motor functions as well as ADL functions to test whether the correlations existed. All clinical covariates that might affect the autonomic outcome variables were adjusted in partial correlation, such as demographic data (age) and vascular risk factors, including hypertension, Diabetes, etc. All statistical analyses were performed using SPSS version 25.0 (SPSS, Inc., Chicago, Illinois, USA). $P < 0.05$ was considered statistically significant.

5 Result

Among the stoke patients admitted to Beijing Bo'ai Hospital from October 2015 to October 2016, excluding those with paroxysmal atrial fibrillation, previous stroke, brain stem infarction and hemorrhage, and multiple infarction, we collected data of 64 patients who met our criteria (45 males, accounting for 70.3%), and the age range was 59.05 ± 10.76 years. Among them, there were 39 cases of cerebral infarction, accounting for 60.9%; 25 cases of cerebral hemorrhage, accounting for 39.1%; 27 cases of left hemiparalysis, accounting for 43.8%; 36 cases of right hemiparalysis, accounting for 56.3%; some were complicated with hypertension (79.7%), diabetes (48.4%), coronary heart disease (23.4%), hyperlipidemia (70.3%), or smoking history (51.6%). The HRV parameters, the FMA scores on admission and discharge, and the Barthel Index are shown in Table 1.

Table 1. Baseline characteristics of the patients with chronic stroke enrolled in this study(n = 64)

Characteristics	Values
Gender(male/female), n (%)	45/19(70.3/29.7)
Age (years), mean ± SD	59.05 ± 10.76
Side affected(left/right), n (%)	27/36(43.8/56.3)
Time from stroke (months),median (IQR)	1.50(1.59,2.32)
Type of stroke(ischemic/hemorragic),n (%)	39/25(60.9/39.1)
Medical history (yes/no), n (%)	
Hypertension	51/11(79.7/20.3)
Diabetes	31/33(48.4/51.6)
Coronary heart disease	15/49(23.4/76.6)
Hyperlipidemia	45/19(70.3/29.7)
Smokers	33/31(51.6/48.4)
Time domain parameters	
pNN50(%), median (IQR)	0.65(0.95,2.22)
SDNN(ms), mean ± SD	93.80 ± 31.55
SDANN(ms), mean ± SD	84.59 ± 31.55
RMSSD(ms), median (IQR)	18.55(20.02,30.50)

(continued)

Table 1. (*continued*)

Characteristics	Values
SDSD, median (IQR)	23.00(23.60,34.37)
RR triangular index(ms), median (IQR)	26.75(27.03,32.10)
Frequency domain parameters, median (IQR)	
VLF (ms2)	12286.00(11788.46,19339.82)
LF (ms2)	347.00(307.75,527.94)
HF (ms2)	100.50(123.84,816.41)
LF/HF	3.45(3.00,4.51)
FMA, median (IQR)	
t0	41.00(36.95,48.83)
t1	52.50(45.47,57.16)
Barthel Index, median (IQR)	
t0	47.50(40.86,49.29)
t1	60.00(50.64,60.45)

IQR: interquartile range (25th–75th percentiles); SD: standard deviation; PNN50: NN50 count divided by the total number of all NN intervals; SDNN:standard deviation of all NN intervals; SDANN: standard deviation of the averages of NN intervals in all 5 min segments; RMSSD: square root of the mean of the sum of the squares of differences between adjacent NN intervals; HRV triangular parameter: Total number of all NN intervals divided by the height of the histogram of all NN intervals; VLF: Very low-frequency(0.003–0.04 Hz); LF: Low-frequency(0.04–0.15 Hz); HF: High-frequency(0.15–0.4 Hz); LF/HF: Ratio of LF/HF.

Table 2. Partial correlation analysis for HRV parameters and outcome in chronic stroke (n = 64)

HRV	FMA				Barthel Index			
	t0		t1		t0		t1	
	r	p	r	p	r	p	r	p
Time domain parameters								
pNN50	0.107	0.414	0.036	0.785	0.152	0.241	0.054	0.679
SDNN	0.274	0.032*	0.165	0.204	0.139	0.285	0.128	0.327
SDANN	0.276	0.031*	0.182	0.159	0.11	0.399	0.151	0.244
RMSSD	−0.021	0.875	−0.104	0.424	0.023	0.859	−0.085	0.515
SDSD	−0.009	0.943	−0.098	0.453	0.035	0.792	−0.076	0.562
RR triangular index	0.325	0.011*	0.252	0.05*	0.225	0.082	0.173	0.183
Frequency domain parameters								
VLF	0.358	0.005**	0.302	0.018*	0.183	0.159	0.203	0.116
LF	0.253	0.049*	0.173	0.182	0.212	0.101	0.184	0.155
HF	0.171	0.189	0.125	0.336	0.211	0.102	0.13	0.319
LF/HF	−0.016	0.902	−0.002	0.985	−0.004	0.978	0.033	0.801

Adjusted for gender, diabetes and hyperlipidemia.*p $\leq$ 0.05 significant.

With the variables of age, diabetes history, and hyperlipidemia history controlled, measurement was performed at the baseline in an adjusted correlation analysis which showed that the time domain parameters SDNN(r = 0.274; P = 0.032), SDANN(r = 0.276; P = 0.031), RR triangular index (r = 0.430; P = 0.011) and the frequency domain parameter VLF(r = 0.358; P = 0.005) had significant correlations with the change of motor functions of stroke patients in chronic rehabilitation period. However, in the follow-up period, only the RR triangular index(r = 0.252; P = 0.05) and the VLF(r = 0.302; P = 0.018) showed remarkable correlations with the motor outcomes of stroke patients after their rehabilitation training. All the results were slightly positive correlations. Meanwhile, it is still the above parameters that showed no correlations with the recovery of ADL functions at baseline levels, nor in the follow-up period. See Table 2 and Fig. 1 for details.

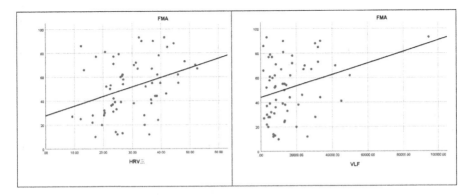

Fig. 1. Association between HRV and motor function outcomes

6 Discussion

The somatic motor nervous system and the autonomic nervous system are simultaneously adjusted by the common neural circuit. These neurons are located in gray matter, hypothalamus and sensorimotor cortex around the aqueduct, and also in the ventromedial medulla, sending multi-synaptic projections to somatic motor and autonomic nerve target areas. The sensorimotor cortex and corticospinal cord pathways directly or indirectly regulate the vagus nerve, and initiate and control movements of upper and lower limbs [24, 25]. Therefore, when stroke damages sensorimotor cortex and corticospinal cord pathway, it may damage vagus nerve activity and reduce heart rate. The exact mechanism by which the autonomic nervous system regulates limb movements is still unclear. There is an overlap between the corticospinal pathway that controls upper limb movements and the vagus nerve that provides the cardiac parasympathetic nerves. Lower limb movements are also controlled by several nonspecific interspinal neurons that coexist with the autonomic nervous system and lower limb movements [26, 27], which may explain the relationship between HRV and the condition of upper and lower limb movements 3 months after stroke.

In our study, we used Holter, a long-term HRV testing tool for more than 24 h to collect HRV data of patients with convalescence, and analyzed the motor function and daily life ability outcomes after the patient's post-hospital rehabilitation follow-up. We found that the HRV parameter level of patients admitted to hospital has a synchronous relationship with the recovery of motor function of stroke patients. Particularly, SDNN (r = 0.274; P = 0.032) and SDANN(r = 0.276; P = 0.031) are supportive to the evaluation and judgement of the motor functions of stroke patients in chronic rehabilitation period. This result is similar to that of Sethi et al. [22] in the study of post-stroke motor outcomes. For patients with acute stroke due to unilateral motor weakness, he found that their time domain HRV(SDNN) was significantly correlated with the recovery of their limb motor function after 3 months of follow-up, especially for patients with severe motor function impairment upon admission. It is worth mentioning that this study did not include patients with acute stroke episodes. Compared with HRV parameters in acute period, the HRV parameters in rehabilitation period have a stronger correlation with motor functions. Some studies show that 76.5% of patients with acute ischemic stroke suffer from autonomic nerve dysfunction and related dysfunction prognosis for more than six months after the onset of the stroke [13, 28]. However, the cardio-cerebral vessels of patients with acute stroke are still under stress, and the autonomic nervous function is more likely to be disordered. When the vital signs of patients become stable, the autonomic nervous function will slowly transit from drastic oscillation to a steady state, which makes the indication of prognosis of motor outcomes more reliable.

It was also found in the follow-up survey of our study that only the RR triangular index (r = 0.252; P = 0.05) in the time domain and the VLF(r = 0.302; P = 0.018) in the frequency domain had remarkable correlations with motor function levels of patients in the survey and were thus retained. Previous studies of Graff et al. [18] have found that HRV complexity indicators and non-linear indicators are more predictive of acute functional outcomes of stroke, such as nonlinear entropy methods (ApEN, SampEn, and FuzzyEn). The traditional frequency domain HRV parameters have good long-term (90-day follow-up) prognostic value, such as absolute VLF power, absolute LF power, HF%, LFnu, HFnu and LF/HF. The experiment has once again substantiated the correlation between VLF and the change of motor functions, and the correlation exists from the admission to about 3–4 months after onset of the stroke(the time of the follow-up survey). Although we excluded posterior circulation vascular lesions from our experiment, the type of the stroke was not limited. Because of the different mechanisms of cerebral hemorrhage and cerebral infarction, the prognosis is different, which may have an impact on the final outcomes. In addition, whether these parameters are related to the time of initial infarction, we should strengthen the follow-up of HRV parameters, and make it clear that it is the rule of HRV evolution and the best period and parameters related to functional prognosis.

Previous studies on RR triangular index are few. Gujjar et al. [15] applied short-term HRV parameters to analyze 25 patients with severe stroke, and found that LFnu, VLF percentage, absolute power rate, and TINN (triangular parameter of NN interval histogram) were related to the morality of patients, though only the LFnu parameter was retained by the regression after adjusting the model with multiple logistic regression. Through this experiment, we found that after rehabilitation training, the RR triangular index of stroke patients were still correlated to their motor functions: the decrease of RR triangular index may be related to the mortality of patients in acute phase, while the increase of RR triangular index may be relevent to the prognosis of motor function in chronic rehabilitation period. Whether HRV parameters are independent predictors of prognosis in acute and chronic strokes requires further validation.

Many experiments have found that the time domain and frequency domain indicators (SDNN, RMSSD, LF, HF) in the HRV parameters of Katz-Leurer and Shochina [21] are related to the functional independence assessment (FIM) scale. This relationship was found to exist in the acute phase (within 2 weeks after stroke) and lasted until 3 months later. Despite the effect that motor functions and ADL abilities vary synchronously, and that the HRV parameters were not sampled in the acute period, our experimental result did not show a correlation between HRV parameters and the variation of ADL abilities, which suggests that HRV does little help to the assessment of the patients' ADL abilities and their dependence on external assistance. Therefore, HRV can be seen as a very promising marker and indicator for the judgement of the motor function recovery of stroke patients. Further research needs to be conducted on the correlation between HRV and the function-independent abilities, especially in the time domain.

This study has several limitations: First, the sample size is small and comes from one hospital. The second is that the cerebral hemorrhage and cerebral infarction have not been studied separately, and the cardiovascular autonomic dysfunction is more obvious when the island leaves are involved. This experiment did not exclude insular stroke damage [29, 30]. The third is that the application of angiotensin converting enzyme inhibitor, β receptor blocker and calcium antagonist drugs is not excluded, and there are related ethical problems in interrupting drug use. The baseline characteristics of the control group have no difference, which can eliminate this error. Fourthly, our study was not long enough to observe the long-term (6 months, 1 year, or even longer) recovery of motor function and HRV changes. Fifth, due to the insufficient number of cases included, it is impossible to conduct a stratified analysis according to the severity of the patient's stroke. Since HRV modulation is considered to be a non-stationary process of nonlinear processes, multi-scale entropy (MSE) of HRV has been shown to assess early prognosis and potential stroke progression in patients with acute ischemic stroke [31]. The next step is to introduce this nonlinear method to quantify the HRV for evaluation. Sixth, we did not choose the control participants, which may enlarge our research results on HRV differences. Next time, healthy people or stroke patients in sequelae period can be recruited as control. In the next step, the sample can be expanded, the follow-up time can be prolonged, the motor function such as lower limb function and walking ability can be further refined, the severity of the patient's initial motor function can be analyzed hierarchically, and comprehensive functional evaluation such as NIHSS classification can be added, which is helpful to establish HRV parameter prediction models for specific populations and specific obstacles.

In summary, this study has once again verified that there is a certain correlation between autonomic nervous disorder in rehabilitation period and the prognosis of motor disorder after stroke. HRV parameters in chronic rehabilitation period (RR triangle index in the time domain and VLF parameter in the frequency domain) are significantly related to motor function recovery. Non-invasive monitoring of HRV may be an optional method to judge the prognosis of cerebrovascular diseases. However, there are still some limitations in this study. The correlation study is still in the preliminary stage, and the correlation between HRV and clinical results needs to be further verified.

Acknowledgement. Our work was supported by Independent Scientific Research Project of China Rehabilitation Research Center (2016ZX—22). This work was also supported by NSFC (91646202), National Key R&D Program of China(2018YFB1404400,2018YFB1402700).

References

1. Dutsch, M., Burger, M., Dorfler, C., Schwab, S., Hilz, M.J.: Cardiovascular autonomic function in poststroke patients. Neurology **69**, 2249–2255 (2007)
2. McLaren, A., Kerr, S., Allan, L., et al.: Autonomic function is impaired in elderly stroke survivors. Stroke **36**, 1026–1030 (2005)
3. Kocan, M.J.: Cardiovascular effects of acute stroke. Prog. Cardiovasc. Nurs. **14**, 61–67 (1999)
4. Task Force of the European Society of Cardiology and the North American Society of Pacing and Electrophysiology: Heart rate variability: standards of measurement, physiological interpretation and clinical use. Circulation **93**(5), 1043–1065 (1996)
5. Akselrod, S., Gordon, D., Ubel, F.A., Shannon, D.C., Berger, A.C., Cohen, R.J.: Power spectrum analysis of heart rate fluctuation: a quantitative probe of beat-to-beat cardiovascular control. Science **213**(4504), 220–222 (1981)
6. Dawson, S.L., Manktelow, B.N., Robinson, T.G., Panerai, R.B., Potter, J.F.: Which parameters of beat-to-beat blood pressure and variability best predict early outcomes after acute ischemic stroke? Stroke **31**, 463–468 (2000)
7. Heart rate variability: standards of measurement physiological interpretation and clinical use: Task Force of the European Society of Cardiology and the North American Society of Pacing and Electrophysiology. Circulation **93**, 1043–1065 (1996)
8. Rovere, M.T.L., Bigger, J.T., Marcus, F.I., Mortara, A., Schwartz, P.J.: Baroreflex sensitivity and heart-rate variability in prediction of total cardiac mortality after myocardial infarction. The Lancet. **351**, 478–484 (1998)
9. Stein, P.K., Domitrovich, P.P., Huikuri, H.V., Kleiger, R.E.: Traditional and nonlinear heart rate variability are each independently associated with mortality after myocardial infarction. J. Cardiovasc. Electrophysiol. **16**, 13–20 (2005)
10. Thayer, J.F., Yamamoto, S.S., Brosschot, J.F.: The relationship of autonomic imbalance, heart rate variability and cardiovascular disease risk factors. Int. J. Cardiol. **141**, 122–131 (2010)
11. Xiong, L., Leung, H.W., Chen, X.Y., Leung, W.H., Soo, O.Y., Wong, K.S.: Autonomic dysfunction in different subtypes of post-acute ischemic stroke. J. Neurol. Sci. **337**, 141–146 (2014). https://doi.org/10.1016/j.jns.2013.11.036
12. Chen, P.L., Kuo, T.B., Yang, C.C.: Parasympathetic activity correlates with early outcomes in patients with large artery atherosclerotic stroke. J. Neurol. Sci. **314**, 57–61 (2012). https://doi.org/10.1016/j.jns.2011.10.034
13. Xiong, L., et al.: Comprehensive assessment for autonomic dysfunction in different phases after ischemic stroke. Int. J. Stroke **8**, 645–651 (2013). https://doi.org/10.1111/j.1747-4949.2012.00829.x

14. Naver, H.K., Blomstrand, C., Wallin, B.G.: Reduced heart rate variability after rightsided stroke. Stroke **27**, 247–251 (1996)
15. Gujjar, A.R., Sathyaprabha, T.N., Nagaraja, D., Thennarasu, K., Pradhan, N.: Heart rate variability and outcomes in acute severe stroke: role of power spectral analysis. Neurocrit. Care **1**, 347–354 (2004)
16. He, L., Li, C., Luo, Y., Dong, W., Yang, H.: Clinical prognostic significance of heart abnormality and heart rate variability in patients with stroke. Neurol. Res. **32**, 530–534 (2010)
17. Arad, M., Abboud, S., Radai, M.M., Adunsky, A.: Heart rate variability parameters correlate with functional independence measures in ischemic stroke patients. J. Electrocardiol. **35**, 243–246 (2002)
18. Graff, B., Gsecki, D., Rojek, A., et al.: Heart rate variability and functional outcomes in ischemic stroke: a multiparameter approach. J. Hypertension. **31**, 1629–1636 (2013)
19. Tang, S.-C., Jen, H.-I., Lin, Y.-H., et al.: Complexity of heart rate variability predicts outcomes in intensive care unit admitted patients with acute stroke. J. Neurol. Neurosurg. Psychiat. **86**(1), 95–100 (2015)
20. Wei, L., Zhao, W.-B., Ye, H.-W., et al.: Heart rate variability in patients with acute ischemic stroke at different stages of renal dysfunction: a cross-sectional observational study. Chinese Med. J. **130**, 652–658 (2017)
21. Katz-Leurer, M., Shochina, M.: Heart Rate Variability (HRV) parameters correlate with motor impairment and aerobic capacity in stroke patients. Neurorehabilitation **20**, 91–95 (2005)
22. Sethi, A., Callaway, C.W., Sejdić, E., Terhorst, L., Skidmore, E.R.: Heart rate variability is associated with motor outcomes 3-months after stroke. J. Stroke Cerebrovasc. Dis. **25**, 129–135 (2016)
23. Al-Qudah, Z., Yacoub, H.A., Souayah, N.: Serial heart rate variability testing for the evaluation of autonomic dysfunction after stroke. J. Vasc. Intervent. Neurol. **7**, 12–17 (2014)
24. Sequeira, H., Viltart, O., Ba-M'Hamed, S., et al.: Cortical control of somato-cardiovascular integration: neuroanatomical studies. Brain Res. Bull. **53**, 87–93 (2000)
25. Keizer, K., Kuypers, H.G.: Distribution of corticospinal neurons with collaterals to lower brain stem reticular formation in cat. Exp. Brain Res. **54**, 107–120 (1984)
26. Kerman, I.A.: Organization of brain somatomotorsympathetic circuits. Exp. Brain Res. **187**, 1–16 (2008)
27. Hung, C.Y., Tseng, S.H., Chen, S.C., et al.: Cardiac autonomic status is associated with spasticity in post-stroke patients. Neurorehabilitation **34**, 227–233 (2014)
28. Xiong, L., Leung, H., Chen, X.Y., et al.: Preliminary findings of the effects of autonomic dysfunction on functional outcomes after acute ischemic stroke. Clin. Neurol. Neurosurg. **114**, 316–320 (2012)
29. De Raedt, S., De Vos, A., De Keyser, J.: Autonomic dysfunction in acute ischemic stroke: an underexplored therapeutic area? J. Neurol. Sci. **348**, 24–34 (2015). https://doi.org/10.1016/j.jns.2014.12.007
30. Te Benarroch, E.E.: central autonomic network: functional organization, dysfunction, and perspective. Mayo Clinic proc. **68**, 988–1001 (1993)
31. Costa, M., Goldberger, A.L., Peng, C.K.: Multiscale entropy analysis of biological signals. Phys. Rev. E, Stat., Nonlinear Softw. Matter Phys. **71**, 021906 (2005). https://doi.org/10.1103/PhysRevE.71.021906

Document Recommendation Based on Interests of Co-authors for Brain Science

Han Zhong[1(✉)] and Zhisheng Huang[2]

[1] College of Information Technology and Network Security, People's Public
Security University of China, Beijing 100038, China
z.h0912@163.com
[2] Knowledge Representation and Reasoning Group,
Vrije University Amsterdam, 1081 HV Amsterdam, The Netherlands
huang@cs.vu.nl

Abstract. Personalized knowledge recommendation is an effective measure to provide individual information services in the field of brain science. It is essential that a complete understanding of authors' interests and accurate recommendation are carried out to achieve this goal. In this paper, a collaborative recommendation method based on co-authorship is proposed to make. In our approach, analysis of collaborators' interests and the calculation of collaborative value are used for recommendations. Finally, the experiments using real documents associated with brain science are given and provide supports for collaborative document recommendation in the field of brain science.

Keywords: User and co-author · Interests · Recommendation · Semantic technology · Brain science

1 Introduction

With the development of big data and artificial intelligence, the field of brain science based on digital resources has become a hot topic in recent years [1]. The style of people's life and knowledge renewal speed are accelerated with the ever-growing of brain science data. How to make the users to find interesting contents from large scale of data resources quickly and accurately has become an inevitable problem in the development of brain science. However, personal recommendation of data and interests provides an ideal way to solve this problem. Personalized recommendation is a mode of information service to provide information for users based on the needs of users [2, 3]. Establishing the interest model of author-topic and analyzing the interest degree of co-author' topics is a hot research interest to predict that the target users may be interested in the theme of resources.

There are many recommendation methods such as recommendation algorithm based on contents, recommendation algorithm based on rules [4] and collaborative recommendation algorithm [5]. Despite there are advantages and disadvantages, these algorithms are capable of mining users' potential interests and providing new

© Springer Nature Switzerland AG 2019
H. Wang et al. (Eds.): HIS 2019, LNCS 11837, pp. 108–118, 2019.
https://doi.org/10.1007/978-3-030-32962-4_11

learning resources. Shehata et al. [6] discovered users' interests and model to study the semantic relations between sentences through the concept map of ontology. Zhang et al. gave a kind of interest points of attention degree from semantic and structural features [7]. Chen et al. realized the theme recommendation based on the users' interests through the combination of the graph abstract method with the similarity algorithm based on the contents [8]. Cai et al. introduced the mechanism of trust of collaborative filtering to make the recommendation [9]. Guo et al. gave a novel social recommendation method and incorporate item relations using a probabilistic matrix factorization framework from the items' perspective [10]. Chen et al. introduced a novel attention mechanism in collaborative filtering to address the challenging item- and component-level implicit feedback in multimedia recommendation [11]. Jiang et al. proposed an author topic model-based collaborative filtering method to facilitate comprehensive points of interest recommendations for social users [12]. However, existing recommendation approaches often ignored the relationship between users and recommended objects. There are some problems among the literature recommendation because many users have access to record data in large scale. At the same time, the results need to be sorted and optimized based on a huge number of results from the reasoning relationships.

Meanwhile, knowledge service based on the semantic technology is becoming a new technology of information system from new generation of Web and many systems of semantic technology have been put into applications [13]. We are interested in a series of semantic technology application systems based on the platform of LarKC, especially based on the platform of brain informatics knowledge service. The platform of LarKC is the major semantic technology research and development project in the European Union's seventh research framework project. The name LarKC stands for the Large Knowledge Collider, which commits to develop a platform for massive semantic data processing and reasoning [14, 15]. It is important to use the method of recommendation systems among the process of personalized recommendation. This paper introduced the method of calculating co-author' interests and constructed the model of authors - topic interests.

The remainder of this paper is organized as follows. Sections 2 and 3 describe the model of interests between authors and topics and the model of interests between co-author and topics, respectively. Section 4 describes the model of interests between author and co-author. Section 5 provides an experiment and discussion. Section 6 discusses the knowledge service system of brain science based on semantic technology. Finally, Sect. 7 gives conclusions and future work.

2   The Model of Interests Between Authors and Topics

Users' interests on the topic of the literature can be understood that providing appropriate resources and content services is important for users. Selecting the topics of possible interests is the most favorable way for recommendation systems [16, 17, 18]. In this paper, we provide potential interests based on the interests of author and co-author.

In this paper, we consider that the authors interested in the topics instead of the relationship between the documents' topics in order to describe the model of interests. The user-topic model reflects the degree of interests in different concept topics.

A document can be described through some attributes, such as the title of a document, authors, the date of publication, the press, the form of document and so on. We simplified this document into a kind of three basic attributes of DOI, the author (authors) and topic (Topics) to identify it in this paper. So, some definitions are made as follows:

Definition 1 (Document). *A document d = <DOI, Authors, Topics> where Authors are a sequence of <author$_1$, author$_2$, ..., author$_n$> , Topics = {topic$_1$, topic$_2$, ..., topic$_m$}*

A document is composed of classification number, author and topics in general. The authors of a document constitute a sequence according to the order of authorship and the topic is the set of the keywords. However, one document usually owns more than one author. So the collection consisting of some documents is defined as follows:

Definition 2 (Document Repository). *A document repository D is a set of documents {d$_1$, d$_2$, ..., d$_k$}, among them, di ∈ D*

Each document includes some authors in the collection of documents. So, the set of all authors in a document is defined as follows:

Definition 3 (Author Set). *Given a document repository D, the author set of D is defined as:*

$$Author\ Set\ (D) = \{author_i | \exists d = <DOI, Authors, Topics> \in D, \exists i, Authors = <\ldots, author_i, \ldots> \}$$

Each document includes some topics. So, the set of topics among the documents is defined as follows:

Definition 4 (Topic Set). *Given a topic repository D, the topic set of D is defined as:*

$$Topic\ Set\ (D) = \{topic_i | \exists d = <DOI, Authors, Topics> \in D, \exists i, topics = <\ldots, topic_i, \ldots> \}.$$

The interest degree of topic can be measured by the number of the topic publication and this kind of measure does not take new interests and the order of this author into account. Because the first author and the last author of this paper may be different on the level of interests in the topics. We will discuss other forms of improvements in this metric mode. So, the interest of topics among the authors is defined as follows:

Definition 5 (Interest). *A set of documents is D, the interest of topics of an author is defined as follows:*

$$Interest\ (author, topic) = \frac{|\{d : d = <DOI, <\ldots, author, \ldots> , \{\ldots, topic, \ldots\} > \}|}{|All\ Published\ Papers|} \tag{1}$$

Among them, |AllPublishedPapers| refers to the number of all the published articles, that is All Published Papers = {d : d = <DOI, <..., author, ... >, Topics > ∈ D}.

The value of interest in a topic is actually a regularized (Normalized) value (i.e. it belongs to [0,1]) through above formal definition. It indicates that this author interested in this topic extremely if the value of interests is 1. And it shows that this author is not interested in this topic if the value of interests is 0.

3   The Model of Interests Between Co-author and Topics

The measurement of the author's interest value is often adopted among the literature recommendation. And this simple method can not describe that the author may generate new interests. We believe that a researcher often extended his personal interest to a new topic. A researcher can generate new interests due to the influence of his/her friends, teachers and others. Using the information related to one's social relationships can estimate the new interests.

The relationship of network cooperation is the important part of the social relation network, which has an important significance during the process of the scientific research [19, 20, 21]. The model of author-topic interest is extended to the model of co-author and topics to carry out the recommendation. This paper puts forward the degree of interest of author-topic and finds the topics of co-authors to build the model of interests of co-author-topic.

There are some documents which have more than one authors in one document, the co-author is defined as follows:

Definition 6 (Co-author). *Given a document repository D, Author$_i$ and Author$_j$ are co-author in a D, as Coauthor (D, author$_i$, author$_j$, d), if and only if d = <DOI, Authors, Topics> ∈D and (Authors = <..., author$_i$, ..., author$_j$, ...> or Authors = <..., author$_j$, ..., author$_i$, ...>)*

The co-author refers to the co-author that is described in a specific document. In the same way, there is co-author when not being special documents.

Definition 7 (Co-author without specific document). *Author$_i$ and Author$_j$ have the same interests as Coauthor (D, author$_i$, author$_j$) if and only if ∃d ∈ D such that, Coauthor(D, author$_i$, author$_j$, d).*

The method above defines the common interest of two authors only, which is a partial order relationship. In order to describe the similar degree of the co-author in the same topic, we introduced the co-author's distance, which is defined as follows:

Definition 8 (Authorship distance). *Authorship distance is a partial mapping AD from* Author Set × Author Set → Real Number *which is defined as:*

AD(a, a) = 0;
AD(a, b) = 1; if coauthor(D, a, b)
AD(a, b) = n; if exists an author c such that AD(a, c) = n − 1 and co-author(c, b) and there exists no other c' such that AD(a, c') < n − 1.

There is the nearest distance (distance of 0) between each author and his/her interest. The distance is 1 if two authors were collaborators. Then the distance is 2 if there are other authors, and so on. Above authorship-distance is considered without the number of co-author. If considering the number of co-authors, here is another definition:

Definition 9 (Authorship distance with co-authored number). *Authorship distance is a partial mapping ADN from* Author Set × Author Set → Real Number *which is defined as:*

$ADN(a, a) = 0;$

$ADN(a, b) = \dfrac{1}{|\{d|coauthor(D,a,b,d)\}|};$ *if coauthor (D, a, b)*

$ADN(a, b) = d_1 + d_2;$ *if exists an author c such that ADN (a, c) = d_1 and ADN (c, b) = d_2 and there exists no other c' such that ADN (a, c') < d_1 and ADN (c', b) < d_2.*

Axiom 1. *Authorship distance AD is a metric distance, which owns follow characters:*

(1) *Nonnegativeness: $|AD(a, b)| > = 0$*
(2) *Identity: $AD(a,b) = 0$ if and only if $a = b$*
(3) *Symmetry: $AD(a,b) = AD(b,a)$*
(4) *The triangle inequality: $AD(a,b) + AD(b,c) > = AD(a,c)$*

Axiom 2. *Authorship distance with co-authored number ADN is a metric distance, which owns follow characters:*

(1) *Nonnegativeness: $|ADN(a, b)| > = 0$*
(2) *Identity: $ADN(a,b) = 0$ if and only if $a = b$*
(3) *Symmetry: $ADN(a,b) = ADN(b,a)$*
(4) *The triangle inequality: $ADN(a,b) + ADN(b,c) > = ADN(a,c)$*

4 The Model of Interests Between Author and Co-author

It will makes recommendation by combining the author's interested topics and co-author's interested topics and it is worthy to recommend if there is a close distance between a topic and its own network. Based on this idea, this corresponding recommended formula is defined as follows:

$$recommendationValue(a, topic, p) = Interest(author, topic),$$
$$\text{if } p = \text{my own interest only} \tag{2}$$

$$recommendationValue(a, topic, p) = \sum_{b=1,2,\dots,k} \frac{Interest(b, topic)}{ADN(a, b)}, \text{ if } p = \text{my author network},$$

k is the number of authors

$$\tag{3}$$

The way of single measure can not describe the author's interests. We can combine the topic's interest and co-author's interest to make recommendation. So, the recommended formula is defined as follows:

$$RecommendationValue(a, topic, p) = k_1 \cdot Interest(author, topic) + k_2$$
$$\cdot \sum_{b=1,2,\ldots,k} \frac{Interest(b, topic)}{ADN(a, b)} \tag{4}$$

Here, k is the number of authors. k_1, k_2 is the weight of measurement respectively. Normally $k_1 = k_2 = 0.5$. We do not need to consider the influence of other authors because it requires a lot of overhead in computation. Meanwhile, we need to consider a threshold of an author's distance instead of the author of more distance. The author's influence can be ignored if it is more than the threshold. If the distance of co-author is less than the threshold, the recommended formula with threshold of t is defined as follows:

$$recommendationValue(a, topic, p) = Interest(author, topic),$$
$$\text{if } p = \text{ my own interest only} \tag{5}$$

$$recommendationValue(a, topic, p) = \sum_{b=1,2,\ldots,k} \frac{Interest(b, topic)}{ADN(a, b)},$$
$$\text{if } p = \text{ my author network and AND(a,b)} < t \tag{6}$$

$$RecommendationValue(a, topic, p) = k_1 \cdot Interest(author, topic) + k_2 \cdot \sum_{b=1,2,\ldots,k} \frac{Interest(b,topic)}{ADN(a,b)}$$

(k is the number of authors, $k1 = k2 = 0.5$ and ADN(a, b) < t)

$$\tag{7}$$

5   Experiment and Discussion

For this experiment, the authors' interests of the topics and the co-author's interests of the same topic were represented respectively by using a large number of documents. At the same time, we also needed to calculate the distance of the co-authors to measure the interest value of the recommendation. In the field of brain science, for example, Dr. Liang wants to query the literature or researches about inductive reasoning of human cognitive function. There will be many results of literatures or resources as shown in Table 1 when he queried something in the knowledge service platform of brain science. However, the recommendation of literatures based on the interests of co-authors can improve the search efficiency. The system automatically puts the other two kinds of query conditions as the interests of co-authors when Dr. Liang chooses cognitive function as a query condition. The interest recommendation of topic is shown as Fig. 1. Through some topics of interests, we calculated the value of some topics recommendation. For example, fMRI among the fMRI, ERP, Eye-movement, PET, Behavior has the biggest value of interest recommendation. Healthy college-student among the healthy college-student, healthy young adults, healthy older people, healthy middle-aged, patients have the biggest value of interest recommendation. Inductive reasoning among inductive reasoning, problem-solving, visual research, discovery learning, computation has the biggest value of interest recommendation. In the brain science data system, the redefined query strategy algorithm of using co-author's interest is shown in Table 2 and we got the query results as shown in Table 3.

Table 1. The results of simple query

ID	Title	Cognitive function	Experimental-type	Subjects type
1	ERP characteristics of sentential inductive reasoning in time and frequency domains	Inductive Reasoning	ERP	Normal-Subject
2	An fMRI study of the numerical stroop task in individuals with and without minimal cognitive impairment	Inductive Reasoning	fMRI	Patient-Subject
...	...	...	...	...
35	The Role of Category Label in Adults' Inductive Reasoning	Inductive Reasoning	fMRI	Normal-Subject

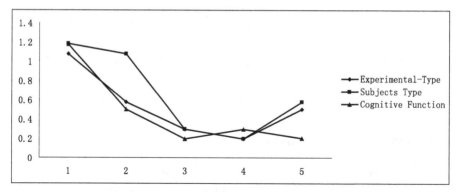

Fig. 1. The recommendation value of interests (the horizontal ordinate indicates the topic of interest and the vertical ordinate indicates the recommended value of interest)

According to the results, it is easy to see that the number of results is 10 when the query is without co-author's interests, however, when the query is defined with co-author's interests, the number of results is 35. In view of the number of results, the co-author recommendation greatly shortens the document filtering process for researchers. And the conclusion of experts' evaluation is that when the query isn't considered with co-author's interests, the accuracy rating is 50.8%; but when the query is refined using co-author's interests, the accuracy rating is 80%. This recommendation method improves the accuracy rating significantly and makes researchers find more suitable literatures and resources.

Table 2. The algorithm of research recommendation

Algorithm of Research Recommendation
Input: username
Output: literatureResults
1. literatures = getLiterature(username)
2. For each topic
3. For each interest of topic and Co-author
4. interests = getInterest(Topics) or [getInterest(Topics)/AND(author and   Co-author)]
5. RecommendationValue = getValue(interests)
6. End For
7. Initialize maxInterestValue(j) = InterestValue(1)
8. For each interest of topic
9. If(InterestValue(i)> InterestValue(i-1)) then
10. maxInterestValue(j) = InterestValue(i)
11. End If
12. End For
13. End For
14. literatureResults = getResult(username, maxInterestValue(1),
15. maxInterestValue(2), maxInterestValue(3))
16. return literatureResults

Table 3. The recommendation results of co-author

ID	Title	Cognitive function	Experimental-type	Subjects type
1	the fMRI research: the inductive reasoning of figure	Inductive Reasoning	fMRI	Normal-Subject
2	Dynamics of frontal, striatal, and hippocampal systems during rule learning	Inductive Reasoning	fMRI	Normal-Subject
…	…	…	…	…
10	The Role of Category Label in Adults' Inductive Reasoning	Inductive Reasoning	fMRI	Normal-Subject

6 The Knowledge Service System of Brain Science Based on Semantic Technology

The knowledge service system of brain science based on semantic technology mainly contains three level called web server, business logic and data process. The architecture of our system is depicted as Fig. 2. In the system, users use the web interface to post operation requirements to the server. The server sends the SPARQL queries to the SPARQL end point, which is launched by the workflow on the LarKC platform. At the same time, the system also permits users to write their own SPARQL queries and submit them by a submitting interface to the server. Meanwhile, the system can carry out the query, reasoning and so on. And a interface of this system is shown as Fig. 3.

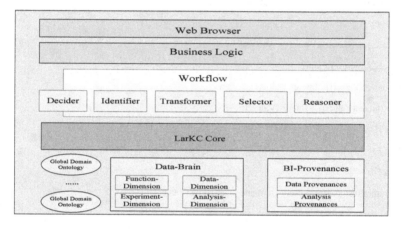

Fig. 2. System architecture

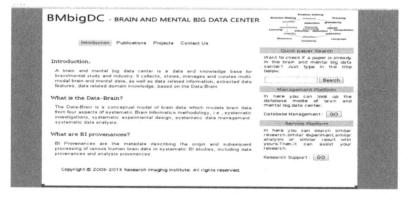

Fig. 3. System interface

Meanwhile, researchers need to query similar studies from internet to understand the development of research in the knowledge service system of brain science. However, the results may be millions among the studies of knowledge service of brain science. It is very difficult to find wanted literature from these results. Therefore, the literature recommendation has an important significance during the system of knowledge service system of brain science. We will put brain science provenances into this platform and conduct the class of data-brain as interests to make recommendations to improve the accuracy for finding similar researches.

7 Conclusions and Future Work

This paper mainly focused on the recommendations for the interesting topics, and put the author's research interest and the co-author's research interest together to research the recommendations. We had been able to quantify the author's interest in a certain topic, which takes a co-author's interest on the same topic and the distance between the co-authors into account. Based on these recommendations in the potential interests, the recommendation algorithm's efficiency and accuracy were improved greatly by combining the co-author's interest on the same topic.

However, we did not take the degree of the author's interest and the co-author's interest changes into consideration in the paper. And in the further study, we will consider to add the author's interest changes into the calculation of interest. It can recommend the interesting topics for researchers in brain science research efficiently.

Acknowledgements. The work is supported by the the JKF program of People's Public Security University of China (2019JKF334), and the National Key Research and Development Plan (2016YFC0801003).

References

1. Lane, R.D., Ryan, L.: Memory reconsolidation, emotional arousal, and the process of change in psychotherapy: New insights from brain science. Behav. Brain Sci. **38**, 1–64 (2015)
2. Ryan, P.B., Bridge, D.: Collaborative recommending using formal concept analysis. Knowl. Based Syst. **19**(5), 309–315 (2006)
3. Sarwa, B.S., Karypis, G., Konstan, J.: Item-based collaborative filtering recommendation algorithms. In: Proceedings of the 10th International Conference on World Wide Web, pp. 285–295. ACM, New York (2001)
4. Ma, H., Zhou, D., Liu, C., et al.: Recommender systems with social regularization. In: Proceedings of the 4th ACM International Conference on Web Search and Data Mining, Hong Kong, China, pp. 287–296 (2011)
5. Adomavicius, G., Tuzhilin, A.: Toward the next generation of recommender systems: a survey of the state-of-the-art and possible extensions. IEEE Trans. Knowl. Data Eng. **17**(6), 734–749 (2005)
6. Berners-Lee, T., Hendler, J., Lassila, O.: The semantic web: a new form of web content that is meaningful to computers will unleash a revolution of new possibilities. Sci. Am. **284**(5), 34–43 (2001)

7. Fensel, D., van Harmelen, F.: Unifying reasoning and search to web scale. IEEE Internet Comput. **11**(2), 94–95 (2007)
8. Dan, B., Guha, R.V, Brian, M.: RDF Vocabulary Description Language 1.0: RDF Schema, W3C Recommendation, 10 February, 2004
9. Hao, C., Yubo, J., Chengwei, H.: Research of collaborative filtering recommendation based on user trust model. Comput. Eng. Appl. **46**(35), 148–151 (2010)
10. Guo, L., Ma, J., Chen, Z., Jiang, H.: Incorporating item relations for social recommendation. Chin. J. Comput. **37**(1), 219–228 (2014)
11. Chen, J., Zhang, H., He, X., Nie, L., Liu, W., Chua, T.-S.: Attentive collaborative filtering: multimedia recommendation with item- and component-level attention. In: Proceedings of the 40th International ACM SIGIR Conference on Research and Development in Information Retrieval, pp. 335–344. ACM, New York (2017)
12. Jiang, S., Qian, X., Shen, J., Yun, F., Mei, T.: Author topic model-based collaborative filtering for personalized POI recommendations. IEEE Trans. Multimedia **17**(6), 907–918 (2015)
13. Efthymiou, K., Sipsas, K., Mourtzis, D.: On knowledge reuse for manufacturing systems design and planning: a semantic technology approach. CIRP J. Manuf. Sci. Technol. **8**, 1–11 (2014)
14. Zeng, Y., Zhong, N., Wang, Y., Qin, Y.L., Huang, Z.S., Zhou, H.Y.: User-centric query refinement and processing using granularity based strategies. Knowl. Inf. Syst. **27**(3), 419–450 (2010)
15. Zeng, Y., Zhou, E.Z., Qin, Y.L. Zhong, N.: Research interests: their dynamics, structures and applications in web search refinement. In: Proceeding of the 2010 IEEE/WIC/ACM International Conference on Web Intelligence, pp. 639–646. IEEE Computer Society, Washington, DC, USA (2010)
16. Zhang, J., Tao, X., Wang, H.: Outlier detection from large distributed databases. World Wide Web **17**(4), 539–568 (2014)
17. Li, H., Wang, Y., Wang, H., Zhou, B.: Multi-window based ensemble learning for classification of imbalanced streaming data. World Wide Web **20**(6), 1507–1525 (2017)
18. Khalil, F., Wang, H., Li, J.: Integrating Markov model with clustering for predicting web page accesses. In: Proceeding of the 13th Australasian World Wide Web Conference (AusWeb 2007), pp. 63–74 (2007)
19. Khalil, F., Li, J., Wang, H.: An integrated model for next page access prediction. Int. J. Knowl. Web Intell. **1**(1), 48–80 (2009)
20. Ma, J., Sun, L., Wang, H., Zhang, Y., Aickelin, U.: Supervised anomaly detection in uncertain pseudoperiodic data streams. ACM Trans. Internet Technol. (TOIT) **16**(1), 4–15 (2016)
21. Peng, M., Zeng, G., Sun, Z., Huang, J., Wang, H., Tian, G.: Personalized app recommendation based on app permissions. World Wide Web **21**(1), 89–104 (2018)

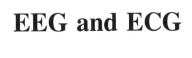

EEG and ECG

Deep Learning for Single-Channel EEG Signals Sleep Stage Scoring Based on Frequency Domain Representation

Jialin Wang[1,3], Yanchun Zhang[2,3,5(✉)], Qinying Ma[4], Huihui Huang[1,3], and Xiaoyuan Hong[1,3]

[1] Shanghai key Laboratory of Data Science, School of Computer Science, Fudan University, Shanghai, China
[2] Institute for Sustainable Industries & Liveable Cities, VU Research, Victoria University, Melbourne, Australia
yanchun.zhang@vu.edu.au
[3] Cyberspace Institute of Advanced Technology, Guangzhou University, Guangzhou, China
[4] The First Hospital of Hebei Medical University, Shijiazhuang, China
[5] Institute of Electronics and Information Engineering of UESTC in Guangdong, Dongguan, China

Abstract. Sleep is vital to the health of the human being. Accurate sleep stage scoring is an important prerequisite for diagnosing sleep health problems. The sleep electroencephalogram (EEG) waveform shows diverse variations under the physical conditions of subjects. To help neurologists better analyze sleep data in a fairly short time, we decide to develop a novel method to extract features from EEG signals. Traditional sleep stage scoring methods typically extract the one-dimensional (1D) features of single-channel EEG signals. This paper is the very first time to represent the single-channel EEG signals as two-dimensional (2D) frequency domain representation. Comparing with similar currently existing methods, a deep learning model trained by frequency domain representation can extract frequency morphological features over EEG signal patterns. We conduct experiments on the real EEG signals dataset, which is obtained from PhysioBank Community. The experiment results show that our method significantly improved the performance of the classifier.

Keywords: Sleep stage scoring · Data representation · Deep learning · EEG · Fourier transform

1 Introduction

In recent years, more and more people have begun to pay attention to sleep health [7]. Sleep stage scoring based on EEG signals, is used to diagnose

Supported by the NSFC (No. 61672161), and the DongGuan Innovative Research Team Program No. 2018607201008).

sleep disorders. It is a time-consuming task for neurologists to read whole night EEG signals in detail and perform sleep stages scoring. The sleep stage scoring is the basis for the diagnosis of many diseases, such as narcolepsy and sleep-disordered breathing syndrome. Sleep stage scoring through EEG-based machine learning methods may improve the diagnostic efficiency of the neurologist.

Accurate sleep stage scoring is a prerequisite for a neurologist to diagnose the sleeping disease of the patient accurately. The methods of collecting EEG signals in different hospitals are different now. There are many differences between the EEG datasets, including electrodes, channel numbers, and sampling frequencies. There are many methods designed according to the characteristics of specific EEG datasets, but in the face of different EEG datasets, the method may fail.

According to the sleep stage scoring standard of Rechtschaffen and Kales (R&K) [23], sleep includes the rapid eye movement (REM) and the non-rapid eye movement (NREM) [2]. In the NREM period, sleep is divided into four stages: N1, N2, N3, and N4. According to the American Academy of Sleep Medicine (AASM) sleep stage scoring method, N3 and N4 were combined in 2007 [19]. The five stages of sleep are the W, N1, N2, N3, and REM. In this paper, our method is to perform sleep stage scoring according to the AASM classification. Different waveform features are included in different sleep stages. For example, an alpha wave that appears in the awake period when the eye is closed, a spike-wave that often occurs in the N1 period, a spindle wave that often occurs in the N2 period, and a slow wave that appears in the N3 period [5].

Currently, with the development of deep learning, it has achieved excellent results in many fields, such as image recognition, speech recognition. Notably, the progress of the convolutional neural network in image recognition has reached the level of human beings and even surpassed human beings in medical imaging [6], and deep learning has also produced many results superior to traditional methods in many EEG datasets [24]. For example, these methods are used in the diagnosis of seizures [1] and sleep stage scoring [3]. We also found that these works require the EEG datasets themselves to meet certain conditions. For example, the EEG datasets are required to have a sufficient number of channels and a sufficiently high sampling frequency. Only if these conditions are met, the EEG datasets can generate enough training data to meet the requirements of the convolutional neural network for large training data. However, this also makes it difficult for the model to classify or predict EEG signals in a single-channel or a few channels. In this paper, we intend to use a single-channel EEG signal for sleep stage scoring to minimize the dependence on the number of EEG signals channels.

The single-channel based neural network model directly analyzes 1D EEG signals in [15,29]. These methods only focus on 1D features, whether using 1D convolution or LSTM is directly using 1D time domain features of EEG signals for analysis [4,8]. The usual method is to input 1D EEG signals directly into the model for training and testing.

The 1D EEG signal is represented on the 2D representation in the form of a curve. The morphological features of the single-channel EEG signals can be obtained intuitively from the 2D representation. The receptive field can obtain the morphological features of EEG signals in different sleep stages, and different morphological features can classify the single-channel EEG signals. The analysis of morphological features is closer to the diagnose method of neurologists.

Taking into account the above factors, we propose a 2D representation based on Fourier transform to perform sleep stage scoring through convolutional neural networks. We represent a 1D EEG signal as a 2D representation to extract the morphological features of the frequency domain of EEG signals.

The structure of this paper is as follows. The second section introduces the existing related EEG signals classification methods and analyzes these methods. The third section introduces data representation and model in detail. The fourth section design experiments to evaluate the representation method proposed in this paper and give the experimental results. The fifth section discusses the advantages and disadvantages of the representation method. The sixth section summarizes the work of this paper.

2   Related Works

Some progress has been made in the sleep stage scoring of the original single-channel EEG. The method [27] constructs a deep 1D convolutional neural network to segment and analyze the single-channel EEG signals according to the label corresponding to the original datasets. In the method [28], the author selects two convolution kernels of different sizes to convolve EEG separately to extract time domain and frequency domain features and uses an LSTM to extract features between different moments. However, the time complexity of the method is very high.

Some work is based on multichannel EEG classification. For example, in work [17], the EEG signal of different channels is convoluted by a plurality of 1D convolutional neural networks. Then, the output of each convolution module is spliced and then fully connected. There are also methods [10,12] for the 2D representation of multichannel EEG signals. The 2D representation of the data is then taken as a training and testing data into a 2D convolutional neural network for classification. These methods are mainly used in the case of collecting a large number of multichannel EEG signals. Some methods [21] rearrange the arrangement of channels in 2D representation to produce different results. The multichannel approach does not handle well the raw EEG signals with fewer channels.

Some methods [18] use the multimodal method to combine EEG signals with eye movement to improve the accuracy of classification. There are also methods to combine sleep EEG signals with ECG signals or body movement data to improve the classification accuracy of sleep stage scoring. Similar to the multichannel approach, the method has a strong dependence on diverse data. However, it is difficult to obtain EEG signals with ECG signals or body movement data at the same time in many datasets [9].

Some analysis of EEG signals by traditional time series methods often extracts the time-frequency features of EEG signals [16,22]. The EEG signals are subjected to the Fourier transform or wavelet transform to extract the time-frequency features of EEG [31]. However, the time-frequency features method requires manual setting of parameters, and the robustness of the method is weak.

In summary, a data representation method for extracting 2D frequency features of single-channel EEG signals can provide a new idea for analyzing sleep stage scoring.

3   Methods

Our goal is to perform accurate sleep stage scoring on sleep EEG signals. We segmented the single-channel EEG signals and performed a Fourier transform on the EEG segment to generate training data. Finally, the training data are represented as 2D images. We use the deep learning model to train and test 2D image representation. The model consists of convolutional modules, and batch normalization is used in the structure to avoid overfitting the model. In particular, datasets with a limited number of channels can also be classified.

3.1   Data Representation

The dataset is segmented by the same number of sampling points according to the classification label of the dataset to generate training data. Each segment has a unique label to indicate its corresponding sleep stage. There is a difference in EEG signals for each individual. Standardizing the EEG signals before training can align the EEG signals formats of different subjects. The standardized formula is as follows:

$$Z(X) = \frac{X - \overline{X}}{\sqrt{\frac{(X-\overline{X})^2}{n-1}}} \tag{1}$$

Where n is the number of training data, X is the original EEG signals, and $\overline{X}$ is the average of the original EEG signals.

1D Representation. After data preprocessing, we segment the EEG signals by the same length. In this paper, we divide the dataset into segments containing 3000 sampling points. Each training data was labeled as a sleep stage given by a medical expert. Let $T = \{X_1, X_2, \ldots, X_m\}$ where m is the number of channels. $X_i = \{X_{i,1}, X_{i,2}, \ldots, X_{i,n}\}$ where i is the EEG signals of the i-th channel. n is the number of sampling points. The label data $Y_i = \{Y_{i,1}, Y_{i,2}, \ldots, Y_{i,n}\}$ is the sleep stage scoring corresponding to the i-th channel EEG signals. The goal is to create a mapping from X to Y.

2D Time Domain Representation. In order to extract the 2D features of single-channel EEG signals, we represent a 1D array as a sparse 2D representation to extract the morphological features of EEG, in Fig. 1. According to the ECG signals inspiration [13], the EEG signals segment is represented as a sparse

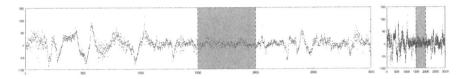

Fig. 1. We segment EEG signals in same length and finally represent it into an image. In this example, each image contain 3000 sampling points.

2D representation with the horizontal axis as the sampling point, and the vertical axis is the fluctuation amplitude. Since EEG signals are different from ECG signals, there is no obvious periodic feature. Only the same length of time can be used as the segmentation strategy. Each 2D representation denotes a segment of sleep EEG signals that includes 30 s.

2D Frequency Domain Representation. Both the 1D representation and the 2D representation are a representation of the time domain features of the EEG signals mentioned above. To extract the frequency domain features of the single-channel EEG signal, we perform the discrete fast Fourier transform on the segmented EEG signals. The frequency of the EEG signals is 100 Hz.

$$Z_i(k) = \sum_{x=0}^{L-1} X_i(x)e^{-jx\frac{2\pi}{L}k} \tag{2}$$

Where X_i is EEG signals in channel i. k and x are discrete. It means that the time and the frequency are discrete.

3.2   Models

1D Convolutional. We build the model based on the original single-channel EEG signals. The formula is as follows:

$$y_1 = \sum_{v=1}^{n} \omega_v \cdot Z_{i-v+1} + b_v \tag{3}$$

Where ω_v is the weight parameter b_v is the bias parameter. In the model are parameters that can be trained.

2D Convolutional. The 2D representations can be trained through a 2D convolutional neural network. This paper uses 2D convolutional network based on the VGG [26] as shown in Fig. 2. A 2D convolutional neural network was established to extract morphological features from the 2D representation of EEG. The formula is as follows:

$$y_2 = \sum_{u=1}^{m} \sum_{v=1}^{n} \omega_{u,v} \cdot Z_{i-u+1,j-v+1} + b_{u,v} \tag{4}$$

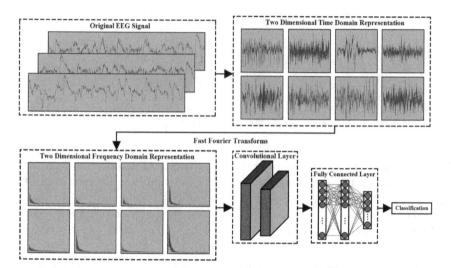

Fig. 2. Illustration of 2D representation for sleep stage scoring problem. We segment EEG signals in same length and finally represent it into an 2D representation. In this example, the 2D representation represents an EEG signals segmentation, each 2D representation contain 3000 sampling points. We use a convolutional neural network model to extract frequency domain features.

The convolution kernel size we use for 1D convolution is 1×3. The convolution kernel size used in 2D convolution is 3×3. We can use a 3×3 convolution kernel multiple times to perceive a larger area of the image. In the convolution process, we use the method of zero-padding the input data to achieve the same output and input size.

We avoid overfitting by using batch normalization [11]. Batch normalization re-normalizes the distribution of output values for each layer of neural networks to a case where the mean is 0, and the variance is 1. Batch normalization returns the input value of the activation function to the response interval of the activation function. We are thereby avoiding the phenomenon that the gradient disappears.

The optimization strategy we chose was Adam with an initial learning rate of 0.001 [25,30].

4   Experiments

To evaluate the performance of the method we proposed, we designed some experiments on the public dataset. Our experiment was to analyze the performance of different data representation of single-channel EEG signals. These data representations include 1D representation, 2D time domain representation, and 2D frequency domain representation. We compare the methods in this paper with different methods.

The method was implemented using the python language and the TensorFlow framework. The experiments were run on a machine with four Nvidia Titan X Pascal GPUs.

4.1   Datasets

In this paper, We choose sleep-EDF [14] as the experimental dataset[1]. The dataset contains 197 overnight polysomnographic records which include EEG, EOG, chinEMG and event tags. At the same time, the dataset also includes sleep stage scoring tags based on R&K by medical professionals. A total of 153 healthy subjects who did not take any sleep-related medications were included in the Cassette dataset, with age distribution between 25 and 101 years of age. The EEG and EOG have a sampling frequency of 100 Hz, and the EEG contains two channels. Following the Deepsleepnet [28], we used 39 nights of sleep EEG signals from 20 subjects. We generated a 2D grayscale image according to the label of the dataset sleep stage scoring, and each image contains 3000 sampling points that do not overlap each other. A total of 42308 images were generated. During the training and testing, we use one subject as testing data and validation data, which is referenced to the comparison method, and the other subjects as training data.

4.2   Evaluation

We first experimented with a 1D convolutional neural network on a 1D array of 3000 sampling points. We compare the experimental results of the two methods, and we also compared other methods that use a single-channel EEG with our approach.

This section introduces the methods of this article. All methods are trained and tested on the Sleep-EDF dataset.

The 1D CNN model classifies EEG by constructing multiple layers of convolutional layers in [27].

The training and testing with single-channel EEG signals are the same with [28]. The method was performed by convolution kernel and LSTM.

The 1D convolution integration model obtains the final classification result by splicing the multichannel CNN model through the fully-connected layer [17].

The total amount of EEG signal segments we entered for all models is the same. According to the structure of different models, the EEG signals data is adjusted separately according to different forms.

4.3   Results

Select the number of sampling points for the input data. When the number of sampling points of the EEG signals exceeds 3000, the excess is not guaranteed

---

[1] http://www.physionet.org/physiobank/database/sleep-edfx/.

to belong to the same sleep stage. Therefore, the choice of EEG signal segments size cannot be greater than 3000 sampling points.

The 3000 sampling points are the experts as the smallest unit of the mark and fragments contained therein belong to one sleep stage. Therefore, selecting the number of sampling points less than 3000 can ensure that each sampling point in the segment belongs to the same sleep stage. At this point, the total number of EEG signal segments increases as the EEG signal is subdivided, and the information contained in a single EEG signal segment reduce. Finding a balance between the number of segments and the information of EEG signals that does not affect the classification results is the goal of rationally selecting the number of sampling points.

At this point, we have selected several options for the number of sampling points, which are 1000, 1500, and 3000, respectively, to ensure that the EEG signals segment is equally divided and belongs to the same sleep stage.

Table 1. Accuracy on different sampling points.

Method	Sampling points								
	1000			1500			3000		
	Accuracy	Precision	Recall	Accuracy	Precision	Recall	Accuracy	Precision	Recall
2DCNN	0.74	0.58	0.62	0.74	**0.63**	0.65	**0.78**	0.62	**0.66**

It can be seen from Table 1 that the classification accuracy is the highest when the input data contains 3000 sampling points. Because each segment contains a small amount of information, increasing the number of segments does not improve classification accuracy. However, reducing the number of sampling points for a single segment reduces the classification accuracy.

To select the image size, we designed the experiment to select 3000 sampling points as the number of sampling points in a 2D representation of a single segment and then to select different sizes as the size of the input data. Smaller pictures take up less memory space and are less computationally intensive, but only fewer features can be described. Larger images take up more memory space, but more EEG signals segment detail features can be described. The specific situation we design input image size is 128×128, 256×256, 384×384 in Table 2.

Table 2. Accuracy on different image size.

Method	Image sizes								
	128			256			384		
	Accuracy	Precision	Recall	Accuracy	Precision	Recall	Accuracy	Precision	Recall
2DCNN	0.78	0.62	0.66	**0.84**	**0.65**	**0.70**	0.83	0.65	0.66

We also consider activation functions such as CReLU, ELU, and ReLU in the selection of the activation function in Table 3.

Table 3. Accuracy on different activation functions.

Method	Activation functions								
	CReLU			ELU			ReLU		
	Accuracy	Precision	Recall	Accuracy	Precision	Recall	Accuracy	Precision	Recall
2DCNN-F	0.78	**0.76**	**0.71**	0.82	0.63	0.64	**0.84**	0.65	0.70

In this paper, we consider the computational overhead of the experiment. We select the image size as 256×256 and the activation function as ReLU.

We also considered the accuracy of data representation in different dimensions. For the 1D case, we directly input the EEG signal segments containing 3000 sampling points into the 1D convolutional neural network. For the 2D case, we carry out a 2D representation of the EEG signal segments of 3000 sampling points into a 2D convolutional neural network.

In Table 4, T is the 2D representations of time domain EEG signal segments, and F is the 2D representations of frequency domain EEG signal segments.

Table 4. Accuracy on different methods.

Methods	Accuracy	Precision	Recall
SyncNet [17]	0.33	–	–
1DCNN [27]	0.68	–	–
CRF [20]	0.70	–	–
DeepsleepNet [28]	0.82	0.76	**0.79**
2DCNN-T	0.75	0.66	0.67
2DCNN-F	**0.85**	**0.77**	0.75

We compare the method proposed in this paper with other methods. The results of our data representation method are better than the results of 1D representation. Explain that the features contained in the 2D representation of the EEG signal segments can improve the accuracy of the classification. In Table 4, our fusion method accuracy has a 3% improvement over other methods.

5   Discussion

In the experiment, the 2D representation of single-channel EEG signal segments is an effective solution to promote accuracy. The predicted results are highly consistent with the labeling of the 2D representation of single-channel EEG signal segments. In the case of a limited number of channels, such an approach can effectively reduce the dependence on the number of EEG signal channels. Moreover, this method can extract features from frequency domain representation. The result of our method is improved compared to previous work.

The significance of our method is to represent the 1D EEG signals to 2D frequency domain representation. To the best of our knowledge, this is the first time that a single-channel sleep EEG signal is represented in this way. This representation reflects the 2D nature of the single-channel EEG signal. The difficulty in sleep stage scoring is that there are differences in sleep EEG signals between different individuals. The morphological features of sleep EEG signals of the same individual at the same sleep stage are diverse. These two factors make the sleep stage scoring of humans a challenging problem. The approach we have proposed provides a new way of thinking about this issue.

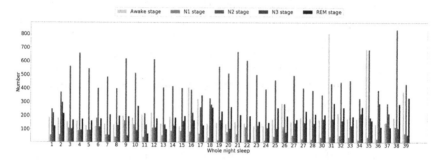

Fig. 3. The distribution of different sleep stages during all-night sleep is unbalanced.

The problems affecting the accuracy of classification mainly include the following four aspects. (1) The proportion of each sleep stage is different during the all-night sleep. For example, the N2 period accounts for a large proportion, while the N1 period accounts for a tiny proportion, which makes the entire dataset unbalanced, as shown in Fig. 3. Category imbalances can affect the accuracy of classification results. (2) There were significant differences in the same category in EEG signals, such as a significant change in frequency during a sleep phase. These changes affect the results of the classification. (3) The segmentation with 3000 sampling points results in less EEG signals information being lost, but the total number of EEG signals 2D representation generated by an entire night record of the subject is less than 1000. Limited training data also affects the accuracy of the classification results. (4) Noise data have a significant impact on the training of the model. We found that there were wrong labels in the dataset. For example, the W period contains some EEG signal segments of the N1 period, which can be misleading to the model. Incorrect EEG signal segments labels can mislead the model.

There are some limitations in our research: (1) The standardization approach does not eliminate the interference caused by individual differences; (2) There is no pre-processing of noise contained in the EEG signals such as blinks, EMG. In future work, we will use our method to analyze more sleep EEG datasets.

6   Conclusion

In this paper, we use a convolutional neural network to classify the 2D representation of the frequency domain of the single-channel sleep EEG signals. This new data representation is analyzed for the effect of sleep stage scoring. The 2D representation of the single-channel EEG signal reduces the dependence of the convolutional neural network model on the number of EEG channels. Due to the small dependence on the number of EEG channels, the model can be applied to more cases. Through experiments, we found that the 2D representation of the frequency domain of the single-channel EEG signals has a positive effect on the accuracy of model classification. In the experiment, by comparing with the classification results of the other representations, our representation significantly improved the performance of the classifier. Experiments have shown that our method can assist neurologists in the diagnosis of sleep stage scoring of EEG signals.

References

1. Akut, R.: Wavelet based deep learning approach for epilepsy detection. Health Inf. Sci. Syst. **7**(1), 8 (2019)
2. Aserinsky, E., Kleitman, N.: Regularly occurring periods of eye motility, and concomitant phenomena, during sleep. Science **118**(3062), 273–274 (1953)
3. Biswal, S., Sun, H., Goparaju, B., Westover, M.B., Sun, J., Bianchi, M.T.: Expert-level sleep scoring with deep neural networks. J. Am. Med. Inform. Assoc. **25**(12), 1643–1650 (2018)
4. Chen, W., et al.: EEG-based motion intention recognition via multi-task RNNs. In: Proceedings of the 2018 SIAM International Conference on Data Mining, SDM 2018, San Diego Marriott Mission Valley, San Diego, CA, USA, pp. 279–287 (2018)
5. Fraiwan, L., Lweesy, K., Khasawneh, N., Wenz, H., Dickhaus, H.: Automated sleep stage identification system based on time-frequency analysis of a single EEG channel and random forest classifier. Comput. Methods Programs Biomed. **108**(1), 10–19 (2012)
6. He, K., Zhang, X., Ren, S., Sun, J.: Deep residual learning for image recognition. In: 2016 IEEE Conference on Computer Vision and Pattern Recognition, CVPR 2016, Las Vegas, NV, USA, pp. 770–778 (2016)
7. Hor, H., Tafti, M.: How much sleep do we need? Science **325**(5942), 825–826 (2009)
8. Hsu, Y., Yang, Y.C., Wang, J., Hsu, C.: Automatic sleep stage recurrent neural classifier using energy features of EEG signals. Neurocomputing **104**, 105–114 (2013)
9. Hwang, S., et al.: Sleep period time estimation based on electrodermal activity. IEEE J. Biomed. Health Inform. **21**(1), 115–122 (2017)
10. Ieracitano, C., Mammone, N., Bramanti, A., Hussain, A., Morabito, F.C.: A convolutional neural network approach for classification of dementia stages based on 2D-spectral representation of EEG recordings. Neurocomputing **323**, 96–107 (2019)
11. Ioffe, S., Szegedy, C.: Batch normalization: Accelerating deep network training by reducing internal covariate shift. In: Proceedings of the 32nd International Conference on Machine Learning, ICML 2015, Lille, France, pp. 448–456 (2015)

12. Jiao, Z., Gao, X., Wang, Y., Li, J., Xu, H.: Deep convolutional neural networks for mental load classification based on EEG data. Pattern Recogn. **76**, 582–595 (2018)
13. Jun, T.J., Nguyen, H.M., Kang, D., Kim, D., Kim, D., Kim, Y.: ECG arrhythmia classification using a 2-D convolutional neural network. CoRR abs/1804.06812 (2018)
14. Kemp, B., Zwinderman, A.H., Tuk, B., Kamphuisen, H.A.C., Oberye, J.J.L.: Analysis of a sleep-dependent neuronal feedback loop: the slow-wave microcontinuity of the EEG. IEEE Trans. Biomed. Eng. **47**(9), 1185–1194 (2000)
15. Lederman, R.R., Talmon, R., Wu, H., Lo, Y., Coifman, R.R.: Alternating diffusion for common manifold learning with application to sleep stage assessment. In: 2015 IEEE International Conference on Acoustics, Speech and Signal Processing, ICASSP 2015, South Brisbane, Queensland, Australia, pp. 5758–5762 (2015)
16. Li, X., Cui, L., Tao, S., Chen, J., Zhang, X., Zhang, G.: HyCLASSS: a hybrid classifier for automatic sleep stage scoring. IEEE J. Biomed. Health Inform. **22**(2), 375–385 (2018)
17. Li, Y., et al.: Targeting EEG/LFP synchrony with neural nets. In: Advances in Neural Information Processing Systems 30: Annual Conference on Neural Information Processing Systems 2017, Long Beach, CA, USA, pp. 4623–4633 (2017)
18. Lu, Y., Zheng, W., Li, B., Lu, B.: Combining eye movements and EEG to enhance emotion recognition. In: Proceedings of the Twenty-Fourth International Joint Conference on Artificial Intelligence, IJCAI 2015, Buenos Aires, Argentina, pp. 1170–1176 (2015)
19. Luana, N., Raffaele, F., Oliviero, B.: Sleep classification according to AASM and Rechtschaffen and Kales: effects on sleep scoring parameters of children and adolescents. J. Sleep Res. **19**(1p2), 238–247 (2010)
20. Luo, G., Min, W.: Subject-adaptive real-time sleep stage classification based on conditional random field. In: AMIA Annual Symposium Proceedings, vol. 2007, p. 488. American Medical Informatics Association (2007)
21. Moon, S., Jang, S., Lee, J.: Convolutional neural network approach for EEG-based emotion recognition using brain connectivity and its spatial information. In: 2018 IEEE International Conference on Acoustics, Speech and Signal Processing, ICASSP 2018, Calgary, AB, Canada, pp. 2556–2560 (2018)
22. Munk, A.M., Olesen, K.V., Gangstad, S.W., Hansen, L.K.: Semi-supervised sleep-stage scoring based on single channel EEG. In: 2018 IEEE International Conference on Acoustics, Speech and Signal Processing, ICASSP 2018, Calgary, AB, Canada, pp. 2551–2555 (2018)
23. Rechtschaffen, A.: A manual for standardized terminology, techniques and scoring system for sleep stages in human subjects. Brain Information Service (1968)
24. Ren, Y., Wu, Y.: Convolutional deep belief networks for feature extraction of EEG signal. In: 2014 International Joint Conference on Neural Networks, IJCNN 2014, Beijing, China, pp. 2850–2853 (2014)
25. Ruder, S.: An overview of gradient descent optimization algorithms. CoRR abs/1609.04747 (2016)
26. Simonyan, K., Zisserman, A.: Very deep convolutional networks for large-scale image recognition. CoRR abs/1409.1556 (2014)
27. Sors, A., Bonnet, S., Mirek, S., Vercueil, L., Payen, J.: A convolutional neural network for sleep stage scoring from raw single-channel EEG. Biomed. Signal Proc. Control **42**, 107–114 (2018)
28. Supratak, A., Dong, H., Wu, C., Guo, Y.: DeepSleepNet: a model for automatic sleep stage scoring based on raw single-channel EEG. IEEE Trans. Neural Syst. Rehabil. Eng. **25**(11), 1998–2008 (2017)

29. Tsinalis, O., Matthews, P.M., Guo, Y., Zafeiriou, S.: Automatic sleep stage scoring with single-channel EEG using convolutional neural networks. CoRR abs/1610.01683 (2016)
30. Wilson, A.C., Roelofs, R., Stern, M., Srebro, N., Recht, B.: The marginal value of adaptive gradient methods in machine learning. In: Advances in Neural Information Processing Systems 30: Annual Conference on Neural Information Processing Systems 2017, Long Beach, CA, USA. pp. 4151–4161 (2017)
31. Yuan, Y., Xun, G., Jia, K., Zhang, A.: A novel wavelet-based model for EEG epileptic seizure detection using multi-context learning. In: 2017 IEEE International Conference on Bioinformatics and Biomedicine, BIBM 2017, Kansas City, MO, USA, pp. 694–699 (2017)

Improving Understanding of EEG Measurements Using Transparent Machine Learning Models

Chris Roadknight[✉], Guanyu Zong, and Prapa Rattadilok

University of Nottingham Ningbo Campus, Ningbo, China
{chris.roadknight, zyl9656,
prapa.rattadilok}@nottingham.edu.cn

Abstract. Physiological datasets such as Electroencephalography (EEG) data offer an insight into some of the less well understood aspects of human physiology. This paper investigates simple methods to develop models of high level behavior from low level electrode readings. These methods include using neuron activity based pruning and large time slices of the data. Both approaches lead to solutions whose performance and transparency are superior to existing methods.

Keywords: Deep Learning · Physiological data · CAPing

1 Introduction

1.1 Physiological Data

With the rise in popularity of smart devices such as smart watches, fitness trackers and EEG monitoring devices, high quality, high frequency physiological data is easier than ever to collect. With the promise of improving health, fitness and/or sleep this trend shows no sign of abating. They capture large amounts of high frequency data that largely goes unused. With the rise of availability of all forms of personal healthcare related data comes the requirement to do something with it. The desired output includes an understanding of the current and future state of the individual recording the data. This physiological data can come in the form of static values such as weight, height, gender and data that has more short term time dependence such as temperature, sweat levels and respiratory rate. There are also a range of measurements that vary rapidly in short time frames, these include electrical activity in the brain or heart.

The EEG signal is a voltage that can be measured on the surface of the head, this signal is related to coordinated neural activity. This is particularly powerful when groups of neurons fire at the same time. Neural activity varies depending on the patient's mental state and the EEG signal can detect such variation with a degree of noise.

© Springer Nature Switzerland AG 2019
H. Wang et al. (Eds.): HIS 2019, LNCS 11837, pp. 134–142, 2019.
https://doi.org/10.1007/978-3-030-32962-4_13

1.2   Machine Learning

Machine learning takes many forms and means different things to different people. For the purposes of this research we will deem it any process where we use computational algorithms to learn relationships between causal data and resulting effects. By modelling these cause-effect relationships we can make predictions about labels associated with a range of causal data. This is also deemed 'supervised learning' as we supervise the training of a model until we can no longer improve its accuracy. This trained model is then evaluated on data that was not used to train it, giving us an idea on how well the model generalized. Many machine learning techniques exist, this research uses some well-known methods such as Gradient Boosting and Deep Learning.

1.3   Deep Learning

Deep learning is an extension of classic single hidden layer neural networks. One form of deep learning is based on a multi-layer feedforward artificial neural network that uses backpropagation for stochastic gradient descent training. The network can contain a large number of hidden layers consisting of neurons. Adaptive learning rates, rate annealing, momentum training and regularization enable high prediction accuracy in many complex prediction scenarios. This kind of feed-forward ANN model is the most common type of deep neural network and will be used in this research

Within a practical problem-solving context using conventional machine learning techniques, researchers have discovered that although the existing models could perform well on synthetic or well-structured datasets, when working with raw natural data, like processing an image pixel-wise in a pattern recognition task, models often dont reach their optimality unless an extreme amount of effort is spent to convert the raw data into a suitable form of internal representation for the network to process [14]. Besides this, the challenges brought by natural datasets also include the curse of dimensionality, examples of physiological or medical datasets which contain large amount of attributes [15]. When the number of attributes of a dataset rises, the dimensions of data space also rise above conventional intuition and have unfamiliar properties. For networks which are built by human researchers this could be an extra barrier for understanding and analyzing the essence behind data [9]

The deep learning methodology aims to solve these two problems by both providing a simpler way to convert high-dimensional, raw data into feature vectors or other internal representations that has lower data dimensions, and, under some conditions, boosting the computational power of the model itself by allowing more computing units in the process.

Deep learning models can be difficult to interpret, due to their non-linearity. It is important to make these models as simple as possible while still retaining performance so as to be more human readable, this is sometimes called Mimic Learning [5]. The basic premise is to first ensure you have the simplest version of your model and then convert the underpinning complex mathematical processes into more understandable forms [7, 8] The approach here is based on a method used for single hidden layer neural networks [9] but modifications have been made to enact the process on a deep neural network

2 Experimental Design

2.1 Dataset

EEG data has been widely used in machine learning-based classification problems. This research uses a publically available dataset [4]. In this data 10 college students were asked to wear a wireless single channel 'MindSet' EEG device [10] that measured activity over the frontal lobe. They were then asked to watch ten 2-min long videos that ranged in complexity and then decide if they were confusing or not. This dataset contains 11 EEG based metrics:

a. The raw EEG measurement itself (Raw)
b. 8 frequency based transformation (Delta, Theta, Alpha 1, Alpha 2, Beta 1, Beta 2, Gamma 1, Gamma 2)
c. 2 proprietary functions (Attention, Mediation)

It also contains a label that is a subjectively assigned decision as to whether the video was confusing or not. This was largely ignored in this research. The data is collected for 2 min but only the middle minute is deemed usable. The data is binned at one sample every 0.5 s Even though the EEG is measured at a 512 Hz (Table 1).

Table 1. Features generated from EEG data.

Features	Description	Sampling rate	Statistic
Attention	Proprietary measure of mental focus	1 Hz	Mean
Meditation	Proprietary measure of calmness	1 Hz	Mean
Raw	Raw EEG signal	512 Hz	Mean
Delta	1–3 Hz of power spectrum	8 Hz	Mean
Theta	4–7 Hz of power spectrum	8 Hz	Mean
Alpha 1	Lower 8–11 Hz of power spectrum	8 Hz	Mean
Alpha 2	Higher 8–11 Hz of power spectrum	8 Hz	Mean
Betal	Lower 12–29 Hz of power spectrum	8 Hz	Mean
Beta 2	Higher 12–29 Hz of power spectrum	8 Hz	Mean
Gamma 1	Lower 30–100 Hz of power spectrum	8 Hz	Mean
Gamma 2	Higher 30–100 Hz of power spectrum	8 Hz	Mean

There are 8 attributes based on different power spectrums, 2 proprietary measurements and a 2 Hz mean of the 512 Hz raw sample. Preprocessing this kind of data is always a key step in gaining an understanding of cause-effect relationships. This is usually carried out using statistical or time series approaches to smooth out unwarranted variation and noise. This step is hugely important as models need to be developed for underlying processes and not the overlaying noise.

In addition to the transformations of the raw EEG data detailed in the previous paragraph, we log transformed some of the attributes based on their distribution.

2.2   Machine Learning Approaches

The current 'best' performance of this dataset is yielded using 2 different types of Long Short Term Memory (LSTM) Recurrent Neural Networks [2, 16]. These approaches build on the back propagation algorithm that passes through layers, each layer summating to a transfer function. During the training process, error sent backward through the network can be amplified, which may lead to instability, oscillating weights, or vanishing gradients. Exploding gradients can be mitigated via truncation with correct transfer functions. Vanishing gradients are addressed using the Long Short-Term Memory RNN (LSTM) approach, introducing memory units to RNNs. The memory units help stop the error signal vanishing so that it is large enough to be back.

We compare the current leading methods discussed in the previous paragraph with 2 more sets of approaches: Flat Time Segmentation and Batch Processing. The 'Flat Time Segment' approach takes raw 0.5 s time slices of data and uses them as time independent training data. This method has no knowledge of whether the 0.5 s of data is the first, second or last time segment. This removes possibly useful temporal information but makes the resulting models somewhat simpler to understand.

The Batch processed approach takes a larger time segment and performs statistical analysis on the data producing static values such as mean, median and standard deviation of the metric over a 1 min time period. This is a simpler way of retaining memory than the LSTM approach

The machine learning algorithms are all publically available approaches, largely used 'out-of-the-box' with little or no tuning. This means subsequent researchers should easily be able to reproduce our results. We use the H2o [6] and R [17] platforms. In H20 we use the Random Forest, Gradient Boosting, Naïve Bayes and Deep Learning algorithms and within R we use the e1071 [18] package for SVM and the CARET [19] package for Classification Trees

2.3   Correlated Activity Pruning

There has been some success in optimizing deep and shallow neural networks using a pruning approach, whereby less useful links and nodes are removed. The most popular is the pruning method of Han et al. [11] which works by first training a network, setting all the weights to zero based on a fixed threshold, are then fine-tuning the remaining connections. An alternative method reduces values of trained weights by applying vector quantization techniques [12]. A distillation approach can be used to train a separate smaller network that imitates the original one [13]. Correlated activities can be used to condense networks [8–10]. A 'brain damage' approach can be used that makes use of second-order information on the gradient of the cost function to remove connections [14]. Simpler approaches include using limited numerical precision [15] (eg. single bit per weight [16]) and lossy hash functions to force weight sharing [17].

The correlated activity approach has been applied to deep networks in a whole node merging manner [20] but this approach fails to simplify for correlations in activity profiles for single connections between layers. For this work we applied a piecewise approach to the process. After the initial training and testing of the deep learning network, connections between all the nodes in layer n − 1 to layer n were examined and a Pearson correlation coefficient taken, the connections with the highest correlation coefficient were merged, the network was retrained and as long as the resulting accuracy was not significantly affected this was repeated (Fig. 1).

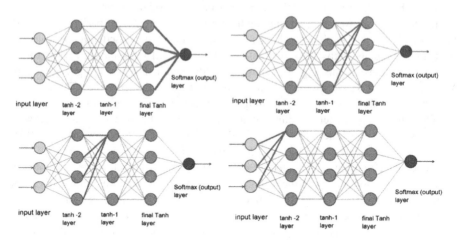

Fig. 1. Schematic of correlated activity pruning process

3   Results

The results presented here will show how well different groups of methods compare to the existing 'leading' approaches. Accuracy is a suitable measure here as there is a balanced target ratio. Qualitatively we have assessed how difficult the machine learning approach is to apply and subsequently understand, this makes up our 'Complexity' metric. This is used for information only and it allows the reader an insight into our opinion on the difficulty (application and interpretation) each method brings. Figure 2 and Table 2 shows the performance of different methods. It can be seen that the three groups of methods discussed previously group together into three clear groups. The flat time segment approaches has a range of lower complexity methods but accuracy is inferior to the published 'best'. The memory enabled LSTM have relatively high complexity and better accuracy. The batch processed approach has the highest range of accuracy but also 5 methods that clearly outperform the LSTM approaches.

Different deep learning methods exhibit a range of accuracies (Fig. 3). We manually prune the training attributes so that 'No AMR' means no Attention, Mediation or Raw values were used. 'No Pre' means that the preassigned confusion value was not used (unused in any of the previous models). It can be seen that deep learning performance can vary between 56 to 81% depending on the attributes used, with our CAPed approach giving a reasonable 75% accuracy with a minimal architecture.

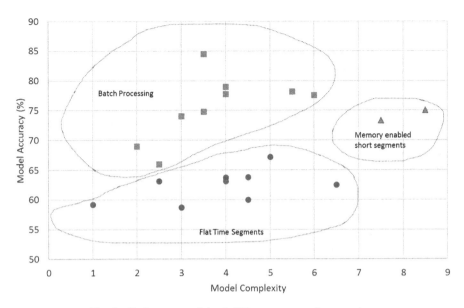

Fig. 2. Performance of the 3 different groups of approaches.

Table 2. Qualitative and quantitative performance of models

Model	Accuracy (%)	Complexity (model)	Complexity (process)	Complexity (combined)
LSTM approaches				
CF-Bi-LSTM (Ni et al 2017)	73.3	7	8	7.5
Bi-LSTM (Wang et al 2018)	75	8	9	8.5
Flat time segmented				
SVM (LibSVM)	67.2	6	4	5
Gradient Boosting (H2o)	63.7	5	3	4
MLP (neuralnet)	63.1	3	5	4
Naïve bayes (H2o)	58.7	5	1	3
SVM (e1071)	60	5	4	4.5
Random Forest (H2o)	63.8	4	5	4.5
Classification Tree (CARET)	63.1	2	3	2.5
Logistic Regression (R)	59.2	1	1	1
Deep Learning (H2o)	62.5	6	7	6.5
Batch processed				
Gradient Boosting (H2o)	84.5	4	3	3.5
NaïVe bayes (H2o)	66	4	1	2.5
Random Forest (H2o)	79	3	5	4
Deep Learning (H2o)	77.6	5	7	6
Classification Tree (CARET)	76	2	3	2.5

(continued)

Table 2. (*continued*)

Model	Accuracy (%)	Complexity (model)	Complexity (process)	Complexity (combined)
Gradient Boosting - Only Power Spectrum data	74.03	3	3	3
NaiVe bayes (H2o) - Only Power Spectrum data	69	3	1	2
Random Forest (H2o) – Only Power Spectrum data	74.8	2	5	3.5
Deep Learning (H2o) – Only Power Spectrum data	78.2	4	7	5.5
CAPed Deep Learning (H2o) - Only Power Spectrum data	75	2	6	4
Classification Tree (CARET) - Only Power Spectrum data	73	1.5	2.5	2

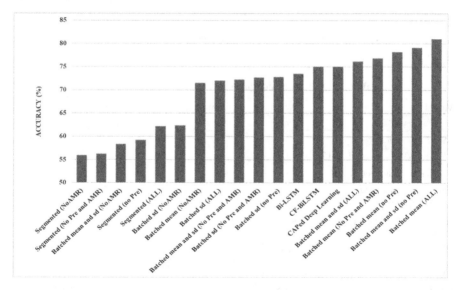

Fig. 3. Accuracy of a range of Deep Learning approaches

4   Conclusions

Modelling physiological data is a growing and important area of data modelling. Within this area, brain behavior and function is still poorly understood. This research shows that an understanding of what is happening when we observe different media of different complexity is more accurately model-able than previously thought. It appears that using publically available modelling tool we can achieve in excess of 80% accuracy in predicting if someone is 'confused' or not based on power spectrum values from a single EEG reading. Using a complicated memory based approach to weight optimization appears to be unnecessary if the correct window size for data aggregation statistical transformations are chosen. Further to this, by taking a small reduction in accuracy we can produce a minimal solution using pruning and merging of links with correlated activity.

This is the first publication to outline a correlated activity pruning approach based on link merging rather than whole node merging. This allows for more fine-tuned pruning of a deep learnt network. Secondly, this paper demonstrates that while the LSTM approach offers a performance improvement over crude time-slice segmentation, correctly dimensioned time slicing can offer both a simpler and more accurate solution for modelling the temporal EEG data used in this paper.

Acknowledgements. This work is supported by Ningbo Municipal Bureau of Science and Technology (Grant No. 2017D10034).

References

1. https://www.kaggle.com/wanghaohan/confused-eeg
2. Yin, Z., Zhao, M., Wang, Y., Yang, J., Zhang, J.: Recognition of emotions using multimodal physiological signals and an ensemble deep learning model. Comput. Methods Programs Biomed. **140**, 93–110 (2017)
3. Wang, H., Li, Y., Hu, X., Yang, Y., Meng, Z., Chang, K.M.: Using EEG to improve massive open online courses feedback interaction. In AIED Workshops, June 2013
4. Ni, Z., Yuksel, A.C., Ni, X., Mandel, M.I., Xie, L.: Confused or not confused?: disentangling brain activity from eeg data using bidirectional lSTM recurrent neural networks. In Proceedings of the 8th ACM International Conference on Bioinformatics, Computational Biology, and Health Informatics, pp. 241–246. ACM, August 2017
5. Ba, J., Caruana, R.: Do deep nets really need to be deep? In: Advances in Neural Information Processing Systems, pp. 2654–2662 (2014)
6. H2o.ai Company: H2o home - open source leader in AI and ML. https://www.h2o.ai/. Accessed 27 Apr 2019
7. Roadknight, C., Palmer-Brown, D., Al-Dabass, D.: Simulation of correlation activity pruning methods to enhance transparency of ANNs. Int. J. Simul. **4**, 68–74 (1997)
8. Roadknight, C.M., Palmer-Brown, D., Mills, G.E.: Correlated activity pruning (CAPing). In: Reusch, B. (ed.) Fuzzy Days 1997. LNCS, vol. 1226, pp. 591–592. Springer, Heidelberg (1997). https://doi.org/10.1007/3-540-62868-1_176
9. Roadknight, C.M., Balls, G.R., Mills, G.E., Palmer-Brown, D.: Modeling complex environmental data. IEEE Trans. Neural Netw. **8**(4), 852–862 (1997)
10. NeuroSky: NeuroSky's eSense meters and detection of mental state (2009)
11. Han, S., Pool, J., Tran, J., Dally, W.: Learning both weights and connections for efficient neural network. In: Advances in Neural Information Processing Systems, pp. 1135–1143 (2015)
12. Gong, Y., Liu, L., Yang, M., Bourdev, L.: Compressing deep convolutional networks using vector quantization. arXiv preprint arXiv:1412.6115 (2014)
13. Hinton, G., Vinyals, O., Dean, J.: Distilling the knowledge in a neural network. arXiv preprint arXiv:1503.02531 (2015)
14. LeCun, Y., Bengio, Y., Hinton, G.: Deep learning. Nature **521**(7553), 436 (2015)

15. Minli, Z., Shanshan, Q.: Research on the application of articial neural networks in tender offer for construction projects. Phys. Procedia **24**, 1781–1788 (2012)
16. Wang, H., Wu, Z., Xing, E.P.: Removing confounding factors associated weights in deep neural networks improves the prediction accuracy for healthcare applications. arXiv preprint arXiv:1803.07276 (2018)
17. RC Team: R: a language and environment for statistical computing (2013)
18. Dimitriadou, E., Hornik, K., Leisch, F., Meyer, D., Weingessel, A., Leisch, M.F.: Package 'e1071'. R Software package (2009). http://cran.rproject.org/web/packages/e1071/index.html
19. Kuhn, M.: Building predictive models in R using the caret package. J. Stat. Softw. **28**(5), 1–26 (2008)
20. Babaeizadeh, M., Smaragdis, P., Campbell, R.H.: A simple yet effective method to prune dense layers of neural networks (2016)

Automatic Identification of Premature Ventricular Contraction Using ECGs

Hao Chen, Jiaqi Bai, Luning Mao, Jieying Wei, Jiangling Song, and Rui Zhang$^{(\boxtimes)}$

The Medical Big Data Research Center, Northwest University, Xi'an, China
{haochen,bjq,maoluning,201620507,sjl}@stumail.nwu.edu.cn,
rzhang@nwu.edu.cn

Abstract. Premature ventricular contraction (PVC) is one of the most common arrhythmia diseases. The traditional diagnosis of PVC by visual inspection of PVC beats in electrocardiogram (ECG) is a time-consuming process. Hence, there has been an increasing interest in the study of automatic identification of PVC using ECGs in recent years. In this paper, a novel automatic PVC identification method is proposed. We first design a new approach to detect peak points of QRS complex. Then nine features are extracted from ECG according to the detected peak points, which are used to measure the morphological characteristics of PVC beats from different points of view. Finally, the key features are selected and fed into back propagation neural network (BPNN) to differentiate PVC ECGs from normal ECGs. Simulation results on the China Physiological Signal Challenge 2018 (CPSC2018) Database verify the feasibility and efficiency of the proposed method. The average accuracy attains 97.46%, as well as the average false detection rate and omission ratio are 3.41% and 1.37% respectively, which implies that the proposed method does a good job in identifying PVC automatically.

Keywords: ECG · Premature ventricular contraction (PVC) · QRS complex · R peak detection · Back propagation neural network (BPNN)

1 Introduction

Premature Ventricular Contraction (PVC) is one of the most common arrhythmia diseases [1], which is caused by the ventricular activation in advance [18]. In clinics, PVC typically manifests in palpitations, dizziness, sweating and dyspnea, accompanied with coronary heart disease, rheumatic heart disease, hypertensive heart disease etc [17]. More seriously, the frequent occurring of PVC may result in syncope, angina pectoris, heart failure and even death. Therefore, the timely and accurate diagnosis of PVC plays a crucial role in the early warning and treatment of these diseases.

Electrocardiogram (ECG) is the recording of bioelectrical signals produced by activating of cardiac myocyte. It has been verified that ECG is a common and

© Springer Nature Switzerland AG 2019
H. Wang et al. (Eds.): HIS 2019, LNCS 11837, pp. 143–155, 2019.
https://doi.org/10.1007/978-3-030-32962-4_14

important way to diagnose cardiovascular diseases including PVC [4]. Figure 1 illustrates an ECG segment with PVC beats. Compared with normal heart beats, the characteristics of PVC beats can be stated as follows: (1) an advanced QRS-T complex without ectopic P wave appears; (2) the QRS complex looks broader and malformed, as well as its duration generally lasts more than 0.12 s; (3) T wave has an opposite direction with QRS's main wave; (4) there exist compensatory pauses [5]. In the traditional way, PVC beats are inspected visually from an ECG recording by experienced physicians. However, such traditional way is a time-consuming process. In generally, it takes at least 1–2 h to detect a 24-h ECG recording even by a very experienced physician [10], which means that one physician could only complete 4–6 ECG recordings in a whole working day. Based on such situation, the study of the automatic identification of PVC, which will be very helpful to increase the inspection efficiency, has been attracted more and more researchers in recent years.

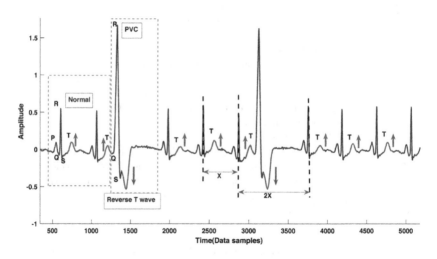

Fig. 1. Comparison of normal and PVC morphologies.

Various methods on identifying PVC using ECGs have been presented [6]. Bhardwaj et al. [3] extracted nine features of PVC beats in time domain, and then fed them into the support vector machine to recognize five classes of ECG beats (i.e. normal, ventricular beat, premature beat, ventricular out-of-phase beat and ventricular fibrillation beat). Liu et al. [9] proposed an adaptive approach for PVC detection based on personalized template matching. In [4], a PVC detection algorithm was designed according to the relative amplitude of R waves' troughs and peaks. Zhou et al. [18] applied deep neural networks to learn features from the ECG signal, and then combined rules reference to complete PVC detection. Liu et al. [11] developed a deep-learning-model-based PVC detection approach by combining waveform image data and time-series data with convolutional neural networks. Pachaur [13] et al. described a wavelet-energy-based technique for detecting PVC ECGs. In [10], Liu et al. extracted two ECG features using Lyapunov exponents, and then fed them into learning vector quantization (LVQ) neural network to detect PVC, Premature Atrial Contraction (PAC) and normal beats. Bazi [2] et al. presented an efficient Bayesian classification system based on Gaussian process classifiers (GPC) for detecting PVC beats in ECG signals.

In this paper, we will propose an automatic PVC identification method using ECGs. Firstly, a new approach is designed to detect the peak points of QRS complex. In detail, ECG signals are decomposed and reconstructed according to the wavelet transform. The reconstructed ECGs are then applied to find R peaks, Q peaks and S peaks respectively by designing an adaptive threshold method and quantifying the time-domain characteristics of QRS complex. Secondly, nine features are extracted for measuring the morphological characteristics of PVC beats from different points of view, where the key ones are further selected to be the final PVC-ECG features. Thirdly, the extracted PVC-ECG features are fed into BP neural network (BPNN) to differentiate PVC ECGs and normal ECGs. Finally, performances of the proposed automatic PVC identification method is verified on CPSC2018 Database.

2   Methods

In this section we will first describe the automatic QRS complex peak points detection method. Then the nine morphological ECG feature extraction methods will be proposed according to the detected QRS complex peak points.

2.1   Automatic Detection of Peak Points of QRS Complex

QRS complex is the main characteristics of the ECG waveforms, which reflects the ventricular activity. This section introduces a novel method for detecting QRS peaks points (i.e. R peak, Q peak and S peak) automatically. It can be summarized as algorithm I.

Algorithm I: Given an ECG signal $\mathbf{X} = \{X(1), X(2), \cdots, X(N)\}$ with sampling rate f_s, the length of signal N.

Step 1. The wavelet transform with $\mathbf{J}$ scale is applied to reconstruct $\mathbf{X}$ and denote the reconstructed signal as $\overline{\mathbf{X}}$. Here, $\overline{\mathbf{X}} = \{\overline{X(1)}, \overline{X(2)}, \cdots, \overline{X(N)}\}$. In order to better strengthen the information of the R peaks, we use $|\overline{\mathbf{X}}|$ instead of $\overline{\mathbf{X}}$ itself in our method.

Step 2. The edge peak points in $|\overline{\mathbf{X}}|$ are selected, and which are applied to obtain the fitted curve $\hat{\mathbf{X}}$. Then, all local extreme points' positions in $\hat{\mathbf{X}}$ are computed, whose corresponding values in $\mathbf{X}$ are denoted by $\tilde{\mathbf{X}} = \{X_{j_1}, \cdots, X_{j_m}\}$.

Step 3. A series of ECG segments are constructed on the basis of $\tilde{\mathbf{X}}$, denoted by $\tilde{\mathbf{X}}_l = \{X_{j_l - v_1}, \cdots, X_{j_l + v_1}\}, l = 1, \cdots, m$. Here, v_1 is the window width.

Step 4. The maximum value point in each ECG segment $\tilde{X}_l$ is taken as the candidate R peaks, denoted by $\mathbf{F_r} = \{F_r(1), F_r(2), \cdots, F_r(m)\}$ and $\mathbf{F_r^*} = \{F_r^*(1), F_r^*(2), \cdots, F_r^*(m)\}$, $F_r^*(i) < F_r^*(i+1)$. The corresponding locations are denoted as $\mathbf{R} = \{R(1), R(2), \cdots, R(m)\}$.

Step 5. Determine the accurate position of R peaks.

(i) The RR intervals (i.e. the time between two adjoining R peaks) are calculated according to the following formula:

$$\mathbf{RR} = \{RR(i)|RR(i) = R(i+1) - R(i), i = 1, \cdots, m-1\}.$$

Then, $\mathbf{RR^*} = \{RR^*(1), RR^*(2), \cdots, RR^*(m-1)\}, RR^*(i) \leq RR^*(i+1)$.

(ii) The three adaptive thresholds are defined according to the obtained $\mathbf{RR^*}$ and $\mathbf{F_r^*}$ as follows

$$\mathbf{THR_{rr1}} = \alpha_1 \times mean(\sum_{i=k+1}^{m-1-k} RR^*(i)),$$

$$\mathbf{THR_{rr2}} = \alpha_2 \times mean(\sum_{i=k+1}^{m-1-k} RR^*(i)),$$

$$\mathbf{THR_f} = \beta \times mean(\sum_{i=k+1}^{m-k} F_r^*(i)),$$

Here, $\alpha_1, \alpha_2, \beta$ are parameters.

(iii) The final R peaks are calculated by comparing $\mathbf{RR}$ and $\mathbf{F_r}$ with above adaptive thresholds. That is,

(a) If $RR(i) > \mathbf{THR_{rr1}}$, one missing R peak is existed in $(R(i), R(i+1))$. Then we define a new R peak $R_{new1} \in (R(i), R(i+1))$. At the same time, we can get a new sequence of R peak, denoted by $\mathbf{R_{new1}}$.

(b) If $RR(i) \leq \mathbf{THR_{rr2}}$, one false detected R peak is existed in $[R(i), R(i+1)]$. Then we tune the $\mathbf{R_{new1}}$ to obtain the new R peaks as follows,

$$\mathbf{R_{new2}} = \begin{cases} null, & \text{if } F_r(i) \leq \mathbf{THR_f} \\ R_{new1}(i), & \text{if } F_r(i) > \mathbf{THR_f}. \end{cases}$$

Then $\mathbf{R_{new2}}$ is taken as the final accurate location of R peaks (shown in Fig. 4). For convenience, we still denote it as $\mathbf{R} = \{R(1), R(2), \cdots, R(m^*)\}$, and the corresponding amplitude sequence is $\mathbf{F'} = \{F'(k_1), F'(k_2), \cdots, F'(k_{m^*})\}$.

Step 6. Determine the location of Q peak and S peak.

For $F'(k_j) \in \mathbf{F'}$, the segment $\mathbf{F}_{j,left} = \{F'(k_j - v2), \cdots, F'(k_j)\}(j = 1, \cdots, m^*)$ is constructed. Here, v_2 is the window width. Then the position of the local minimum in each $\mathbf{F}_{j,left}$ is defined as the jth Q peak point location. If the local minimum cannot be detected by the method of minimum value detection, we set $R(j) - t_4$ is the jth Q peak point location. All detected Q peak point locations are denoted by $\mathbf{Q} = \{Q(1), Q(2), \cdots, Q(m^*)\}$.

Similarly, the position of the local minimum in each $\mathbf{F}_{j,right}$ is defined as the jth S peak point location. Here, $\mathbf{F}_{right} = \{F'(k_j), \cdots, F'(k_j + v3)\}$, and v_3 is the window width. If the local minimum cannot be detected by the method of minimum value detection, we set $R(j) + t_4$ is the jth S peak point location. All detected S peak point locations are denoted by $\mathbf{S} = \{S(1), S(2), \cdots, S(m^*)\}$.

The procedures of QRS complex peak points detection method can be summarized as Fig. 2.

2.2   Morphological ECG Feature Extraction

In this subsection, we introduce nine extracted ECG features based on the detected QRS complex peak points, which are amplitude of R peaks ($\mathbf{F'}$), amplitude variation of R peaks ($\mathbf{DF'}$), duration of QRS complex ($\mathbf{D_{qrs}}$), area of QRS complex ($\mathbf{S_{qrs}}$), major axis ($\mathbf{a}$) and area ($\mathbf{S_p}$) of lag-T Poincare plots, RR interval ($\mathbf{RR}$), RR interval ratio ($\mathbf{IR}$) and the proportion of negative points of RR interval ($\mathbf{NR}$).

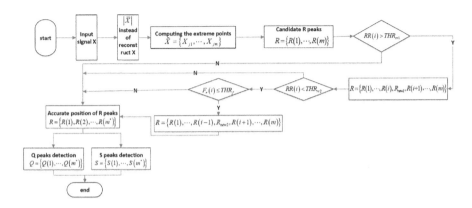

Fig. 2. The flowchart of automatic detection of peak points of QRS complex method

(A) R-Peak-Based Feature Extraction

The R wave is the most obvious waveform in QRS complex [14], which is weakly affected by most of the artifacts. It is known that the R peak of PVC beats is strongly higher than that of normal beats. Therefore, the amplitude ($\mathbf{F'}$) and amplitude variation ($\mathbf{DF'}$) of R peaks could be applied to differentiate PVC beats and normal beats, which can be calculated as follows.

(i) According to algorithm I, the amplitude sequence of R peaks is defined as

$$\mathbf{F'} = \{F'(k_1), F'(k_2), \cdots, F'(k_{m^*})\}.$$

(ii) The amplitude variation of R peaks ($\mathbf{DF'}$) is calculated by the first-order derivative of $\mathbf{F'}$ as follows:

$$\mathbf{DF'} = \{DF'(k_j) | DF'(k_j) = F'(k_j + 1) - F'(k_j)\}, j = 1, \ldots, m^* - 1.$$

(B) QRS-Complex-Based Feature Extraction

According to [18], the duration of QRS complex in PVC ECGs (PVC QRS complex) was larger than that of normal ECG (normal QRS complex), as well as, the amplitude of PVC QRS complex is higher than that of normal QRS complex (as shown in Fig. 3(a)), which is measure by the area of QRS complex. Therefore, we take the duration of QRS complex ($\mathbf{D_{qrs}}$) and area of QRS complex ($\mathbf{S_{qrs}}$) as two ECG features to differential PVC beats and normal beats. The lag-T Poincare plot is a geometric representation of signals in phase space [12], which allows a signal to be analyzed in its behaviour in different phases along its evolution in time. Figure 3(b) describes the lag-T Poincare plots of normal and PVC QRS complexes in Fig. 3(a), where the F_{qrs}^h and $F_{qrs}^{h+T}(T = 3)$ are the horizontal coordinate and vertical coordinate of the h-th point in lag-T Poincare plot. Here, F_{qrs}^h and F_{qrs}^{h+T} represent the amplitudes of the h-th and $(h + T)$-th points in QRS complexes respectively. In visualization, we can observe that the Poincare plot of PVC complexes is more scattered than that of normal complexes. Therefore, we define the major axis (**a**) and area ($\mathbf{S_p}$) of lag-T Poincare plots to measure such differences. Based on this, an algorithm II is proposed to characterize these features as follows:

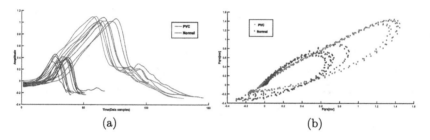

(a)   (b)

Fig. 3. (a) The QRS complexes of normal beats and PVC beats; (b) lag-T Poincare plots of the normal QRS complexes and PVC QRS complexes.

Algorithm II: Given an ECG signal $\mathbf{X}$, which sampling rate is f_s.

Step 1. A series of QRS complexes are extracted from $\mathbf{X}$, denoted as $\mathbf{X_{qrs}} = \{X_{qrs}(1), X_{qrs}(2), \cdots, X_{qrs}(m^*)\}$. Here, $X_{qrs}(k)$ is the kth QRS complex, and the amplitude sequence is $F_{qrs}(k) = \{F_{qrs}^h(k)\}_{h=1}^{M_k}$, where M_k is the sample number of $X_{qrs}(k)$.

Step 2. According to the algorithm I, the Q peak point location and S peak point location of $X_{qrs}(k)(k = 1, \cdots, m^*)$ could be detected, denoted by $Q(k)$ and $S(k)$ respectively. Then the duration of $X_{qrs}(k)$ is defined as

$$D_{qrs}(k) = S(k) - Q(k).$$

We write $\mathbf{D_{qrs}} = \{D_{qrs}(k), k = 1, \cdots, m^*\}$.

Step 3. The area of $X_{qrs}(k)(k = 1, \cdots, m^*)$ is calculated by the Riemann sum method, that is

$$S_{qrs}(k) = \sum_{h=1}^{M_k} F_{qrs}^h(k) \cdot \Delta X_{qrs},$$

where ΔX_{qrs} is the slip length. We write $\mathbf{S_{qrs}} = \{S_{qrs}(k), k = 1, \cdots, m^*\}$.

Step 4. The Poincare plot of $F_{qrs}(k)$, denoted by $P_{F_{qrs}(k)}$, is consisted of pair of points $\{(F_{qrs}^h(k), F_{qrs}^{h+T}(k))\}$. Then the two features, the major axis $a(k)$ and the area $S_p(k)$ of $P_{F_{qrs}(k)}$ are computed respectively as follows:

$$a(k) = \max(d(h)) - \min(d(h)), \qquad d(h) = \sqrt{(X_{qrs}^h(k))^2 + (X_{qrs}^{h+T}(k))^2},$$

$$S_p(k) = \tfrac{\pi}{4}a(k)b(k), \qquad b(k) = \max(d^*(h)) - \min(d^*(h)),$$

$$d^*(h) = \sqrt{(\widetilde{X}_{qrs}^h(k))^2 + (\widetilde{X}_{qrs}^{h+T}(k))^2}, \qquad \widetilde{X}_{qrs}(k) = \begin{bmatrix} \cos\theta & -\sin\theta \\ \sin\theta & \cos\theta \end{bmatrix} X_{qrs}(k),$$

where $h = 1, 2, \cdots, M_k$, $b(k)$ is the short axis of $P_{F_{qrs}(k)}$. We write $\mathbf{a} = \{a(k), k = 1, \cdots, m^*\}$, $\mathbf{S_p} = \{S_p(k), k = 1, \cdots, m^*\}$.

(C) Compensatory-Pause-Based Feature Extraction
It is known that PVC beats often start with a compensatory pulse, which is the advanced QRS complex. It means the interval between PVC beat and the former normal beat is smaller than the mean RR interval, as well as, the interval between PVC beat and next normal beat is lager than the mean RR interval [5]. Here, the mean RR interval is the average value of all beats intervals in ECG signals.Therefore, the RR interval (**RR**) and RR interval ratio (**IR**) can be extracted to describe such characteristics, which can be summarized as follows:

(i) Given an ECG signal $\mathbf{X}$, the sequence of R peak $(\{R(1), \cdots, R(m^*)\})$ and RR interval (**RR**) can be obtained by algorithm *I*.

$$\mathbf{RR} = \{RR(j)|RR(j) = R(j+1) - R(j), j = 1, \cdots, m^* - 1\}.$$

(ii) The RR interval ratio (**IR**) represents the deviation from the constant heart rate [15], which is given by

$$\mathbf{IR} = \{IR(j), j = 1, 2, \cdots, m^* - 1\}, IR(j) = \frac{RR(j)}{mean(\sum_{j=1}^{m^*-1} RR(j))}.$$

(D) T-Wave-Based Feature Extraction
In normal ECG, the direction of T-wave and ST segment are consistent with the direction of the QRS complex. However, in PVC ECGs, the direction of T-wave and ST segment are converse with the main wave of QRS complex, which implies the magnitude of T-wave and ST segment are smaller than zero. In such situation, the number of negative points of RR interval in PVC beats is more than that of RR interval in normal beats. Based on this, a novel feature is proposed to characterize the negative points of RR interval and to discriminate PVC beats and normal beats, which can be summarized in algorithm *III*.

Algorithm *III*:

Step 1. Given an ECG signal $\mathbf{X}$, a RR interval sequence is extracted according to algorithm I, denoted as $\mathbf{RR} = \{RR(1), RR(2), \cdots RR(m^* - 1)\}$. Here, $RR(j)$ is the jth RR interval, and the corresponding amplitude is $F_{rr}(j) = \{F_{rr}^l(j)\}_{l=1}^{L_j}$, where L_j is the sample number of $RR(j)$.

Step 2. Due to the existing of shift in $\mathbf{X}$, the baseline of $\mathbf{X}$ is calculated firstly, which are denoted by $\mathbf{X}^* = \{X^*(1), \cdots, X^*(N)\}$. For $F_{rr}(j)(j = 1, \cdots, m^*-1)$, corresponding baseline is $F_{X^*}(k_j) = \{F_{X^*}^l(k_j)\}_{l=1}^{L_j}(j = 1, \cdots, m^* - 1)$ and we define as $\mathbf{e_{rr}(j)} = \{e_{rr}^{(1)}(j), e_{rr}^{(2)}(j), \cdots, e_{rr}^{(L_j)}(j)\}$, where

$$e_{rr}^{(l)}(j) = \begin{cases} 1, & d_{rr}^{(l)}(j) \leq 0 \\ 0, & d_{rr}^{(l)}(j) > 0, \end{cases}$$

and $d_{rr}^{(l)}(j) = F_{rr}^l(j) - F_{X^*}^l(k_j)$.

Step 3. Calculate the ratio $\mathbf{NR}$ as follow:

$$\mathbf{NR(j)} = \frac{\sum_{l=1}^{L_j} e_{rr}^{(l)}(j)}{L_j},$$

which represents the proportion of negative points of RR interval.

3   Experiments and Results

3.1   Database

The ECG recordings applied in this study are taken from the China Physiological Signal Challenge 2018 (CPSC2018) database. It contains 6877 patients (female: 3178; male: 3699) and 8 types of arrhythmic ECG recordings with 12 leads, which were collected from 11 hospitals. All ECG recordings were sampled as 500 Hz, and which lasting from 6 s to just 60 s.

3.2   Experimental Results

In this subsection, we will verify the performance of the proposed methods, including the peak points detection method, feature extraction method and PVC identification method, which integrates the proposed features with the classifier BPNN.

(1) Preprocessing. The ECG signals applied in our work contain a large variety of artifacts, which will cover up some useful information. Therefore, denoising is the first and necessary step. The common artifacts are power frequency interference, electromyographic noise and baseline wander [9], which are mainly caused by the action of electromagnetic field between human body and lead, respiration, electrode impedance change due to body movement etc. In this paper, a method based on wavelet transform [16] is applied to de-noise the artifacts in ECGs. Figure 4 illustrates the raw ECG signal and de-noised signal with a duration of 12 s.

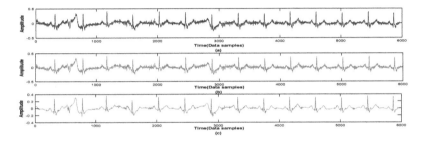

Fig. 4. The raw ECG and de-noised ECG. (a) Raw ECG signal. (b) ECG signal with removed baseline drift. (c) De-noised ECG signal.

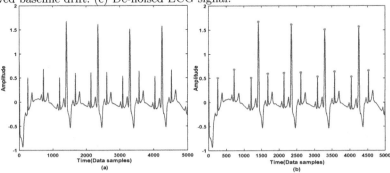

Fig. 5. R peak detection. (a) De-noised ECG signal; (b) Detected R peaks.

(2) Verification of the Automatic Peak Detection Method. In this part, we will verify the performance of the proposed peak detection algorithm (that is algorithm I). The corresponding results are shown in Fig. 5. Figure 5(a) is the raw ECG signal $\mathbf{X}$. The detected R peaks are shown in Fig. 5(b). We can see that the accurate R peak locations are labeled by the proposed method. Here, the parameter J in wavelet transform is 4. Besides, the parameters $v_1 = 20$ (that is 0.04 s), $\alpha_1 = 1.65$, $\alpha_2 = 0.7$, $\beta = 0.513$. Based on the obtained R peaks, the corresponding Q peak and S peak are also detected, which are shown in Fig. 6. Here, the parameters $v_2 = v_3 = 60$ (that is 0.12 s), and $t_4 = 30$ (that is 0.06 s). It can be observed the proposed method could detect Q and S peaks accurately. Besides, we also verify that the proposed method not only suitable for R peak detection of PVC ECG, but also suitable for R detection of other types (normal ECG, atrial fibrillation (AF), first-degree atrioventricular block (I-AVB) and ST-segment elevated (STE)) of ECGs with arrhythmia diseases.

(3) Verification of Automatic PVC Detection Method. We randomly select 500 PVC beats and 2000 normal beats from CPSC2018 database to construct our training data set, and the 336 PVC ECG recordings and 200 normal ECG recordings to constitute our testing data set. The 100 trails have been conducted with training and testing data sets randomly generated for each trail.

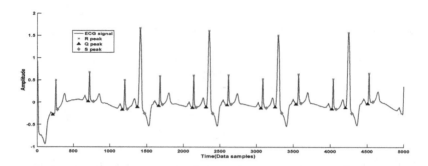

Fig. 6. Q peak points and S peak points detection.

Table 1. The ROC area of each feature.

Features	NR	RR	DF′	D_{qrs}	F′	a	S_{qrs}	S_p	IR
AUC (%)	81.60	84.53	97.79	96.13	89.98	91.92	97.68	76.88	98.12

For training data set, 9 features are computed for all ECG beats and to train the back-propagation neural network (BPNN) to discriminate the PVC beats and normal beats. The discriminative capability of BPNN with different features can be shown through the Receiver Operating Characteristic (ROC) Curve analysis, which gives us an intuitive view of whole spectrum of sensitivity against 1-specificity [8]. Corresponding results are shown in Fig. 7. It is noticed that evident different performances among different features. In order to reduce the complexity of computation of features and elevate the identification performances, we conduct the feature selection and feature fusion. We choose the features that the Area Under ROC Curve (AUC) is over 0.90 as the key features. The AUC of each feature is shown in Table 1. In the final, the RR interval ratio (**IR**), the area of QRS complex ($\mathbf{S_{qrs}}$), the amplitude differences (**DF′**), the major axis of the ellipse (**a**) and the width of QRS complex ($\mathbf{S_{qrs}}$) are selected and applied to construct the final PVC-ECG features. Then the final PVC-ECG features combined with BPNN are applied in testing data set to further verify the proposed method. In clinic, if there are one or more PVC beats in an ECG signal, then it will be classified into the PVC. Thus, in our work, the ECG signal is identified as PVC signal if at least one PVC beat could be detected. The classification performance is evaluated using formulas as following:

$$\mathbf{FDR} = \frac{FP}{TN+FP} \times 100\%.$$

$$\mathbf{O} = \frac{FN}{FN+TP} \times 100\%.$$

$$\mathbf{Acc} = \frac{TP+TN}{TP+FN+TN+FP} \times 100\%.$$

Here, TP, FP, TN and FN are true positive, false positive, true negative, and false negative respectively [7].

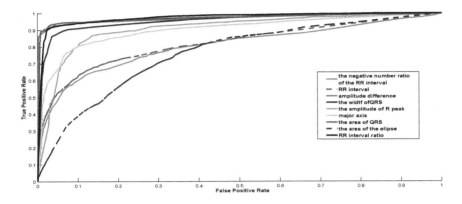

Fig. 7. ROC curves of nine features.

For de-noised testing data set, the final PVC-ECG features are computed for all recordings. We used the average results of 100 trails as the final results to measure the classification performance. The false detection rate, omission ratio and accuracy of the average results reach 3.41%, 1.37% and 97.46%.

Finally, we compare the proposed PVC identification method with six existing methods where the same performance measurements are applied. It is shown in Table 2, where the authors, the methods and corresponding accuracies are listed. We can see that, except the works of Zhou et al., the proposed method performs better than others. Although the accuracy of the work of Zhou et al. is slightly higher than that of ours, their omission ratio (1.94%) and false detection rate (3.76%) are much poor.

Table 2. A comparison between the proposed methods in this paper and the methodologies in other literatures.

Methods	Omission ratio	False detection rate	Accuracy
Zhou et al. [18]	1.94%	3.76%	98.03%
Bazi et al. [2]	4%	3.34%	96.72%
Bhardwaj et al. [3]	10.85%	–	95.21%
Chang et al. [4]	–	–	94.73%
Liu et al. [11]	–	–	88%
Pachauri et al. [13]	–	–	86.48%
This paper	1.37%	3.41%	97.46%

4   Conclusion

In this paper, we have proposed an automatic PVC identification method using ECGs. Firstly, we have designed a novel approach to detect peak points of QRS complex. Then the nine features have been extracted for measuring the morphological characteristics of PVC beats from different points of view. Furthermore, we have selected key features according to the training accuracy. Finally, the final PVC-ECG features have been fed into BPNN to differentiate PVC ECGs from normal ECGs. The performance of the proposed method has been verified on CPSC2018 Database. All the experimental results have demonstrated that the proposed method does a good job in the automatic PVC identification.

Acknowledgement. This work was supported by the Innovative Talents Promotion Plan of Shaanxi Province under Grant 2018TD-016.

References

1. Ebrahimzadeh, A., Khazaee, A.: Detection of premature ventricular contractions using MLP neural networks: a comparative study. Measurement **43**, 103–112 (2010)
2. Bazi, Y., Hichri, H., Alajlan, N., Ammour, N.: Premature ventricular contraction arrhythmia detection and classification with Gaussian process and S transform. In: 2013 Fifth International Conference on Computational Intelligence, pp. 36–41. IEEE (2013)
3. Bhardwaj, P., Choudhary, R.R., Dayama, R.: Analysis and classification of cardiac arrhythmia using ECG signals. Int. J. Comput. Appl. **38**, 37–40 (2012)
4. Chang, C.H., Lin, C.H., Wei, M.F.: High-precision real-time premature ventricular contraction (PVC) detection system based on wavelet transform. J. Signal Process. Syst. **77**, 289–296 (2014)
5. Cuesta, P., Lado, M.J., Vila, X.A.: Detection of premature ventricular contractions using the RR-interval signal: a simple algorithm for mobile devices. Technol. Health Care Off. J. Eur. Soc. Eng. Med. **22**, 651–656 (2014)
6. Deutsch, E., Svehlikova, J., Tysler, M.: Effect of elimination of noisy ECG leads on the noninvasive localization of the focus of premature ventricular complexes. In: Lhotska, L., Sukupova, L., Lacković, I., Ibbott, G. (eds.) World Congress on Medical Physics and Biomedical Engineering 2018, vol. 68. Springer, Singapore (2019). https://doi.org/10.1007/978-981-10-9035-6_14. ISBN 978-981-10-9034-9
7. Jung, Y., Kim, H.: Detection of PVC by using a wavelet-based statistical ECG monitoring procedure. Biomed. Signal Process. Control. **36**, 176–182 (2017)
8. Lee, J., Mcmanus, D., Chon, K.: Atrial fibrillation detection using time-varying coherence function and shannon entropy. IEEE Eng. Med. Biol. Soc. **104**, 4685–4688 (2011)
9. Liu, C.Y., Li, P., Zhang, Y.T., Zhang, Y., Liu, C.C., Wei, S.S.: A construction method of personalized ECG template and its application in premature ventricular contraction recognition for ECG mobile phones. Expert. Syst. Appl. **24**, 85–92 (2012)
10. Liu, X.L., Du, H.M., Wang, G.L.: Automatic diagnosis of premature ventricular contraction based on Lyapunov exponents and LVQ neural network. Comput. Methods Progams Biomed. **122**, 47–55 (2015)

11. Liu, Y., Huang, Y., Wang, J.: Detecting premature ventricular contraction in children with deep learning. J. Shanghai Jiaotong Univ. (Sci.) **23**, 66–73 (2018)
12. Mabrouki, R., Khaddoumi, B., Sayadi, M.: Atrial fibrillation detection on electrocardiogram. In: International Conference on Advanced Technologies for Signal and Image Processing, vol. 34, pp. 268–272 (2016)
13. Pachauri, A., Bhuyan, M.: Wavelet and energy based approach for PVC detection. In: 2009 International Conference on Emerging Trends in Electronic and Photonic Devices and Systems, pp. 257–261. IEEE (2010)
14. Sun, Y., Chan, K.L., Krishnan, S.M.: Characteristic wave detection in ECG signal using morphological transform. BMC Cardiovasc. Disord. **5**, 28 (2005)
15. Tsipouras, M.G., Fotiadis, D.I., Sideris, D.: An arrhythmia classification system based on the RR-interval signal. Artif. Intell. Med. **33**, 237–250 (2005)
16. Wei, J.Y., Wang, D., Sun, Y.N., Zhang, R.: A novelfusion feature extraction method for atrial fibrillation detection. J. Northwest Univ. **49**, 19–26 (2019)
17. Winkens, R.A.G., Höppener, P.F., Kragten, J.A.: Are premature ventricular contractions always harmless? Eur. J. Gen. Pract. **20**, 134–138 (2014)
18. Zhou, F.Y., Jin, L.P., Dong, J.: Premature ventricular contraction detection combining deep neural networks and rules inference. Artif. Intell. Med. **79**, 42–51 (2017)

Automated Detection of First-Degree Atrioventricular Block Using ECGs

Luning Mao, Hao Chen, Jiaqi Bai, Jieying Wei, Qiang Li, and Rui Zhang[⊠]

The Medical Big Data Research Center, Northwest University, Xi'an, China
{maoluning,haochen,bjq,201620507,lqlq}@stumail.nwu.edu.cn,
rzhang@nwu.edu.cn

Abstract. Automated detection of first-degree atrioventricular block (I-AVB) using electrocardiogram (ECG) has been paid more and more attraction since it is very helpful for the timely and efficient diagnosis and treatment of AVB-related heart diseases. In this paper, a novel automated I-AVB detection method FPR_{dur}-SVM is proposed, where the I-AVB feature FPR_{dur} is extracted from ECGs and then fed into the support vector machine (SVM) to differentiating I-AVB ECG from normal ECG. Performances of the proposed method FPR_{dur}-SVM are verified on the China Physiological Signal Challenge 2018 Database (CPSC2018). Simulation results show that the accuracy, sensitivity and specificity are reached 98.5%, 98.7% and 98.3%.

Keywords: First-degree atrioventricular block (I-AVB) ·
Electrocardiogram (ECG) · P peak detection · PR duration · Feature
extraction · Support vector machine (SVM)

1 Introduction

Atrioventricular block (AVB) is a type of arrhythmia which is caused by deficient electrical conduction between the atria and the ventricle during cardiac electrical stimulation [11]. AVB can be divided into three classes, that is, the first-degree block (I-AVB), the second-degree block (II-AVB) and the third-degree block (III-AVB). I-AVB is a benign finding in the early stage, however, if there lacks the timely and efficient control, it may grow worse into II-AVB or III-AVB, even leading to the loss of consciousness, convulsions and sudden death. Therefore, the accurate diagnosis of I-AVB is the first and necessary step for the follow-up treatment of AVB-related heart disease.

As an important tool of recording the heart electrical activity, electrocardiogram (ECG) has been widely used in the diagnosis and treatment of AVB. Clinically, the I-AVB can be identified in ECG signals by experienced physicians, but it still has some drawbacks, like costly, inefficient, and subjective [1]. Hence, the way detecting I-AVB automatically using ECGs has attracted more and more attention in recent years. To this end, extracting proper features from ECGs,

© Springer Nature Switzerland AG 2019
H. Wang et al. (Eds.): HIS 2019, LNCS 11837, pp. 156–167, 2019.
https://doi.org/10.1007/978-3-030-32962-4_15

which are then fed into an efficient classifier, is the key point for completing the automatic detection of I-AVB.

There are many works regarding the feature extraction from time domain and frequency domain. In the case of time-domain analysis, the RR intervals between two successive R waves, PP intervals between two successive P waves and PR intervals between P wave and QRS complex were applied as inputs to the CNN and MLP in the [12]. Kerthi et al. [8] has presented an efficient and flexible software tool based on MATLAB GUI to analyze ECG, extracted features like PR, RR interval and QRS width using Discrete Wavelet transform, that could distinguish between I-AVB and normal ECG. In the case of frequency-domain analysis, a method based on the cancellation of QT segment, and the P wave detection using spectrogram in the obtained residual signal was proposed in [6]. Norhashimah et al. [15] used periodogram power spectrum estimate to discern the I-AVB ECG, but it could not distinguish the I-AVB and the II-AVB. Viola et al. [19] compared the absolute HRV indexes and low frequency during sleep stages in 9 healthy controls and one subject with second degree atrioventricular blocks (AVB). From these research, it can be observed that the detection of P peak is a key point to achieve the task of automatic AVB detection. The most common way detecting P wave can be found by: wavelet analysis [3], wavelet transform and neural network [10,17], morphological transform [18], a combination of Hidden Markov model and wavelet [5], syntax template recognition method [16], function approximation method [13], esophageal electrocardiogram [7].

In this study, we developed a novel automated I-AVB detection method where the feature FPR_{dur} is extracted from ECG signals and then fed into SVM to complete the detection. The key idea can be summarized as follows. First, we detect the R peaks of a given ECG signal by applying the modulus maximum method and wavelet transform. Then, a new P detection algorithm is designed according to the detection of local maximum point on the left side of R peak. Next, PR duration of an ECG signal is defined and fusion feature is calculated to be the extracted features on the basis of several statistics of the sequence of PR duration, denoted by FPR_{dur}. Finally, we employ SVM to accomplish the task of differentiating I-AVB ECG and normal ECGs.

The rest of this paper is organized as follows. Section 2 describes the R and P peak detection algorithm, as well as the FPR_{dur}-based feature extraction method. The ECG database and validation of the proposed automatic I-AVB detection method FPR_{dur}-SVM are presented in Sect. 3. Finally, some conclusions are summarized in the last section.

2   Methods

2.1   R Peak Detection

Since the ECG signals are susceptible to a variety of noise during the acquisition, like baseline drift, power line interference, and muscle tremors, we firstly denoise the original ECG by using discrete wavelet transform [14].

The R peak is the highest peak in the QRS complex, represents early ventricular depolarization, as shown in Fig. 1.

Here, we employ the modulus maximum of wavelet transform [9] to detect R peak in this work. The R peak sequence is recorded as

$$R = \{R(1), R(2), \cdots, R(m)\}.$$

In addition, the RR interval is the duration between two consecutive R peaks, denoted by

$$RR(i) = RR(i+1) - RR(i), i = 1, 2, \cdots, m-1.$$

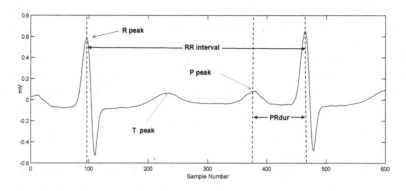

Fig. 1. P, R, T peak and RR interval, PR$_{dur}$ in an ECG segment (Color figure online)

2.2   P Peak Detection

The right and left atrial waveforms summate to form the P wave. The P wave is the first positive deflection on the ECG and represents atrial depolarization, and it is a small, positive and smooth wave. The first 1/3 of the P wave corresponds to right atrial activation, the final 1/3 corresponds to left atrial activation, the middle 1/3 is a combination of the two. The P peak appears about 0.2 s before the R peak and it's amplitude value is lower than 0.25 mV in general, as shown in Fig. 1.

Motivated by this fact, a new P peak detection algorithm is developed as follows.

Algorithm I: Given an ECG signal s.

Step 1. Add a window before each R peak, which is represented by

$$W(i) = [t_R(i) - k_1, t_R(i) - k_2], \delta > k_1 > k_2, i = 2, 3, ...m,$$

where $t_R(i)$ is the time point of the i-th R peak in s, and k_1, k_2 is time of searching forward. m is the number of the window. In order to avoid the inference of the high T wave as Fig. 1 shows (yellow arrow indication), the size of the window

$W(i)$ is set within the duration time between T wave and R peak, which is denoted by δ.

Step 2. In every $W(i)$, the point of the maximum value of signal is defined as the candidate P peak, which is recorded as $\bar{P}(i)$.

Step 3. Determine the final P peaks on **s**, the specific process of the P peak detection is as follows:

(i) If the amplitude value of $\bar{P}(i)$ is greater than 0.25 mV and the duration time between $\bar{P}(i)$ and R(i) is longer than 0.5 s, the edge point is considered to be falsely detected as the P peak. Then we correct the P peak by add a window $W'(i)$, whose start point is on the right of $\bar{P}(i)$. The $W'(i)$ is denoted by

$$W'(i) = [t_{\bar{P}}(i) + k_3, t_R(i) - k_2],$$

(ii) If the amplitude value of $\bar{P}(i)$ is greater than 0.25 mV and the duration time between $\bar{P}(i)$ and R(i) is shorter than 0.08 s, the edge point is considered to be falsely detected as the P peak. Then we correct the P peak by add a window $W''(i)$, whose end point is on the left of $\bar{P}(i)$. The $W''(i)$ is denoted by

$$W''(i) = [t_R(i) - k_1, t_{\bar{P}}(i) - k_3],$$

where $t_{\bar{P}}(i)$ is the time of the i-th $\bar{P}(i)$ in an ECG segment, and k_3 is the variety size of the window $W'(i)$ and $W''(i)$.

Finally, we define the maximum value in $W'(i)$ or $W''(i)$ as the final P peak, and denote the corresponding P peak sequence by

$$P = \{P(2), P(3), \cdots, P(m)\}.$$

2.3 Feature Extraction Method

Firstly, the definition of PR_{dur} is given. We name the duration time between P and R peak as PR_{dur}, as shown in Fig. 1, which can be calculated by the following way.

$$PR_{dur}(i) = t_R(i) - t_P(i-1), i = 2, 3, \cdots, m,$$

we record the PR_{dur} sequence as:

$$PR_{dur} = \{PR_{dur}(2), PR_{dur}(3), \cdots, PR_{dur}(m)\}.$$

The PR_{dur} is a important indicators of I-AVB identification. Because when the I-AVB appears, the distance is longer than normal people's. So we calculate three statistical features on the basis of PR_{dur} sequence obtained above. In following process, it should be noted that the points between 10th percentile and 90th percentile are selected to improve the robustness, denoted by

$$\bar{PR}_{dur} = \{\bar{PR}_{dur}(2), \bar{PR}_{dur}(3), \cdots, \bar{PR}_{dur}(m')\}$$

Secondly, calculate the statistics of $\bar{PR}_{dur}$ sequence that are shown as follows:

(1) The median of the $\bar{PR}_{dur}$ sequence, which is obtained by

$$MDPR_{dur} = median(\bar{PR}_{dur}).$$

(2) Calculate the mean value of $\bar{PR}_{dur}$ sequence as

$$MAPR_{dur} = mean(\bar{PR}_{dur}).$$

(3) Define the mean value of the ratio of each RR interval to the PR_{dur} in an ECG signal as

$$RAPR_{dur} = mean\left(\frac{PR_{dur}(i)}{RR(i-1)}\right), i = 2, 3, \cdots, m-1.$$

Thirdly, we constitute a fusion feature FPR_{dur} by combining $MDPR_{dur}$, $MAPR_{dur}$, and $RAPR_{dur}$ together, which is formulated by

$$FPR_{dur} = \begin{bmatrix} MDPR_{dur} \\ MAPR_{dur} \\ RAPR_{dur} \end{bmatrix}^{T}.$$

2.4 Automated I-AVB Detection Method

Finally, according to the previous desorption, the automated I-AVB detection method can be summarized as the flowchart depicted in Fig. 2.

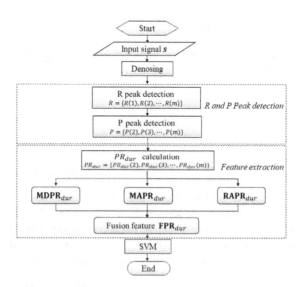

Fig. 2. The flowchart of automated I-AVB detection method

3   Experiments and Results

3.1   Database

The ECG database used in this study is taken from the China Physiological Signal Challenge 2018 database (CPSC2018). The database contains 6877 (female: 3178; male: 3699) ECG recordings with 12 leads, lasting from 6 s to 60 s, and the sample rate is 500 Hz. All data are provided in MATLAB format (each recording is a .mat file containing the ECG data, as well as the patient sex and age information). The details of CPSC2018 Database can be found in Table 1. Aim to verify the performance of the automated I-AVB detection method FPR_{dur}-SVM, we select the set 1 (918 normal ECG signals) and set 3 (704 I-AVB ECG signals) with lead II as the experimental data in this study. Figure 3 illustrates two ECG segments in set 1 and set 3 respectively.

Table 1. Detail ECG information of $CPSC$ database

Dataset	ECG type	Recording	Mean length
1	Normal	918	15.43
2	Atrial fibrillation (AF)	1098	15.01
3	First-degree atrioventricular block (I-AVB)	704	14.32
4	Left bundle branch block (LBBB)	207	14.92
5	Right bundle branch block (RBBB)	1695	14.42
6	Premature atrial contraction (PAC)	556	19.46
7	Premature ventricular contraction (PVC)	672	20.21
8	ST-segment depression (STD)	825	15.13
9	ST-segment elevated (STE)	202	17.15

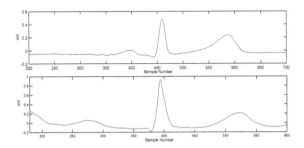

Fig. 3. The ECG segments of the set 1 (normal) and set 3 (I-AVB)

3.2   Experimental Results and Discussion

This subsection verifies the performance of the proposed method from four aspects: (1) R and P peak detection; (2) the practicability of features $MDPR_{dur}$, $MAPR_{dur}$ and $RAPR_{dur}$; (3) performance comparison of three single features and the fusion feature with SVM; (4) performance comparison of the SVM, k-Nearest Neighbors (KNN) and logistic regression with the fusion feature FPR_{dur}.

We describe the calculation way and values of the parameters used in this work. In R and P peak detection, the window parameters $k_1 = 0.05$ s, $k_2 = 0.01$ s, $k_3 = 0.02$ s are determined respectively by many times experiments and we let the δ less than 0.7 s in this study. In SVM, the LIBSVM software package 3.22 version is applied with the radial base function (RBF) as the kernel function, the regularization parameter C and the kernel width g are selected by the grid search method. In KNN, the Euclidean distance is applied and the parameter k is chosen by ten-fold cross validation. In logistic regression, the parameter $theta$ is determined by glmfit function of MATLAB. All of the specified parameters are summarized in Table 2.

Table 2. Specified parameters in the experiment

Methods	Symbol	Description	Values
SVM	C	Regularization parameter	2^5
SVM	g	Kernel width	2
KNN	k	Number of nearest neighbors	10
Logistic regression	θ	Regression coefficients	$1.3549, 0.1258, 1.236, 1.498$

First, Fig. 4 shows the R and P peak detection result, as depicted by black and green point respectively. The red points represent the edge points detected as candidate P peak. Obviously, our P detection algorithm can restrain the edge errors effectively.

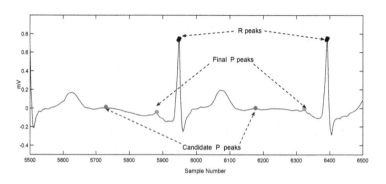

Fig. 4. The P, R peak and candidate P peak in an ECG signal (Color figure online)

Second, Fig. 5(a) shows the scatter plot of three features MDPR$_{dur}$, MAPR$_{dur}$ and RAPR$_{dur}$, the red '▲' represents the feature of the I-AVB ECG, and the blue '•' represents the feature of the normal ECG. It can be seen that all features are effective in distinguishing the I-AVB and normal ECG. Similar results can be observed from the boxplot of three features, as shown in Fig. 5(b). Here, it should be noted that only 50 ECG signals are randomly selected from the set1 and set3 respectively to observe the difference between features more clearly.

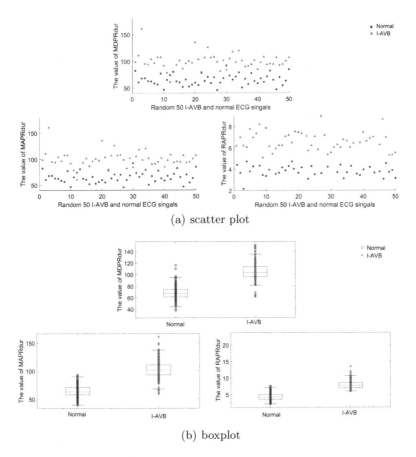

(a) scatter plot

(b) boxplot

Fig. 5. The scatter plot and boxplot of MDPR$_{dur}$, MAPR$_{dur}$ and RAPR$_{dur}$ (Color figure online)

Next, we compare the classification performance between three single features and fusion feature with the same SVM. Table 3 shows the experiment results including accuracy (ACC), sensitivity (SEN) and specificity (SPE), which are used to measure the performance of classifiers and calculated by the following way.

$$ACC = \frac{TP + TN}{TP + FN + TN + FP} \times 100\%,$$

$$SEN = \frac{TP}{TP + FN} \times 100\%,$$

$$SPE = \frac{TN}{FP + TN} \times 100\%.$$

where the TP (true positive) denotes the number of the positive tuples that were correctly labeled by classifier, TN (true negatives) denotes the number of the negative tuples that were correctly labeled by classifier, FP (false positive) denotes the number of the negative tuples that were incorrectly labeled as positive, FN (false negative) denotes the number of the positive tuples that were incorrectly labeled as negative [4].

As observed from Table 3, the performance of the fusion features FPR_{dur} has been greatly improved comparing with the three single features. The classification accuracy obtained by FPR_{dur} increases from 94.0% to 98.5%. In addition, the ability of different features to discriminate the I-AVB ECG and normal ECG can also be revealed by the Receiver Operating Characteristic Curve (ROC), whose evaluation depends on the area under ROC curve (abbreviated by AUC)[2]. The larger AUC is, the better classification performance will be.

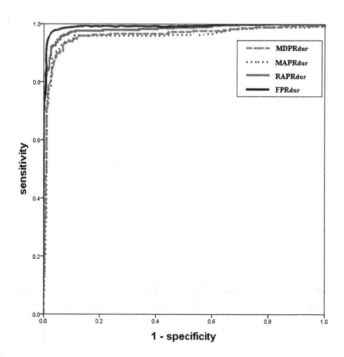

Fig. 6. ROC curve of four features $MDPR_{dur}$, $MAPR_{dur}$, $RAPR_{dur}$ and FPR_{dur}

Table 3. Performance comparison of all features by SVM

Methods	ACC (%)	SEN (%)	SPE (%)	AUC (%)
MDPR$_{dur}$+SVM	92.2	92.0	92.3	94.0
MAPR$_{dur}$+SVM	92.5	91.0	94.0	96.2
RAPR$_{dur}$+SVM	94.0	93.3	95.0	97.0
FPR$_{dur}$+SVM	**98.5**	**98.7**	**98.3**	**99.2**

Figure 6 shows the ROC of three features and fusion feature. Apparently, the fusion feature FPR$_{dur}$ has the better performance than other three single features MDPR$_{dur}$, MAPR$_{dur}$ and RAPR$_{dur}$.

Finally, we compare the performance of SVM with other classifiers using the same fusion feature FPR$_{dur}$. The corresponding results are given in Table 4. Clearly, the classification accuracy by SVM is higher than KNN and logistic regression. Meanwhile, the time spent by SVM is much shorter than others. All experimental results provide a strong evidence for that a better and stabler performance of I-AVB detection can be achieved by using the method FPR$_{dur}$-SVM proposed in this study.

Table 4. Performance comparison among classifiers with the fusion feature FPR$_{dur}$

Methods	ACC (%)	SEN (%)	SPE (%)	Time(s)
SVM+FPR$_{dur}$	**98.5**	**98.7**	**98.3**	**0.9672**
KNN+FPR$_{dur}$	97.5	96.3	97.5	1.9854
Logistic Regression+FPR$_{dur}$	96.1	95.3	97.2	6.4607

4   Conclusion

In this study, we proposed a novel automatic I-AVB detection method FPR$_{dur}$-SVM, which combines the FPR$_{dur}$ feature with SVM effectively. In order to describe the changes of morphological characteristics of the ECG segment between P and R wave, we firstly detected the R and P peak by using the modulus maximum method and wavelet transform. Then, a new P detection algorithm is designed according to the detection of local maximum point on the left side of R peak. Secondly, the definition of PR$_{dur}$ is presented and the corresponding statistics of PR$_{dur}$ sequence are calculated as the features (MDPR$_{dur}$, MAPR$_{dur}$, RAPR$_{dur}$). Then the fusion feature FPR$_{dur}$ is defined by combining MDPR$_{dur}$, MAPR$_{dur}$ and RAPR$_{dur}$ together. Finally, an automated I-AVB detection method FPR$_{dur}$-SVM has been built, which is integrated between the novel fusion feature FPR$_{dur}$ and Support Vector Machine (SVM). The performance of the proposed method FPR$_{dur}$-SVM has been verified with CPSC2018

Database from two aspects: (1) performance comparison of the fusion feature FPR_{dur} and other three single features with the same classifier SVM; (2) performance comparison of SVM, KNN and logistic regression with same fusion feature FPR_{dur}. Experimental results reveal that our FPR_{dur}-SVM method does a good job in the I-AVB detection.

Acknowledgement. This work was supported by the Innovative Talents Promotion Plan of Shaanxi Province under Grant 2018TD-016.

References

1. Ferlitsch, A., et al.: Bradycardia and sinus arrest during percutaneous ethanol injection therapy for hepatocellular carcinoma. Eur. J. Clin. Investig. **34**, 218–223 (2004)
2. Alcaraz, R., Sandberg, F., Sörnmo, L.: Classification of paroxysmal and persistent atrial fibrillation in ambulatory ECG recordings. IEEE Trans. Bio-Med. Eng. **58**, 1441–1449 (2011)
3. Almeida, R., Martinez, J.P., Olmos, S., Rochal, A., Laguna, P.: Automatic delineation of T and P wave using a wavelet-based multiscale approach. In: International Congress on Computational Bioengineering, vol. 13, pp. 243–247 (2003)
4. Francois, P.: P wave detector with PP rhythm tracking: evaluation in different arrhythmia contexts. Physiol. Meas. **29**, 145–155 (2008)
5. Graja, S., Boucher, J.M.: Hidden markov tree model applied to ECG delineation. IEEE Trans. Instrum. Meas. **54**, 2163–2168 (2005)
6. Gurrero, J., Marntize, M., Magdalena, R., Munoz, J., Bataller, M., Rosado, A.: P and R wave detection in complete congenital atrioventricular block. Ann. Biomed. Eng. **37**, 94–105 (2009)
7. Hernandez, A., Carrault, G., Mora, F.: Multisensor fusion for atrial and ventricular activity detection in coronary care monitoring. IEEE Trans. Biomed. Eng. **46**, 1186–1190 (1999)
8. Keerthi, P., Umamaheswara, G.R.: Matlab based GUI for arrhythmia detection using wavelet transform. Comput. Biomed. Res. **27**, 45–60 (1994)
9. Legarreta, I.R., Addison, P.S., Reed, M.J., Grubb, N., Clegg, G.R., Robertson, C.E.: Continuous wavelet transform modulus maxima analysis of the electrocardiogram: beat characterisation and beat-to-beat measurement. Int. J. Wavelets Multiresolution Inf. Process. **03**, 19–42 (2005)
10. Li, X.Y., Wang, T., Feng, H.Q.: Adaptive filter based on wavelet transform eliminates baseline drift in ECG. J. Univ. Sci. Technol. China **30**, 3450–454 (2000)
11. Li, Y., Chen, Y., Xin, J.: A diagnostic analysis on dynamic ECG for II AVB in patients with atrial fibrillation. Pract. J. Card. Cereb. Pneumal Vasc. Dis. **12**, 7–10 (2004)
12. Meghriche, S., Boulemden, M., Amer, D.: Two neural networks architectures for detecting AVB, vol. 7, pp. 193–198 (2008)
13. Murthy, S., Rangaraj, M.R., Udupa, K.J.: Homomorphic analysis and modeling of ECG signals. IEEE Trans. Biomed. Eng. **26**, 330–344 (1979)
14. Quiroga, R.: Single-trial event-related potentials with wavelet denoising: method and applications. Int. Congr. **1278**, 429–432 (2005)
15. Saad, N.M., Abdullah, R., Low, Y.F.: Detection of heart blocks in ECG signals by spectrum and time-frequency analysis. In: IEEE Conference on Research and Development, vol. 5, pp. 61–65 (2006)

16. Skordalakis, E.: Syntactic ECG processing: a review. Pattern Recogn. J. Pattern Recogn. Soc. **19**, 305–313 (1986)
17. Sternickel, K.: Automatic pattern recognition in ECG time series. Comput. Methods Programs Biomed. **68**, 109–115 (2002)
18. Sun, Y., Chan, K.L., Krishnan, S.M.: Characteristic wave detection in ECG signal using morphological transform. BMC Cardiovasc. Disord. **5**, 1–7 (2005)
19. Viola, A.U., et al.: Abnormal heart rate variability in a subject with second degree atrioventricular blocks during sleep. Clin. Neurophysiol. Off. J. Int. Fed. Clin. Neurophysiol. **115**, 946–950 (2004)

A New Automatic Detection Method for Bundle Branch Block Using ECGs

Jiaqi Bai, Luning Mao, Hao Chen, Yanan Sun, Qiang Li, and Rui Zhang[✉]

The Medical Big Data Research Center, Northwest University, Xi'an, China
{bjq,maoluning,haochen,ynsun,lqlq}@stumail.nwu.edu.cn, rzhang@nwu.edu.cn

Abstract. The automatic detection of bundle branch block (BBB) using electrocardiogram (ECG) has been attracting more and more attention, which is recognized to be helpful in the diagnosis and treatment of BBB-related heart diseases. In this paper, a novel automatic BBB detection method is developed. We first propose a new R peak detection algorithm which is able to detect both single R peak and multiple R peaks in one ECG beat. Then the number of R peaks and the length of RR interval are calculated to be the extracted features. Finally, linear classification is implemented to differentiate BBB ECG from normal ECG. Simulation results on CPSC2018 Database show that the average accuracy, sensitivity and specificity attain 96.45%, 95.81% and 96.80% respectively, demonstrating that the presented method of automatic BBB detection works well in distinguishing the normal ECG signals and the BBB ECG signals. This research thus provides insights for the automatic detection of BBB.

Keywords: Bundle branch block · Electrocardiogram · Feature extraction · R peak detection

1 Introduction

Bundle branch block (BBB) is a type of ventricular block resulting from the damage of bundle in ventricle [14,19]. Depended on the block occurring in the left or right ventricle, there include left BBB (LBBB) and right BBB (RBBB) [3,18]. For patients with BBB, the heart is difficult to pump blood so that it may further cause fainting and lead to serious complications, even sudden cardiac death [4,17].

Electrocardiogram (ECG) is the signal recording the myocardium electrical activity by placing electrodes on body surface [1,16]. Since ECG contains a lot of physiological and pathological information about heart, it is an indispensable tool for the diagnosis and treatment of heart diseases [2,12]. A normal ECG beat is composed of P wave, QRS complex and T wave (see Fig. 1(a)). Differently,

Supported by the Innovative Talents Promotion Plan of Shaanxi Province under Grant 2018TD-016.

in a BBB ECG beat, the QRS complex may exhibit abnormal waveforms which includes rsR' type, rSR' type, rsr' type and M type [10]. That is to say, multiple R peaks will appear in one QRS complex (see Fig. 1(b)) [11]. In this paper, we focus on the study of automatically detecting such malformed QRS complex in BBB ECG recordings.

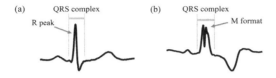

Fig. 1. Example of ECG signals. (a) Normal ECG wave. (b) Abnormal ECG wave with BBB in precordial lead.

The automatic detection of BBB using ECG is considered to be important for the diagnosis and treatment, and its key point lies in designing appropriate feature extraction method. Various feature extraction methods have been developed from the perspectives of frequency domain and time domain in recent years. From the frequency domain, Huptych et al. [20] proposed a method of feature extraction based on wavelet packets transform. Yildirim [9] employed the wavelet sequences layer to conduct feature extraction. Khalaf et al. [7] presented an approach of extracting features by calculating spectral correlation coefficients. Sahoo et al. [13] utilized multiresolution wavelet transform to detect QRS complex features which are used to classify four types of ECG beats. However, above methods based on frequency domain are not intuitive and time consuming, and such drawbacks can be overcame by the feature extraction methods on time domain. Feature extraction methods based on the time domain analysis can be listed as follows. An adaptive bacterial foraging optimization algorithm for obtaining important features from each ECG beat based on its waveform characteristics was introduced by Kora et al. [8]. But, the optimization algorithm is easy to get stuck at the local optimal value, thus the method of feature extraction without optimization algorithm has been developed. Higher order statistics of ECG signals combined with three timing interval features containing R-R time interval ratio (IR) and two R-R time intervals were extracted by Ebrahimzadeh et al. [5]. Yeh et al. [21] extracted statistical features by utilizing the morphological characteristics of QRS complex such as the width of QRS complex, the time duration between Q and T, etc. These two methods extracted features based on the morphological characteristics of the ECG signal, which can provide desirable performance of classification. Thus, in this work, we will design feature extraction methods according to the morphological characteristics.

In this paper, an automatic BBB detection method using ECGs will be developed. First, we propose a new R peak detection algorithm based on the morphological characteristics of QRS complex, which is able to detect both single R peak and multiple R peaks in one ECG beat. Then, the number of R peaks and the length of RR interval are calculated to be the extracted features. Finally, linear classification is employed to differentiate BBB ECG from normal ECG to complete the automatic detection of BBB.

The rest of this paper is organized as follows. The second section presents the methods to detect R peak and extract features, respectively. The third section demonstrates the validity of the proposed features for automatic BBB detection by linear classification. Finally, a brief conclusion is given in the last section.

2   Methods

2.1   Detection of R Peak

This subsection proposes a novel R-peak detection algorithm based on the morphological characteristics of QRS complex, and such detection algorithm can be used to detect both single R peak and multiple R peaks in one ECG beat. The key idea can be summarized as follows: (1) In each ECG beat, taking the variation of amplitude into consideration, the single R peak is initially detected by employing a differential signal in *step 1*; (2) Next, we detect the other R peaks locating in the k-th beat of the given ECG signal by *step 2*; (3) At last, if the other R peaks in the k-th beat is not detected, we save the single R peak detected in *step 1*; otherwise, the sequence of R peaks on y are detected by *step 3*.

R-peak detection algorithm: Given an ECG signal $y = \{y(n)\}_{n=1}^{N}$ (Fig. 2(a)).

(1) *Step 1.*

Step 1.1. Obtain a differential ECG signal y_d (Fig. 2(b)) by Eq. (1).

$$y_d(n) = y(n+1) - y(n), n = 1, 2, ..., N - 1. \tag{1}$$

Step 1.2. Gain y_s (Fig. 2(c)) by simplifying y_d through Eq. (2) [22].

$$y_s = \begin{cases} 0 & if\ 0 \leq y_d < th^+,\ or\ th^- < y_d \leq 0, \\ y_d & if\ y_d \geq th^+,\ or\ y_d \leq th^-, \end{cases} \tag{2}$$

where th^+ and th^- are the thresholds set by taking the δ-percentile from the positive and negative parts of y_d, respectively.

Step 1.3. Add $\alpha\%$ - overlapping moving window on y_s, find the local maximum point and local minimum point in each window and form binary pair set $\{(p_i, q_i)|p_i > 0, q_i < 0, i = 1, ..., m \leq T\}$, which is shown in Fig. 2(c) with red circles. Here, T is the number of the windows. The width of the moving window is denoted as l_1.

Step 1.4. Obtain the single R peaks sequence $\{R_1, ..., R_P\}$ from y by utilizing binary pair set, where P is the number of ECG beats in y. There are two situations involved.

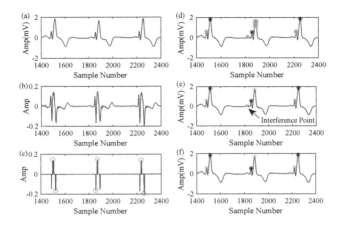

Fig. 2. The illustration of the procedures to detect R peaks for a segment of ECG signal. (a) y; (b) y_d; (c) y_s, marking binary pair set in *step 1.3* on y_s; (d) marking $\{r_k\}_{k=1}^{Q_1}$ obtained from *step 2.1* on y; (e) marking $\{r_k\}_{k=1}^{Q_2}$ obtained from *step 2.2* on y; (f) marking $\{r_k\}_{k=1}^{Q_3}$ obtained from *step 2.3* on y.

(a) If p_i appears firstly, we need to match the location of p_i and q_i in y_s to y, and R peak is the point with the largest amplitude between the two points on y;

(b) If q_i appears firstly, we need to match the location of q_i in y_s to y, and windowing forward from the matched point on y with width of l. R peak is the point with the largest amplitude in the window.

(2) *Step 2.*

Step 2.1. Determine sequences of the other candidate R peaks within a window whose center is the position of R_k and width is l_2, and the sequences is denoted by $r_k = \{r_k(1), ..., r_k(Q_1)\}$. Here, in Fig. 2(d), the purple stars denote the determined r_k and the black star in k-th ECG beat of y denotes the detected R_k.

Taking the fact that the R peaks must be the local maximum points into consideration, we determine $\{r_k(q)\}_{q=1}^{Q_1}$ by finding the local maximum points in the defined window except R_k. Then separating $\{r_k(q)\}_{q=1}^{Q_1}$ into two parts: $\{r_k^{left}(h)\}_{h=1}^{H_1}$ and $\{r_k^{right}(t)\}_{t=1}^{T_1}$ denoting the points before R_k and the points after R_k, respectively. Here, $H_1 + T_1 = Q_1$.

Step 2.2. Select points that might be the other R peaks from the r_k by following equation. Here, taking the method in r_k^{left} for example:

$$h_0 = \arg_h \left\{ \max(Amp(r_k^{left}(h)) - Amp(s_k^{left}(h))) \right\}, h = 1, 2, ..., H_1,$$

where $Amp(\alpha)$ denotes the amplitude at point α, $s_k^{left}(h)$ is the position of the point with the smallest amplitude in signal segment $[r_k^{left}(h), R_k]$,

$h = 1, 2, ..., H_1$, $r_k^{left}(h_0)$ denotes the selected point in r_k^{left}, and $s_k^{left}(h_0)$ is the corresponding point within minimum amplitude in $[r_k^{left}(h_0), R_k]$. Besides, if there exists other $r_k^{left}(h)$ between $s_k^{left}(h_0)$ and R_k in r_k^{left}, we further select $r_k^{left}(h)$ closest to R_k. So far, we update r_k^{left} with the selected points data as $\{r_k^{left}(h)\}_{h=1}^{H_2}$, and also update r_k which are shown in Fig. 2(e) with purple stars.

Step 2.3. Update r_k by eliminating interference points.

For the reason that the amplitude of the points in a small interval containing R peaks have rapid amplitude changes, this step eliminates interference points as follows.

We preliminarily calculate the amplitude difference of $\{r_k^{left}(h)\}_{h=1}^{H_2}$ by Eq. (3) written as

$$Amp^{dif}(r_k^{left}(h), L_k^{left}(h)) = Amp(r_k^{left}(h)) - Amp(L_k^{left}(h)), h = 1, ..., H_2, \quad (3)$$

where $\{L_k^{left}(h)\}_{h=1}^{H_2}$ denote the points within smallest amplitude in signal segment $[r_k^{left}(h) - \eta, r_k^{left}(h)], h = 1, ..., H_2$. Furthermore, we need to eliminate the points satisfying the following equation and update r_k^{left} as $\{r_k^{left}(h)\}_{h=1}^{H_3}$:

$$Amp^{dif}(r_k^{left}(h), L_k^{left}(h)) < min(Amp(R_k)/3, th_{amp}),$$

where th_{amp} denotes a threshold value of amplitude. By comparing Fig. 2(e) and (f), it is obvious that the interference point has been eliminated. Similarly, we can apply the above procedure on r_k^{right} to obtain the updated $\{r_k(q)\}_{q=1}^{Q_3}$.

(3) *Step 3.* Determine the sequence of R peaks on y.

To describe the rapid amplitude changes of the signals, we define absolute slope for R_k and $\{r_k(q)\}_{q=1}^{Q_3}$ ($k = 1, ..., P$) by Eq. (4) written as

$$\begin{cases} Slope^+(R_k) = \frac{Amp^{dif}(R_k, L_k)}{Loc(L_k) - Loc(R_k)}, \\ Slope^-(r_k^{left}(h)) = \frac{Amp^{dif}(r_k^{left}(h), L_k^{left}(h))}{Loc(r_k^{left}(h)) - Loc(L_k^{left}(h))}, h = 1, ..., H_3, \end{cases} \quad (4)$$

where $Slope^+(\alpha)$ and $Slope^-(\alpha)$ denote the slope obtained from the right and left segment of point α, respectively. $Loc(\alpha)$ denote the location at point α, L_k denotes the point with the smallest amplitude in signal segment $[R_k, R_k + \eta]$ ($k = 1, ..., P$).

Note that the duration time between two R peaks in the same ECG beat should be less than th_{len}. Thus if the maximum of duration time between r_k^{left} and r_k^{right} is more than th_{len}, we choose r_k^{left} or r_k^{right} with the maximal value of absolute slope as the final r_k ($k = 1, ..., P$). Otherwise, all $r_k(q)$ ($k = 1, ..., P, q = 1, ..., Q_3$) obtained in *step 2* are determined as the other R peaks in k-th ECG beat of y ($k = 1, ..., P$).

After the above procedures in *step 2* and *step 3* are applied on all ECG beats of y, we could obtain $\{r_k(q)\}_{q=1}^{Q_4}$ ($k = 1, ..., P$) that denote the other R peaks on y.

So far, we have completely detected the sequences of R peaks written as $R_s = \{R_s(1), ..., R_s(Q)\}$ by combining $\{r_k(q)\}_{q=1}^{Q_4}$ with R_k $(k = 1, ..., P)$, here, Q is the number of R peaks on y.

2.2 Feature Extraction Methods

In this subsection, according to the detected R peaks, we will introduce two features: the number of R peaks in one ECG beat and the length of RR intervals, respectively.

Number of R Peaks. This part initially counts the total number of R peaks in y based on the detected R peaks. Then, we can attain the mean value of the number of R peaks in an ECG beat by following equation

$$R^{cur} = \frac{1}{P} \times Q,$$

where P is the number of beats of y, Q is the number of the total number of R peaks in y.

Length of RR Intervals. Generally, the length of RR interval is regarded as the time of one ECG beat. On the basis of the detected R peaks, we calculate each length of RR intervals firstly. Then, the standard deviation of RR intervals' length in y is obtained as another feature by following equation:

$$RR = \sqrt{\sum_{j=1}^{Q-1} (RR(j) - RR^{mean})^2},$$

where $RR(j)$ denotes the duration time of j-th RR interval in y, RR^{mean} is the mean value of all $RR(j)$ in y.

3 Experiments

3.1 Database

This work applies the China Physiological Signal Challenge 2018 (CPSC2018) Database collected from 11 hospitals, which contains 6877 (female: 3178; male: 3699) ECG recordings with 12 leads lasting from 6 s to 60 s. The sampling rate is 500 Hz. All data are given in MATLAB format (each recording is a .mat file including the ECG data, the patient sex and age information). A large proportion of the recordings only have one label (denoted as First label). However, the minority of recordings have up to three labels (denoted as First label, Second label and Third label, respectively). All recordings have been divided into 8 data sets according to the First label. We illustrate the performance of the proposed automatic BBB detection method on the data set Normal in leads V1, V2, V5 and V6, data set LBBB in leads V5 and V6, data set RBBB in leads V1 and V2, which are shown in Table 1.

Table 1. Detail ECG information of CPSC2018 Database

Type	Recording
Normal	918
Left bundle branch block (LBBB)	207
Right bundle branch block (RBBB)	1695

3.2   The Experimental Results and Discussions

This subsection will prove the effectiveness of the automatic BBB detection method proposed in our work. The experiments include three parts: R peaks detection, the practicability of the number of R peaks and of the length of RR intervals, and the verification of the automatic BBB detection method. The following experiments are carried out in MATLAB R2016b environment and the same PC with Inter Core i5-4200M CPU and 4 GB RAM.

Firstly, in order to reduce the additional interference, the wavelet transform (WT) [6,15] is employed to denoise the original ECG signals as shown in Fig. 3. Here, an ECG segment from the data sets RBBB (1695) in leads V1 is taken. After that, we detect the R peaks by using R-peak detection algorithm described in Subsect. 2.1, and the corresponding parameters are listed in Table 2. The results of R peak detection are shown in Fig. 4, where both black stars and purple stars denote R peaks. It is obvious that the single R peaks are detected in the normal ECG segment (Fig. 4(a)) and the multiple R peaks are detected in the segment of ECG with RBBB (Fig. 4(b)).

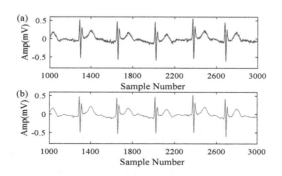

Fig. 3. An ECG segment from lead V1 of RBBB. (a) Original ECG segment; (b) Denoised ECG segment.

Secondly, the number of R peaks and the length of RR interval for LBBB are acquired by taking the maximum values of R^{cur} and RR between lead V5 and lead V6, respectively. The number of R peaks and the length of RR interval for RBBB are acquired by taking the maximum values of R^{cur} and RR between lead V1 and lead V2, respectively. The number of R peaks and the length of

Table 2. Parameters of R-peak detection algorithm

Parameters	Description	Value
δ-percentile	Percentile of the differential signal	2%
$\alpha\%$	Overlap in set window	50%
l_1	The width of moving window	0.14 s
l	The width of the windows forward from q_i	0.05 s
l_2	The width of windows for search the other R peaks	0.09 s
η	The length of signal segment for calculating the amplitude difference	0.02 s
th_{amp}	The minimum amplitude of R peak	0.08 mV
th_{len}	The maximum distance of R peaks in the same beat	0.07 s

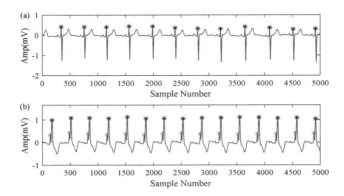

Fig. 4. The results of detecting R peaks in the ECG segments from lead V1. (a) A normal ECG segment; (b) An ECG segment with RBBB.

RR interval for NORM are acquired by taking the maximum values of R^{cur} and RR among lead V1, lead V2, lead V5 and lead V6, respectively. Here, NORM represents a normal ECG signal. Then, by analyzing the range of these two features in box plots shown in Figs. 5 and 6, respectively, we initially ensure that both the number of R peaks and the length of RR interval can be used to classify NORM and LBBB or RBBB because these two features are almost no overlap except some abnormal points. Next, in order to further confirm the practicability of the number of R peaks and the length of RR interval, we plot receiver operating characteristic (ROC) curves shown in Figs. 7 and 8. Here, TPR and FPR denote true positive rate and false positive rate, respectively. The area under the curve (AUC) denotes the area between the ROC curve and the FPR axis. AUC can be employed to evaluate the ability of the features to distinguish between NORM and BBB. The larger value of AUC is expected for a better classification performance of the feature. The values of the AUC for the number of R peaks and the length of RR interval are presented in Tables 3 and 4, respectively. The calculated values of AUC are large, demonstrating the availability of the proposed features.

Finally, the thresholds corresponding to the maximal Youden index in ROC curves are obtained (Table 5) and the linear classification results of the NORM and LBBB or RBBB can be further gained. Here, the red points in Figs. 7 and 8 represent the points with the maximal Youden index. The classification

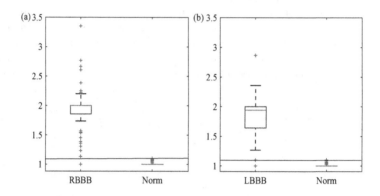

Fig. 5. The box-plots of the number of R peaks on (a) RBBB and Norm, and (b) LBBB and Norm.

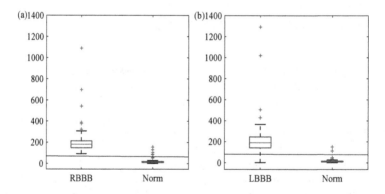

Fig. 6. The box-plots of the length of RR interval on (a) RBBB and Norm, and (b) LBBB and Norm.

Table 3. Experimental results based on the number of R peaks

Indexes	LBBB	RBBB
acc (%)	92.88	96.74
sen (%)	94.48	98.51
spe (%)	91.33	93.37
AUC	0.9753	0.9903

Table 4. Experimental results based on the length of RR interval

Indexes	LBBB	RBBB
acc (%)	94.92	97.97
sen (%)	93.10	98.51
spe (%)	96.67	96.93
AUC	0.9595	0.9897

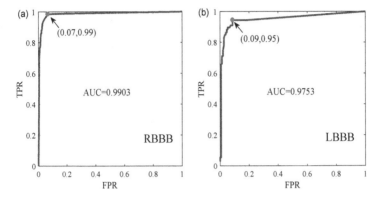

Fig. 7. The ROC curves corresponding to the number of R peaks for (a) RBBB and (b) LBBB, respectively.

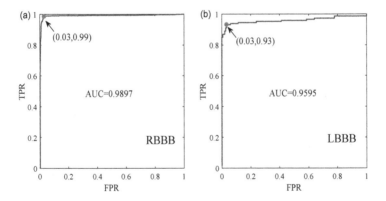

Fig. 8. The ROC curves corresponding to the length of RR interval for (a) RBBB and (b) LBBB, respectively.

indicators containing accuracy rate(Acc), sensitivity(Sen) and specificity(Spe) can be calculated by Eqs. (5)–(7) written as [21]

$$Acc = \frac{TP + TN}{TP + FP + TN + FN} \times 100\%, \tag{5}$$

$$\text{Sen} = \text{TPR} = \frac{\text{TP}}{\text{TP} + \text{FN}} \times 100\%, \tag{6}$$

$$\text{Spe} = 1 - \text{FPR} = \frac{\text{TN}}{\text{FP} + \text{TN}} \times 100\%, \tag{7}$$

where TP, FP, TN and FN are true positive, false positive, true negative and false negative, respectively. Tables 3 and 4 exhibit the results of the classification indicators for the number of R peaks and the length of RR interval, respectively. The indicators of linear classification result demonstrate that the sensitivities of the number of R peaks are 94.48% and 98.51% for the LBBB and RBBB, and the sensitivities of the length of RR interval are 93.10% and 98.51% for the LBBB and RBBB. It can be observed from the experimental results that the proposed automatic BBB detection method perform well for distinguishing the normal ECG signals and the abnormal ECG signals with BBB.

Table 5. Thresholds corresponding to the maximal Youden index in ROC curves

Features	LBBB	RBBB
The number of R peaks	1.09	1.13
The length of RR interval	95.24	83.85

4   Conclusion

In this paper, we proposed a novel automatic BBB detection method based on the morphological characteristics of QRS complex. Specifically, the number of the R peaks and the length of the RR interval are defined to be the features. The corresponding procedures can be summarized as follows. (1) Detect R peak; (2) Count the number of R peaks and calculate its mean value in one ECG beat; (3) Attain each length of RR interval and calculate its standard deviation. The performances of the presented features have been verified from two aspects: (1) the range comparison of the box plot of two features between normal ECG and BBB ECG; (2) the ROC curves of two features. Then the indicators (including Acc, Sen and Spe) of linear classification results obtained by setting threshold values of two features. Experimental results reveal that the proposed BBB detection method have good performance in distinguishing the normal ECG signals and the abnormal ECG signals with BBB. The method of these two extracted features are simple, fast and reliable, and the proposed algorithms require no complex mathematic computations. This research thus provides insights for the automatic detection of BBB and exhibits significance for reference of clinical application.

References

1. Andre, D., Rautaharju, P., Boisselle, E., et al.: Normal ECG standards for infants and children. Pediatr. Cardiol. **1**, 123–131 (1980)
2. Blanco-Velasco, M., Weng, B., Barner, K.E.: ECG signal denoising and baseline wander correction based on the empirical mode decomposition. Comput. Biol. Med. **38**, 1–13 (2008)
3. Brugada, J., Brugada, P.: Further characterization of the syndrome of right bundle branch block, st segment elevation, and sudden cardiac death. J. Cardiovasc. Electrophysiol. **8**, 325–331 (1997)
4. Civelek, A.C., Gozukara, I., Durski, K., et al.: Detection of left anterior descending coronary artery disease in patients with left bundle branch block. Am. J. Cardiol. **70**, 1565–1570 (1992)
5. Ebrahimzadeh, A., Shakiba, B., Khazaee, A.: Detection of electrocardiogram signals using an efficient method. Appl. Soft Comput. **22**, 108–117 (2014)
6. Gilles, J.: Empirical wavelet transform. IEEE Trans. Signal Process. **61**, 3999–4010 (2013)
7. Khalaf, A.F., Owis, M.I., Yassine, I.A.: A novel technique for cardiac arrhythmia classification using spectral correlation and support vector machines. Expert. Syst. Appl. **42**, 8361–8368 (2015)
8. Kora, P., Kalva, S.R.K.: Detection of bundle branch block using adaptive bacterial foraging optimization and neural network. Egypt. Inform. J. **18**, 67–74 (2017)
9. Yildirim, Ö.: A novel wavelet sequences based on deep bidirectional lstm network model for ECG signal classification. Comput. Biol. Med. **96**, 189–202 (2018)
10. Padmavathi, K., Ramakrishna, K.S.: Hybrid firefly and particle swarm optimization algorithm for the detection of bundle branch block. Int. J. Cardiovasc. Acad. **2**, 44–48 (2016)
11. Radovan, S., Ivo, V., Pavel, J., et al.: Fully automatic detection of strict left bundle branch block. J. Electrocardiol. **51**, S31–S34 (2018)
12. Luz Eduardo Jose, da S., Schwartz, W.R., Guillermo, C., et al.: ECG-based heartbeat classification for arrhythmia detection: a survey. Comput. Methods Programs Biomed. **127**, 144–164 (2016)
13. Sahoo, S., Kanungo, B., Behera, S., Sabut, S.: Multiresolution wavelet transform based feature extraction and ECG classification to detect cardiac abnormalities. Measurement **108**, 55–66 (2017)
14. Sgarbossa, E.B., Pinski, S.L., Topol, E.J., et al.: Acute myocardial infarction and complete bundle branch block at hospital admission: clinical characteristics and outcome in the thrombolytic era. J. Am. Coll. Cardiol. **31**, 105–110 (1998)
15. Singh, O., Sunkaria, R.K.: ECG signal denoising via empirical wavelet transform. Australas. Phys. Eng. Sci. Med. **40**, 1–11 (2016)
16. Sun, Y., Chan, K.L., Krishnan, S.M.: ECG signal conditioning by morphological filtering. Comput. Biol. Med. **32**, 465–479 (2002)
17. Vaduganathan, P., He, Z.X., Raghavan, C., et al.: Detection of left anterior descending coronary artery stenosis in patients with left bundle branch block: exercise, adenosine or dobutamine imaging? J. Am. Coll. Cardiol. **28**, 543–550 (1996)
18. Vernooy, K.: Left bundle branch block induces ventricular remodelling and functional septal hypoperfusion. Eur. Hear. J. **26**, 91–98 (2004)
19. Wolff, M.D.L., Parkinson, M.D.J., Paul, D.W.M.D.: Bundle-branch block with short P-R interval in healthy young people prone to paroxysmal tachycardia. Ann. Noninvasive Electrocardiol. **5**, 685–704 (2006)

20. Kutlu, Y., Kuntalp, D.: Feature extraction for ECG heartbeats using higher order statistics of WPD coefficients. Comput. Methods Programs Biomed. **105**, 257–267 (2012)
21. Yeh, Y.C., Chiou, C.W., Lin, H.J.: Analyzing ECG for cardiac arrhythmia using cluster analysis. Expert. Syst. Appl. **39**, 1000–1010 (2012)
22. Yeh, Y.C., Wang, W.J.: QRS complexes detection for ECG signal: the difference operation method. Comput. Methods Programs Biomed. **91**, 245–254 (2008)

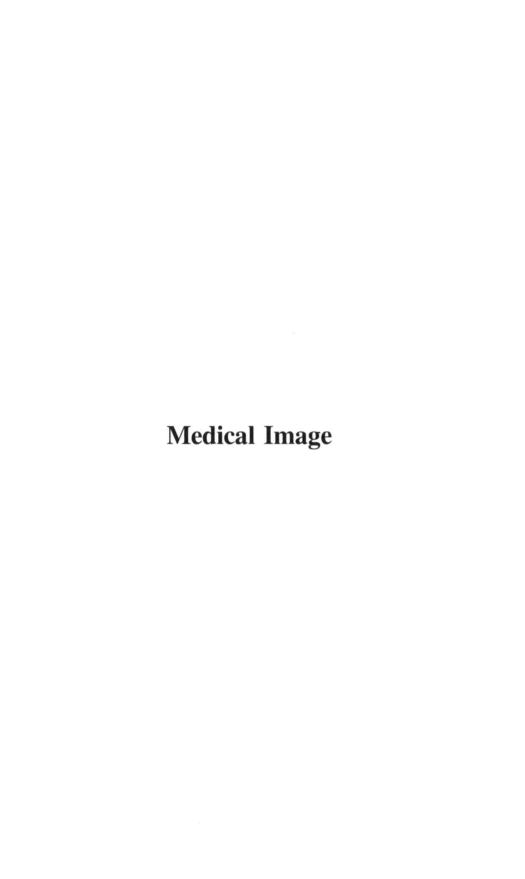

Medical Image

Research and Development of Three-Dimensional Brain Augmented Reality System Based on PACS and Medical Image Characteristics

Yufei Pang[1], Xin Jing[1], and Wang Zhao[2(✉)]

[1] School of Information Management, Zhengzhou University of Aeronautics,
Zhengzhou, China
1319730393@qq.com
[2] School of Information Management, Wuhan University, Wuhan, China
199223263@qq.com

Abstract. With the application of information technology, the scale of various digital image resources is increasing. How to make good use of these digital resources has become a hotspot of hospital management. Because of the use of artificial intelligence technology, the results of automatic recognition and annotation of hospital image resources can be displayed in two-dimensional form. But two-dimensional display, without stereoscopic visual effect, doctors are not easy to observe. In addition, in the real medical environment, it is necessary to combine the virtual information with the real scene, and add some additional information in the real environment to help doctors obtain more useful information. Augmented reality (AR) is a new visualization technology, which can meet the actual business needs mentioned above. In this paper, we focus on brain image, and use PACS as the channel of image acquisition and communication to study the feature extraction of brain image and three-dimensional reconstruction of brain image diseases. Based on the image file, the features of brain image are extracted, and the function module of augmented reality is designed. Unity is used to realize the three-dimensional reconstruction and visualization of brain image features through programming.

Keywords: Augmented reality · Three-dimensional reconstruction · PACS · Unity

1 Introduction

In traditional medical diagnosis, doctors usually judge the condition and identify the lesion according to the two-dimensional medical images (CT, MRI, etc.) obtained by medical equipment scanning and many years of reading experience. The diagnosis results are often accompanied by physician-specific subjective judgments. Under certain circumstances, the scientificity and accuracy of diagnosis results are not good, and misdiagnosis may occur. Medical image three-dimensional visualization technology involves computer graphics, computer vision, image processing and human-computer

© Springer Nature Switzerland AG 2019
H. Wang et al. (Eds.): HIS 2019, LNCS 11837, pp. 183–192, 2019.
https://doi.org/10.1007/978-3-030-32962-4_17

interaction technology. It is a theoretical method of converting two-dimensional medical tomographic image into graphic image on display and interactive processing. Medical data contains the three-dimensional structure of human organs and tissues. The three-dimensional visualization of medical images can vividly show the complex anatomical structure of human organs, which enables physicians to observe the structure of tissues and organs and lesion areas of patients in any angle and direction in an intuitive and three-dimensional way. Three-dimensional visualization of medical images overcomes the shortcomings of traditional physiotherapy diagnosis and treatment, and plays a very important role in accurate and scientific diagnosis of physicians. It plays an increasingly important role in the process of diagnosis and treatment [1].

Three-dimensional reconstruction technology was first proposed by Idesawa [2] in 1973. Hartley [3] and Faugras [4] described the theory of three-dimensional reconstruction in 1992, which shows that the technology of three-dimensional reconstruction has begun to mature, which brings opportunities for the practical application of three-dimensional reconstruction technology in various fields. Three-dimensional reconstruction of medical images refers to the use of computer image processing technology to transform two-dimensional tomographic image sequences such as ultrasound, CT, MRI, tissue and electron microscopy into three-dimensional images with intuitive stereoscopic effect and apply them to three-dimensional reconstruction of medical diagnosis. Because of the three-dimensional shape and spatial relationship of three-dimensional structure [5], three-dimensional reconstruction technology not only provides a complete three-dimensional model, but also interacts with three-dimensional images such as enlargement, reduction, rotation and contrast. It is helpful for doctors to observe areas of interest in detail from multi-level and multi-directional perspectives. These new imaging technologies will continue to make up for the shortcomings of traditional diagnostic methods [6], thus greatly improving the efficiency and accuracy of doctor's diagnosis.

Zhao proposed the texture feature and three-dimensional reconstruction method of brain CT image [7]. Hou studied the precise segmentation and three-dimensional reconstruction of brain tumors [8]. Domestic scholars use relatively old tools to reconstruct the brain in three dimensions. They don't use some of the latest technologies, and they don't have realistic visualizations. At present, doctors urgently need to enhance user interaction after three-dimensional reconstruction. They need better visual and simulation effects to improve user experience and practical application effects.

Now hospitals have used PACS, which is the center of storing medical images. PACS system is the popularization and application of digital technology, multimedia information technology, image processing technology, computer technology and network communication technology in medical imaging [9].

The innovation of this paper is to study the three-dimensional reconstruction and visualization methods of brain image disease features from the perspective of visual human-computer interaction, combined with image segmentation, image three-dimensional reconstruction, visual human-computer interaction and other technologies. In addition, using PACS as the source of image data acquisition and augmented reality technology, a three-dimensional reconstruction and visualization system of brain image disease features based on B/S structure is designed and developed.

2 DICOM and PACS

2.1 DICOM Image File

DICOM Medical Computer Information Protocol, which is jointly formulated by the National Association of Electronic Products Manufacturers and the American College of Radiological Medicine, has been accepted by major medical device manufacturers all over the world and eventually becomes an agreement to be abided by the world. DICOM greatly improves the accuracy and accuracy of medical information storage. There are two main differences between DICOM image format and other image formats. Firstly, the accessory information is complete. It not only stores the image information, but also stores thousands of information about the time, place, way of acquiring the image, as well as the patient's name, number, location and so on. It provides a rich diagnostic basis for doctors. Secondly, the image information contained in the system has high clarity and can directly store all the information of the patient's photographic location. This study is based on medical DICOM radiographic images to achieve and optimize three-dimensional brain imaging.

2.2 Pacs

PACS (Picture Archive and Communication System) is the image archiving and communication system. It is the popularization and application of digital technology, multimedia information technology, image processing technology, computer technology and network communication technology in medical images. The main task of PACS is to digitally store all kinds of medical images (including images generated by magnetic resonance, CT, ultrasound, X-ray machines, infrared instruments, microscopes, etc.) generated in daily life through various interfaces (analog, DICOM, network) in a large amount. When needed, they can be stored under certain authorization. Quickly return to use, while adding some auxiliary diagnostic management functions. It plays an important role in transmitting data and organizing and storing data among various image devices.

2.3 PACS Based on DICOM Standard

The standard DICOM files generated by digital diagnostic equipment and the DICOM files transmitted by HIS system are sent directly to PACS, and then the image files are stored in the database by PACS. The process is shown in Fig. 1.

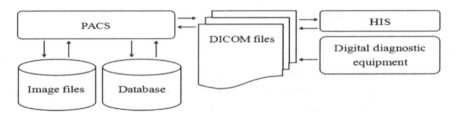

Fig. 1. DICOM and PACS communication processing

3 Feature Extraction and Three-Dimensional Reconstruction of Brain Imaging Diseases

Data processing and three-dimensional reconstruction process includes two processes, forming three files. The first process includes the processing of DICOM files of brain images, including data preprocessing, feature extraction, feature classification and feature marking. The second process includes the reconstruction of brain image features and 3D rendering. The original DICOM image file is processed by the first process and converted into a feature tag file. After the second process, the feature tag file is transformed into a 3D model file. Data processing and three-dimensional reconstruction are shown in Fig. 2.

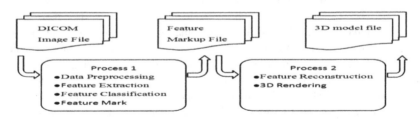

Fig. 2. Data processing and three-dimensional reconstruction

Finally, using 3D model file and augmented reality tools, we can reconstruct the three-dimensional brain and display disease features in the three-dimensional model.

3.1 Feature Extraction of Brain Imaging Diseases

With the development of medical imaging technology, the technology of using computer technology to detect brain structural changes from MRI images to assist early diagnosis and treatment of diseases has been in the practical stage. The steps of feature extraction for brain imaging diseases are shown in Fig. 3.

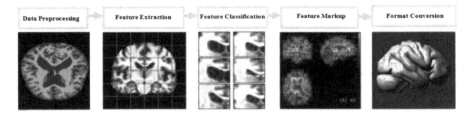

Fig. 3. Feature extraction procedures of brain imaging diseases

Because the results of feature extraction of brain image diseases are still stored in DICOM data format, it is necessary to use medical image development toolkit to transform the format, so as to carry out three-dimensional reconstruction in the next research.

3.2 Three-Dimensional Reconstruction of Brain Image

The research method of medical image three-dimensional reconstruction is mainly realized by ITK + VTK, which mainly deals with medical image data in DICOM format. That is to recognize the boundary of two-dimensional medical images and redraw the three-dimensional images of tissues or organs. Three-dimensional reconstruction methods of medical images can be divided into three categories according to different data description methods in the process of rendering: surface rendering, volume rendering and hybrid rendering [10]. The idea of surface rendering is to recognize and segment boundary from a series of two-dimensional image data, extract human surface information, and use illumination, coloring, and so on. Texture mapping and other methods are used to restore the object's three-dimensional model by rendering algorithm. For example, contour reconstruction method based on fault boundary, line algorithm based on surface reconstruction such as voxels, moving cube algorithm, segmentation cube algorithm, etc. [11], the main idea of volume rendering method is not to generate isosurface, but to give each voxel a certificate. The volume data are projected directly onto the whole image plane, such as the ray projection algorithm in the order of image space, the expansion algorithm in the order of object space, and the shearing and twisting algorithm. The surface rendering algorithm is better than the volume rendering algorithm. In terms of computational efficiency and real-time interaction. The algorithm is simple and occupies less memory resources, but the image details are lost. Volume rendering algorithm contains more details than surface rendering algorithm. Because the purpose of three-dimensional reconstruction is to need rich details, volume rendering algorithm is the preferred algorithm in this study.

There are many tools for 3D image rendering, such as OpenGL, Direct3D, Unity and so on. Considering the support format, rendering time and rendering effect, Unity was selected to render and reconstruct the model [12].

The technical scheme of three-dimensional reconstruction is as follows: Firstly, the image data after feature processing is read, and the input data need to be processed by

ITK and VTK. The OBJ format image needed for three-dimensional reconstruction can be used as input data of API Unity of three-dimensional image processing. Then the whole brain image is preliminarily reconstructed using three-dimensional reconstruction API. The next step is to classify and screen feature slices, which need to be reconstructed in detail and tagged. Finally, the texture mapping and stereo rendering of the model are performed by Unity [13].

Using augmented reality technology, the virtual model obtained from three-dimensional reconstruction of medical images such as CT and MRI is fused into real scene in real time. Enhanced the doctor's visual system, can see the naked eye can not see the internal information of organs. At the same time, accurate organ spatial information related to the patient's body can be obtained [14].

4   Augmented Reality Technology and Its Function Modules

Augmented Reality (AR) is the latest visualization technology. It develops from virtual reality [15]. It superimposes the virtual world constructed by computers in the real world, strengthens users'understanding of reality, and increases various additional information of the real world.

Augmented reality, as the latest visualization technology and method, mainly exists in the form of system function module, and there is data exchange between it and resource database. The function modules of augmented reality system are shown in Fig. 4.

The functional modules of augmented reality system include recognition and matching program and synthesis and interaction program. The recognition and matching program includes three parts: image acquisition, image recognition and image matching. The image acquisition program mainly collects effective recognition images or scene maps, and provides them to image recognition programs for feature extraction. The recognition features are transmitted to image matching programs. The image matching programs retrieve the identical or similar resources from the repository according to the recognition features, and at the same time provide these resources to the synthesis and interaction programs. The synthesis and interaction program includes three parts: virtual and real image synthesis, image projection and human-computer interaction. Firstly, virtual and real image synthesis reads the image or knowledge that needs to be displayed in the resource database, and then fuses the image or knowledge with the real scene to form the target image. Through the image projection program, the target image is projected on the display device to form an augmented reality scene. Doctors and other users can perform various operations through human-computer interaction programs.

Augmented reality function module has good expansibility and stability. Augmented reality module can be used as standard modules for different medical systems or mobile devices.

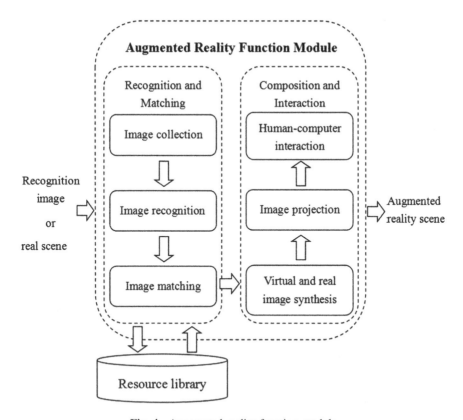

Fig. 4. Augmented reality function module

5 Programming and Core Algorithms

5.1 System Architecture

As shown in Fig. 5, the system is divided into three parts: server side, client side and communication network. On the server side. The client includes importing image, image analysis, feature extraction and three-dimensional reconstruction. The server includes PACS, image file, database, etc.

5.2 Programming of Three-Dimensional Reconstruction

The software is made with Unity tool. The three-dimensional brain model is reconstructed from the previous three-dimensional model file, which can clearly show the detailed features of the brain and display the relevant brain regions.

Figure 6 is the loading material for the model. Different materials can be selected to adjust the visual effect. The material can display information of brain area or the location of disease.

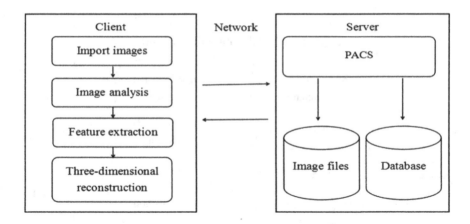

Fig. 5. System architecture

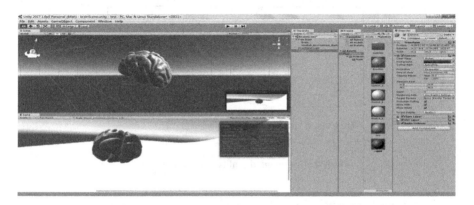

Fig. 6. Loading model material

Figure 7 shows the details of the reconstructed brain tissue. Doctors can see the details of the brain.

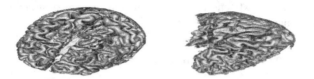

Fig. 7. Details of brain tissue after three-dimensional reconstruction

Figure 8 is a program interface. The three-dimensional model of the brain can be controlled by mouse, including zooming, zooming and moving. Clicking on the brain can display the corresponding two-dimensional disease feature image file, which is convenient for doctors to observe from two-dimensional or three-dimensional perspective.

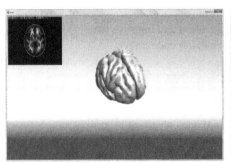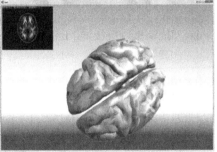

Fig. 8. Program interface

6   Testing and Application

6.1   System Testing

This paper chooses personal computers and servers, as well as two different systems of mobile phones as the test environment, hardware and software environment as shown in Table 1.

Table 1. Testing environment

Testing equipment	Hardware environment	Software environment
OPPO R17 Mobile Phone	CPU: SDM670 RAM: 8 GB	Android
IPhone 8 Mobile Phone	CPU: A11 RAM: 2 GB	iOS
Personal Computer	CPU: Intel i7 RAM: 16 GB	Windows 10
Server	CPU: Intel W2133 RAM: 16 GB	Windows Server 2019

6.2   Application Environment

Because the development tool Unity can release software versions suitable for different application environments, the software can be used in personal computers, servers, mobile phones and other devices, and has the advantages of cross-platform application and good stability.

7   Conclusion

Because of its practicability, augmented reality plays an important role in the three-dimensional reconstruction of brain image features. In this paper, a three-dimensional reconstruction scheme based on augmented reality is preliminarily implemented. It also needs to be tested and applied in the actual scene to improve the function of the program to solve the problem of displaying a large amount of medical information and data. Augmented Reality technology can be used to visualize various medical knowledge. This paper will continue to discuss the application scenarios of Augmented Reality in the construction of hospital informatization and improve medical information display. Show the effect and improve the user experience effect.

References

1. Zhang, C.: Research on GPU-based real-time volume rendering of medical images. Inner Mongolia University of Science and Technology (2014)
2. Idesawa, M.: A system to generate a solid figure from three view. Bull. JSME **16**(2), 216–225 (1973)
3. Hartley, R.I.: Estimation of relative camera positions for uncalibrated cameras. In: Sandini, G. (ed.) ECCV 1992. LNCS, vol. 588, pp. 579–587. Springer, Heidelberg (1992). https://doi.org/10.1007/3-540-55426-2_62
4. Faugeras, O.D.: What can be seen in three dimensions with an uncalibrated stereo rig? In: Sandini, G. (ed.) ECCV 1992. LNCS, vol. 588, pp. 563–578. Springer, Heidelberg (1992). https://doi.org/10.1007/3-540-55426-2_61
5. Rodriguez, J.A., Xu, R., Chen, C.C., et al.: Three-dimensional coherent X-ray diffractive imaging of whole frozen-hydrated cells. IUCrJ **2**(Pt 5), 575–583 (2015)
6. Wang, Y., Du, X., Zhao, S, et al.: Medical Image Processing, pp. 169–202. Tsinghua University Press, Beijing (2012)
7. Zhao, J., Gong, S., Wang, L.: Three-dimensional reconstruction and texture characteristics of brain CT images. Laser Mag. **35**(06), 62–65 (2014)
8. Hou, D., Lu, Y., Wang, Y., Liu, W.: Segmentation and three-dimensional reconstruction of brain tumors on MRI. J. Appl. Sci. **36**(05), 808–818 (2018)
9. Establishment and research of medical image database under Longzhibo. DICOM standard. Jilin University (2009)
10. Wang, R., Zhang, J., Peng, K.: Algorithmic analysis of three-dimensional reconstruction of computer-aided medical images. Tissue Eng. Res. Clin. Rehabil. China **15**(04), 745–748 (2011)
11. Xiong, P., Yang, Y.: Fast three-dimensional surface reconstruction algorithm based on isosurface points. Microcomput. Inf. **26**(14), 6–7+14 (2010)
12. Yuan, Y.: Research on three-dimensional reconstruction technology in augmented reality environment. University of Electronic Science and Technology (2009)
13. Li, C., Liu, S.: Brief analysis of several ways of introducing three-dimensional model formats into Unity3D. New Chin. Technol. Prod. (05), 23–24(2016)
14. Niu, Y.: Augmented Reality Technology in Surgical Navigation. Zhejiang University (2004)
15. Li, Q., Zhang, L.: An empirical study of mobile learning based on augmented reality. Audiov. Educ. China **01**, 116–120 (2013)

Deep Learning in Multimodal Medical Image Analysis

Yan Xu[(✉)]

China Academy of Information and Communications Technology,
Beijing 100045, China
xuyan@caict.ac.cn

Abstract. Various imaging modalities (CT, MRI, PET, etc.) encompass abundant information which is different and complementary to each other. It is reasonable to combine images from multiple modalities to make a more accurate assessment. Multimodal medical imaging has shown notable achievements in improving clinical accuracy. Deep learning has achieved great success in image recognition, and also shown huge potential for multimodal medical imaging analysis. This paper gives a review of deep learning in multimodal medical imaging analysis, aiming to provide a starting point for people interested in this field, and highlight gaps and challenges of this topic. Based on the introduction of basic ideas of deep learning and medical imaging, the state-of-the-art multimodal medical image analysis is given, with emphasis on the fusion technique and feature extraction deep models. Multimodal medical image applications, especially cross-modality related, are also summarized.

Keywords: Deep learning · Medical image analysis · Multimodal

1 Introduction

In recent years, deep learning has seen tremendous growth in its popularity and usefulness, especially image recognition and speech recognition. This is largely due to the development of powerful computers (larger memory and faster graphic processing units), big data resources, and techniques to train deeper networks.

Deep learning is very good at discovering intricate structures in high-dimensional data and is therefore applicable to medical image analysis. Litjens et al. [1] provided a thorough survey on deep learning in medical image analysis. Lundervold et al. [2] focus on MRI image, Liu et al. [3] on ultrasound image. This paper focuses on multimodal medical image analysis.

There exist many medical imaging modalities, including Computed Tomography (CT), Magnetic Resonance Imaging (MRI), Positron Emission Tomography (PET), Single Photon Emission Computed Tomography (SPECT) and Ultra-Sound (US) etc. Various imaging modalities encompass abundant information which is different and complementary to each other. It is reasonable to combine images from multiple modalities to make a more reliable and accurate assessment. For example, PET has certain limitations in accuracy and positioning, therefore PET combines with CT or MRI to improve the accuracy and diagnostic accuracy greatly.

© Springer Nature Switzerland AG 2019
H. Wang et al. (Eds.): HIS 2019, LNCS 11837, pp. 193–200, 2019.
https://doi.org/10.1007/978-3-030-32962-4_18

Medical image fusion [4] is the process of registering and combining multiple images from single or multiple imaging modalities to improve the imaging quality and reduce randomness and redundancy in order to increase the clinical applicability of medical images for diagnosis and assessment of medical problems. Multi-modal medical image fusion algorithms and devices have shown notable achievements in improving clinical accuracy of decisions based on medical images.

This paper gives a review of deep learning in multimodal medical imaging analysis, aiming to provide a starting point for people interested in this field, and highlight gaps and challenges of this topic. The structure of the paper is as follows. In Sect. 2 deep learning for multimodal medical imaging is illustrated from 3 different views: fusion techniques, feature extraction models and applications. Conclusion and outlook for future is given in Sect. 3.

2   Deep Learning in Multimodal Medical Image Analysis

Multimodal medical Imaging can be divided from different views, such as modality used, fusion techniques, feature extraction method, application area, etc. According to the applied modality types, multimodal medical analysis can be classified into two categories: non-image and image included (having one image modality at least). This paper focus on the category of image included.

2.1   Fusion Techniques

The information from multiple modalities can be merged at any point in the deep neural network. According to the merge point in the neural network, multimodal medical imaging can be divided into three categories: feature level fusion, classifier level fusion, and decision-making level fusion.

Feature Level Fusion. Images of multiple modalities are used together to learn a unified image feature set, which shall contain the intrinsic multimodal representation of the data. The learned features are then used to support the learning of a classifier. Feature level fusion may not fully exploit the complementary nature of the modalities involved and may lead to very large input vectors that may contain redundancies. Typically, dimensionality reduction techniques like PCA are applied to remove these redundancies in the input space. Auto encoders, which are nonlinear generalizations of PCA, are popularly used in deep learning to extract a distributed representation from raw data.

Classifier Level Fusion. Images of each modality are used as separate inputs to learn individual feature sets. These single-modality feature sets will be then used to learn a multimodal classifier. Learning the single-modality features and learning the classifier can be conducted in an integrated framework or separately.

Decision-Making Level Fusion. Images of each modality are used independently to learn a single modality classifier (and the corresponding feature set). The final decision of the multimodal scheme is obtained by fusing the output from all the classifiers.

This fusion method is feature independent and the errors from multiple classifiers tend to be uncorrelated. There are various rules for decision making, such as max-fusion, averaged-fusion, or weighted fusion etc.

Fusion Strategies Choice. For deep learning based fusion, the fusion may occur in any depth of the network, and the fusion may occur gradually, one or more modalities merge at one time. Optimizing a method of multimodal image analysis application should consider various fusion architectures and select the most suitable one for a given use case. An intuition would be fusing similar modalities early, and then fusing disparate modalities at a deeper layer. In [9], three fusion strategies for AD (Alzheimer's Disease) classification using SDSAE (Stacked De-noising Sparse Auto-Encoder) were compared: (a) fusing at the SDSAE input layer; (b) fusing at multiple SDSAE output layer; (c) after multiple SDSAE, one or more fully connected fusion layers being applied. Results show that (c) has better performance for AD classification. Recent work of Guo et al. [5] proposed unified framework for multimodal image fusion strategies. An image segmentation system based on CNN was implemented to contour the lesions of soft tissue sarcomas using multimodal images (MRI, CT, and PET). Three fusion strategies were tested. Comparison results show that for the task of tumor region segmentation using CNN, performing fusion within the network (at the convolutional layer or fully connected layer) is generally better than fusing images at the network output (through voting).

2.2 Feature Extraction Deep Model

Feature extraction is a critical step in image analysis. The most commonly used model for medical imaging analysis can be roughly divided into following categories: CNN based, GAN based, SAE based, DBM & DBN based, other layer-wise stacking based and transfer learning based. Recently CNN, GAN and transfer learning have been applied to multimodal medical imaging and shown better performance on medical image classification, segmentation, synthesis etc., which attributes to their abilities of feature extraction from raw images.

CNN Based. Convolutional Neural Networks (CNNs) have gained tremendous popularity within the computer vision community because of their ability to automatically capture high level representations of raw images. Many medical imaging analysis applications are based on CNN. A CNN based sarcomas segmentation system was proposed by using MRI, CT and PET images [5]. Deep CNN [6] and multi-stream FCN (Fully Convolutional Network) [16] were proposed for infant brain tissues segmentation on the basis of multimodal MR images (MRI-T1, MRI-T2, and FA (fractional anisotropy)).

GAN Based. The GANs (Generative Adversarial Networks) is one of the most important developments in deep learning, used in unsupervised machine learning, implemented by a system of two neural networks contesting with each other in a zero-sum game framework. GAN based network has been achieved great success in multimodal medical image synthesis, segmentation etc. Details will be given in Sect. 2.3 (cross-modality image synthesis).

SAE Based. An AE (AutoEncoder) is a neural network that is trained to attempt to copy its input to its output. In this way, the data is projected onto a lower dimensional subspace representing a dominant latent structure in the input. SAE (Stacked AE) are formed by placing AE layers on top of each other. Typically each AE was trained individually after which the full network was fine-tuned. Works in [7] (MRI, PET), [8] (MRI, PET, CSF) and [9] (baseline & longitudinal MRI) are all SAE based neuroimaging feature learning for AD classification.

DBM & DBN Based. RBMs (Restricted Boltzmann Machines) are a type of Markov Random Field, constituting an input layer and a hidden layer that carries the latent feature representation. The connections between the nodes are bidirectional. DBMs are the RBMs with more than one hidden layers. DBNs (Deep Belief Networks) are formed by placing RBMs layers on top of each other. DBM and DBN are unsupervised. They are used to identify latent feature present in the multimodal imaging. Suk et al. [10] used the multimodal DBM to learn features from huge 3D patches in multimodal neuroimaging data for AD/MCI diagnosis. Information from MRI and PET is fused in a hierarchical deep learning approach. Li et al. [11] developed a deep learning framework with PCA, DBM and SVM for multimodal AD diagnosis from MRI and PET scans.

Other Layer-Wise Stacking Based. Inspired by the layer-wise stacking of feature extraction such as DBN, SAE, recently Shi et al. [12] developed a multimodal stacked DPN (MM-SDPN) algorithm, which consists of two-stage SDPNs. In the first stage, two SDPNs are applied to the ROI features of MRI and PET, respectively. In the second stage, both learned features are concentrated and fed to a new SDPN to learn the fused features. It outperforms DBM in [10].

Transfer Learning. Transfer learning is used to improve a learner from one domain by transferring information from a related domain. It could be used to tackle the lack of medical image training sets. Compared to natural images, the amount of medical imaging training data is typically small, and domain-specific pre-trained models that can be used without retraining the network are not available. Transfer learning has been applied to deal with it. Most transfer learning is based on CNNs. Transfer learning can be subdivided into cross domain transfer learning and cross modal transfer learning.

Cross-Domain Transfer Learning. Cross-domain transfer learning is performed by learning from natural images, and then applying to medical images. Gupta et al. [13] used cross-domain features to represent MRI data. They deployed a SAE to learn from natural images and then applied a CNN to obtain a more effective feature representation for AD classification. It showed high classification performance in comparison with contemporary approaches. Carneiro et al. [14] used pretrained CNN (on ImageNet) to classify the risk of breast cancer.

Cross-Modal Transfer Learning. Medical images are typically gray-level, low-contrast and texture-rich, which is different from natural images. Models trained on natural images are not optimal for medical images. Hadad et al. [15] proposes to use cross-modal transfer learning to improve the robustness of the classifiers. They trained a network on mammography images and fine-tuned it to classify breast lesions in MRI images. Comparison between cross-modal and cross-domain transfer learning showed that the former improved the classification performance.

2.3   Applications

Deep Learning in multimodal image analysis has many applications, such as classification [7–12, 14, 15], segmentation [5, 6, 16–19], prediction [20] and image synthesis [21–27] etc. The applications of multimodal image analysis based on deep learning are listed in Table 1. For multimodal, image synthesis refers to cross-modality image synthesis.

Table 1. Deep learning based multimodal image application.

Ref. no	Modality	Model	Application
[7]	MRI, PET	SAE+MKSVM	Classification
[8]	MRI, PET, CSF	SAE-MKL	Classification
[9]	Baseline & Longitudinal MRI	SDSAE	Classification
[10]	MRI, PET	DBM	Classification
[11]	MRI, PET, CSF	PCA, DBM, SVM	Classification
[12]	MRI, PET, CSF	MMSDPN	Classification
[14]	MM-CC, MM-MLO	CNN (transfer)	Classification
[15]	MRI, MM	CNN (transfer)	Classification
[5]	MRI, CT, and PET	CNN	Segmentation
[6]	MRI-T1, MRI-T2, FA	CNN	Segmentation
[16]	MRI-T1, MRI-T2, FA	FCN	Segmentation
[17]	MRI-T1, MRI-T2	FCN (transfer)	Segmentation
[18, 19]	MRI, CT	GAN	Synthesis & Segmentation
[23]	MRI-T1, MRI-T2	LSDN (CNN like)	Synthesis
[24]	MRI-T1, MRI-T2, MRI-DWI	SAE	Synthesis
[25]	MRI-T1, CT	CNN based	Synthesis
[26]	MRI, CT	Fully-CNN, GAN,	Synthesis
[27]	Vessel Trees, Retinal Images	GAN	Synthesis

Cross-Modality Image Synthesis. Multimodal image synthesis referred to as the synthesis being achieved from a cross-modality adaptation model (e.g., from MRI to CT), that is one synthetic image in target imaging modality is synthesized from a real image in source imaging modality. Compared with CT, MRI is safe but cannot be used for either dose calculation or attenuation correction. To reduce unnecessary imaging dose for patients, it is clinically desired to estimate CT images from MR images in many applications. Most cross modality image synthesis related with from MRI to CT by using different deep learning architectures, such as deep embedding CNN [25], CycleGAN [21, 22], context-aware GAN [26] etc. In addition to MRI to CT, there are also some other image synthesis applications. Sevetlidis et al. [24] proposed a SAE to generate T2 scans from T1 scans and DWI scans from T2. Cost et al. [27] proposed a retinal image synthesis method from a binary vessel tree to a new retinal image based on GAN.

Cross-Modality Image Synthetic Segmentation. Cross-modality image synthesis has been shown as a good intermediate presentation for image processing, such as data augmentation, classification and segmentation. Recently end-to-end synthetic segmentation networks are proposed, which leverages both synthesis and segmentation performance simultaneously by using MRI and CT images with manual labels [19] or without [18].

3   Conclusion and Future Challenges

Multi-modal medical imaging has shown notable advantage of improving clinical accuracy. Deep learning is very good at discovering intricate structures in high-dimensional data and is therefore applicable to many domains. This paper gives a review of deep learning in multimodal medical imaging analysis, aiming to provide a starting point for people interested in this field, and highlight gaps and challenges of this topic.

Based on the introduction of basic ideas of deep learning and medical imaging, the state of art of multimodal medical imaging is given, with emphasis on the fusion technique and deep models. Fusion techniques play an important role in the context of multimodal. The fusion techniques are classified as feature level fusion, classifier level fusion and decision-making level fusion. Feature level fusion may not fully exploit the complementary nature of the modalities involved and may lead to very large input vectors that may contain redundancies. The nature of decision level fusion is contrary to feature level fusion, and classifier level fusion is in between them. An intuitional choice would be fusing similar modalities early, and fusing disparate modalities lately. Fusion strategies are application dependent and are very challenge.

Feature extraction, an important part of deep learning, is reviewed in the context of multimodal. Multimodal image features can be learned by classical network models, CNN, SAE, DBM & DBN, and some new stacked method. Multimodal image analysis can be applied in many applications, such as classification, segmentation, annotation, prediction, etc. GAN based network model is also used for cross-modality image synthesis, which has been shown as a good intermediate data for image processing, such as data augmentation, classification and segmentation.

One of the primary challenges in applying deep learning to medical images is the limited number of training samples available to build deep models without suffering from over-fitting. One possible method is transfer learning, which initialize model parameters with those of pre-trained models from nonmedical or natural images, then fine-tune the network parameters with the task-related samples. This has been extend in multimodal medical imaging area and achieved good results.

Multimodal medical image analysis has shown notable advantage of improving clinical accuracy. With the development of deep learning and big data available from medical imaging data, multimodal medical imaging will have a great advance. The years ahead are full of challenges and opportunities to improve multimodal medical image science even further and to bring it to new frontiers.

References

1. Litjens, G., Kooi, T., Bejnordi, B.E., et al.: A survey on deep learning in medical image analysis. Med. Image Anal. **42**, 60–88 (2017)
2. Lundervold, A.S., Lundervold, A.: An overview of deep learning in medical imaging focusing on MRI. https://arxiv.org/abs/1811.10052 (2018)
3. Liu, S., et al.: Deep learning in medical ultrasound analysis: a review, engineering (2019)
4. James, A.P., Dasarathy, B.V.: Medical image fusion: a survey of the state of the art. Inf. Fusion **19**, 4–19 (2014)
5. Guo, Z., Li, X., Huang, H., Guo, N., Li, Q.: Deep learning-based image segmentation on multimodal medical imaging. IEEE Trans. Radiat. Plasma Med. Sci. **3**(2), 162–169 (2019)
6. Zhang, W., Li, R., Deng, H., Wang, L., Lin, W., et al.: Deep convolutional neural networks for multimodality isointense infant brain image segmentation. NeuroImage **108**, 214–224 (2015)
7. Liu, S., et al.: Multimodal neuroimaging feature learning for multiclass diagnosis of Alzheimer's disease. IEEE Trans. Biomed. Eng. **62**(4), 1132–1140 (2015)
8. Suk, H., Shen, D.: Deep learning-based feature representation for AD/MCI classification. In: Proceedings of the International Conference on Medical Image Computing and Computer-Assisted Intervention, pp. 583–590 (2013)
9. Shi, B., Chen, Y., Zhang, P., Smith, C.D., Liu, J.: Nonlinear feature transformation and deep fusion for Alzheimer's disease staging analysis. Pattern Recognit. **63**, 487–498 (2017)
10. Suk, H.I., Lee, S.W., Shen, D.G., ADNI: Hierarchical feature representation and multimodal fusion with deep learning for AD MCI diagnosis. NeuroImage **101**, 569–582 (2014)
11. Li, F., Tran, L., Thung, K.H., Ji, S.W., Shen, D.G., Li, J.: A robust deep model for improved classification of AD/MCI patients. IEEE J. Biomed. Health Inform. **19**(5), 1610–1616 (2015)
12. Shi, J., Zheng, X., Li, Y., Zhang, Q., Ying, S.: Multimodal neuroimaging feature learning with multimodal stacked deep polynomial networks for diagnosis of Alzheimer's disease. IEEE J. Biomed. Health Inform. **22**(1), 173–183 (2018)
13. Gupta, A., Ayhan, M., Maida, A.: Natural image bases to represent neuroimaging data. In: Proceedings of the 30th International Conference on Machine Learning, Atlanta, GA, USA, 16–21 June, pp. 987–994 (2013)
14. Carneiro, G., Nascimento, J., Bradley, A.P.: Unregistered multiview mammogram analysis with pre-trained deep learning models. In: Navab, N., Hornegger, J., Wells, W.M., Frangi, A. F. (eds.) MICCAI 2015. LNCS, vol. 9351, pp. 652–660. Springer, Cham (2015). https://doi.org/10.1007/978-3-319-24574-4_78
15. Hadad, O., Bakalo, R., Ben-Ari, R., et al.: Classification of breast lesions using cross-modal deep learning. In: IEEE International Symposium on Biomedical Imaging. IEEE (2017)
16. Nie, D., Wang, L., Gao, Y., Shen, D.: Fully convolutional networks for multi-modality isointense infant brain image segmentation. In: Proceedings of the 13th IEEE International Symposium on Biomedical Imaging, Washington, DC, pp. 1342–1345 (2016)
17. Zeng, G., Zheng, G.: Multi-stream 3D FCN with multi-scale deep supervision for multi-modality isointense infant brain MR image segmentation. https://arxiv.org/abs/1711.10212, March 2019
18. Huo, Y., Xu, Z., Moon, H., et al.: SynSeg-Net: synthetic segmentation without target modality ground truth. IEEE Trans. Med. Imaging **38**(4), 1016–1025 (2019)
19. Zhang, Z., Yang, L., Zheng, Y.: Translating and segmenting multimodal medical volumes with cycle- and shape-consistency generative adversarial network. https://arxiv.org/abs/1802.09655 (2018)

20. Nie, D., Zhang, H., Adeli, E., Liu, L., Shen, D.: 3D deep learning for multi-modal imaging-guided survival time prediction of brain tumor patients. In: Ourselin, S., Joskowicz, L., Sabuncu, M.R., Unal, G., Wells, W. (eds.) MICCAI 2016. LNCS, vol. 9901, pp. 212–220. Springer, Cham (2016). https://doi.org/10.1007/978-3-319-46723-8_25

21. Wolterink, J.M., Dinkla, A.M., Savenije, M.H.F., Seevinck, P.R., van den Berg, C.A.T., Išgum, I.: Deep MR to CT synthesis using unpaired data. In: Tsaftaris, S.A., Gooya, A., Frangi, A.F., Prince, J.L. (eds.) SASHIMI 2017. LNCS, vol. 10557, pp. 14–23. Springer, Cham (2017). https://doi.org/10.1007/978-3-319-68127-6_2

22. Chartsias, A., Joyce, T., Dharmakumar, R., Tsaftaris, S.A.: Adversarial image synthesis for unpaired multi-modal cardiac data. In: Tsaftaris, S.A., Gooya, A., Frangi, A.F., Prince, J.L. (eds.) SASHIMI 2017. LNCS, vol. 10557, pp. 3–13. Springer, Cham (2017). https://doi.org/10.1007/978-3-319-68127-6_1

23. Van Nguyen, H., Zhou, K., Vemulapalli, R.: Cross-domain synthesis of medical images using efficient location-sensitive deep network. In: Navab, N., Hornegger, J., Wells, W.M., Frangi, A.F. (eds.) MICCAI 2015. LNCS, vol. 9349, pp. 677–684. Springer, Cham (2015). https://doi.org/10.1007/978-3-319-24553-9_83

24. Sevetlidis, V., Giuffrida, M.V., Tsaftaris, S.A.: Whole image synthesis using a deep encoder-decoder network. In: Tsaftaris, S.A., Gooya, A., Frangi, A.F., Prince, J.L. (eds.) SASHIMI 2016. LNCS, vol. 9968, pp. 127–137. Springer, Cham (2016). https://doi.org/10.1007/978-3-319-46630-9_13

25. Xiang, L., et al.: Deep embedding convolutional neural network for synthesizing CT image from T1-weighted MR image. Med. Image Anal. **47**, 31–44 (2018)

26. Nie, D., et al.: Medical image synthesis with context-aware generative adversarial networks. In: Descoteaux, M., Maier-Hein, L., Franz, A., Jannin, P., Collins, D.L., Duchesne, S. (eds.) MICCAI 2017. LNCS, vol. 10435, pp. 417–425. Springer, Cham (2017). https://doi.org/10.1007/978-3-319-66179-7_48

27. Costa, P., et al.: Towards adversarial retinal image synthesis. https://arxiv.org/abs/1701.08974 (2017)

A R-CNN Based Approach
for Microaneurysm Detection
in Retinal Fundus Images

Zihao Wang[1], Ke-Jia Chen[2(✉)], and Lingli Zhang[3]

[1] Bell Honors School, Nanjing University of Posts and Telecommunications,
Nanjing, China
[2] Jiangsu Key Laboratory of Big Data Security and Intelligent Processing,
Nanjing, China
chenkj@njupt.edu.cn
[3] School of Computer Science, Nanjing University of Posts and Telecommunications,
Nanjing, China

Abstract. Diabetic retinopathy (DR) is one of the major diseases causing blindness, and microaneurysms in the fundus are the first reliable lesions in its early stage. This paper proposes an object detection method for microaneurysms based on R-CNN, which consists of five steps: image preprocessing, candidate region generation, feature extraction, classification and non-maximal suppression. First, a fundus image preprocessing method and a candidate region generation algorithm for microaneurysms are proposed. Then, the VGG16 network is trained using the transferred fine-tuning model to extract features from candidate samples. Finally, real aneurysms are selected from candidate regions by a classifier. The experimental results in the internationally published database e-ophtha show that the proposed method outperforms other known related methods on the FROC indicator.

Keywords: Object detection · Microaneurysm · Deep learning ·
Diabetic retinopathy

1 Introduction

Diabetes mellitus is a disease with high incidence in modern people. About 420 million people around the world have been diagnosed with diabetes. In recent years, the population with diabetes mellitus tends to be younger and younger. The prevalence of diabetes has doubled in the past 30 years and is expected to continue increasing [11]. One of the most common complications of vascular injury caused by diabetes mellitus is diabetic retinopathy (DR). It is estimated that about one third of diabetic patients will be diagnosed with diabetic retinopathy, which is a chronic eye disease that causes vision loss and is also one of the major causes of blindness in the world [14]. Experts predict that from 2000 to 2030, with the global prevalence of diabetes increasing from 2.8% to 4.4%, the

H. Wang et al. (Eds.): HIS 2019, LNCS 11837, pp. 201–212, 2019.
https://doi.org/10.1007/978-3-030-32962-4_19

number of patients with DR is expected to increase significantly in the next few years [1].

Ophthalmologists say that most patients with DR can be cured and avoid loss of vision if diagnosed early and treated effectively. Microaneurysms (MAs) are the earliest lesions in fundus images. Doctors can screen DR early according to the condition of microaneurysms in fundus images. Figure 1(a) is an original fundus retinal image, and Fig. 1(b) is a region containing microaneurysms, which are dark and round in shape. Accurate detection and recognition of MAs lesions in fundus images by digital image processing can effectively promote the early screening of DR and greatly reduce the workload of doctors.

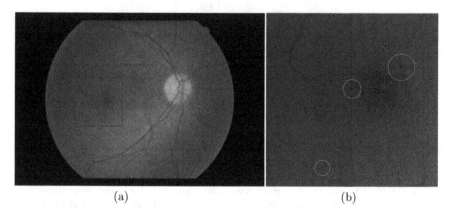

(a)   (b)

Fig. 1. A Fundus image with microaneurysms. This image is one of the images in the e-ophtha database. On the right is the enlarged portion of the green channel image in the blue box on the left image, and the microaneurysms have been marked. (Color figure online)

This paper aims to develop an object detection algorithm based on R-CNN [7] to detect and recognize microaneurysms in retinal fundus images. The main challenge of the study is that the aneurysms are very small and similar to the blood vessels in color. Moreover, since medical images need to be labeled by experts, the cost of data collection is high, so there are fewer retinal images containing microaneurysms in the database [4,8].

The main work and contributions of this paper are as follows:

(1) A candidate region generation algorithm is proposed, which is based on the characteristics of microaneurysms to generate candidate samples of microaneurysms.
(2) A pre-trained convolutional neural network is used to extract the features of candidate regions and the model is fine-tuned for accurate classification.
(3) Experiments on the public database e-ophtha show that the performance in FROC curve of the proposed method is better than the other two state-of-art aneurysm detection methods.

The rest of the paper is organized as follows. Section 2 reviews related work in microaneurysms detection. The proposed method is detailed in Sect. 3. The experimental results are shown and compared in Sect. 4. Section 5 concludes the paper.

2 Related Works

The problem of microaneurysms detection was first raised by Baudoin et al. [3]. They used morphological methods to identify and detect microaneurysms based on angiographic images. Due to the similarity between small vessels and micro-aneurysms, the authors also used top-hat transformation to remove erroneous detection results on blood vessels. Subsequently, on the basis of Baudoin et al.'s work, Frame et al. [6] enhanced the contrast of the image by using shadow correction and matched filtering, which can better distinguished the micro-aneurysm and surrounding background.

Quellec et al. [15] proposed a supervised microaneurysm detection method based on template matching in wavelet-subbands. In the training stage, the lifting scheme framework is used to find the best wavelet transform suitable for the detection of microaneurysms, and the template matching technique in the wave-let domain is used to detect the possible location of microaneurysms. The method needs to give an appropriate threshold to determine the microaneurysms by matching the results. Niemeijer et al. [12] launched the challenge competition of detecting microaneurysms based on color fundus images in 2008, called Retinal Online Challenge (ROC). The goal of ROC competition is to enable different challengers to detect the same dataset, and then to uniformly score the test results and compare the algorithms.

Antal and Hajdu [2] integrated a variety of preprocessing algorithms and microaneurysms detection algorithms in 2012. By choosing the best combination, they get the better results of microaneurysm detection.

Wu et al. [19] proposed an automatic detection method for microaneurysms in fundus images in 2016. In the method, A total of 27 feature features, including local features and contour features, are extracted for KNN classifier to distinguish real aneurysms from false lesions.

Orlando et al. [13] proposed a red lesion detection method in fundus images combining deep learning and domain knowledge in 2017. Red lesions include exudation and microaneurysms. The learning features of convolutional neural network (CNN) are enhanced by combining hand-made features. The set vectors of these features are then used to identify real lesion regions using random forest classification.

Previous methods mostly use manual feature, so it is difficult to further im-prove performance. In Orlando's method, the learning features of CNN are im-proved by adding hand-made features. However, the CNN network structure adopted by Orlando is too simple. Therefore, the proposed method in this paper uses pre-trained VGG16 [18] network for feature extraction. The network structure of VGG16 is a deep convolutional network and the extracted features can be more comprehensive.

3   Proposed Method

3.1   Overview of the Method

The overall detection process of our method is shown in Fig. 2, which consists of three main steps: candidate region generation, feature extraction, classification and detection. Firstly, the fundus image is preprocessed to minimize background noise, and then candidate regions of microaneurysms are extracted by image segmentation. Then, the trained VGG16 network is then used to extract the features of the candidate microaneurysm samples. Finally, the probability of each candidate sample is obtained by using the microaneurysm classifier. In the detection phase, non-maximal suppression is used to preserve the candidate region with the highest probability among several overlapping candidate regions.

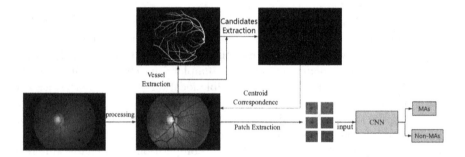

Fig. 2. The overall framework of our MA detection method.

3.2   Detection of Candidate Microaneurysms Regions

There are three main steps in the candidate region generation algorithm for microaneurysms: image preprocessing, vessel segmentation and candidate region generation based on local adaptive threshold segmentation, as shown in Fig. 3. In the preprocessed image, we can distinguish the microaneurysms from the background. The vessel segmentation step can remove the influence of the blood vessels in the fundus image. Finally, the candidate microaneurysms regions can be obtained by locally adaptive threshold segmentation and area screening of the preprocessed image.

Image Preprocessing. Fundus images of diabetic retinopathy have been a hot topic in medical research. However, in the process of obtaining the examiner's fundus image, the difference between the shooting environment results in many noises and shadows in the image. In order to reduce the influence of shadow and noise, we use green channel extraction, region of interest extraction, standardization, contrast-limited adaptive histogram equalization (CLAHE), Gamma adjustment and Gauss filtering to preprocess the fundus image. Microaneurysms can be clearly presented in preprocessed images, as shown in Fig. 3(a).

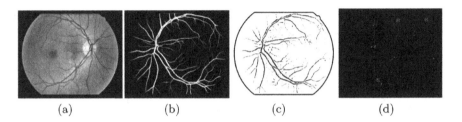

(a)   (b)   (c)   (d)

Fig. 3. The process of generating candidate microaneurysm regions. (a) Preprocessed image; (b) Image after vessel segmentation; (c) Locally adaptive threshold segmented image; (d) Image with candidate microaneurysm regions, and the white boxes are the real microaneurysms.

The RGB color model is often used to decompose the fundus images. Since the microaneurysm is the clearest in the green channel, the gray-scale image of the green channel is extracted and recorded as I_g. Fundus images are always recorded in rectangular form, but the area we focus on is inside the eye contour. In order to better segment the eye region of interest, we use OSTU to calculate the optimal threshold. The OSTU threshold calculation formula is as follows:

$$u = w_0 \times u_0 + w_1 \times u_1 \tag{1}$$

$$g = w_0 \times (u_0 - u)^2 + w_1 \times (u_1 - u)^2 \tag{2}$$

Where T is the segmentation threshold of foreground and background. The proportion of the foreground to the whole image is w_0. The foreground average gray level is u_0. The proportion of the background to the whole image is w_1. The background average gray level is u_1. The average gray level of the whole image is u, and thevariance of the foreground and the background is g. When g reaches the maximum value, the threshold T is the optimal threshold we need.

Then, $I_g(x, y)$ is processed according to the threshold T to obtain the image $I_{ROI}(x, y)$. The calculation formula is as follows:

$$I_{ROI}(x, y) = \begin{cases} I_g(x, y), & I_g(x, y) > T \\ 0, & I_g(x, y) \le T \end{cases} \tag{3}$$

Since the brightness of each fundus image is different, we normalize the images. Let the maximum value of the pixels in $I_{ROI}(x, y)$ image be Max, 0 in gray-scale image be the lowest, and 255 be the highest brightness. $I_{normalized}(x, y)$ denotes the normalized image. The normalization formula is as follows:

$$I_{normalized}(x, y) = \frac{I_{ROI}(x, y)}{Max} \times 255 \tag{4}$$

Next, we choose CLAHE algorithm [16] to enhance the normalized image $I_{normalized}$ and increase the contrast of the image. After the CLAHE algorithm, we can get the enhanced retinal fundus image, recorded as I_{clahe}. For the image

I_{clahe}, we use Gamma transform to correct the shadow part of the image. The calculation formula is as follows:

$$I_{gamma}(x,y) = 255(\frac{I_{clahe}(x,y)}{255})^{\gamma} \tag{5}$$

Finally, we use Gauss filtering to weaken the noise. According to Eq. (6), we calculate the size of the $(2k+1) \times (2k+1)$ Gauss template, and then convolute the template with I_{gamma} image. We define the filtered image as the preprocessed image $I_{preprocessed}$, as shown in Fig. 3(a).

$$H(i,j) = \frac{1}{2\pi\sigma^2}e^{-\frac{(i-l-1)^2+(j-k-1)^2}{2\sigma^2}} \quad i,j = 1,2,3,\cdots,2k+1 \tag{6}$$

Vessel Segmentation. The vessels are very similar to microaneurysms in local fundus images. When generating candidate regions for microaneurysms, many regions will fall near the fundus vessels. Therefore, we use the U-net model [9,10,17] to segment the blood vessel from the preprocessed fundus image. The result of vessel segmentation is shown in Fig. 3(b).

Candidate Region Detection. The preprocessed image is segmented by locally adaptive threshold to get the initial candidate region mask image. Then we subtract the obtained mask image from the vessel segmented image to get the final candidate region mask image after removing the regions larger or smaller than the predetermined region limit. Finally, the candidate regions can be extracted as samples from the preprocessed image based on their corresponding coordinates in the mask image.

3.3 Feature Extraction Based on CNN

The process of feature extraction and sample generation is shown in Fig. 4. Ac-cording to the labeling information of ophthalmologists, the candidate samples that contain real microaneurysm are labeled as positive samples, and vice versa. Since the number of positive and negative samples is imbalanced, the positive samples are expanded by symmetrical transformation, rotation and interception of candidate region samples of different sizes.

Next, the transfer learning method is used to extract features. The desired features are extracted for the new samples based on the feature representation learned from the previous network.

3.4 Classification and Detection

After feature extraction, the full connection layer is added as a classifier. During the training process, the parameters of the classifier are updated fast, but the classification accuracy is low due to the overfitting. Therefore, the fine-tuning

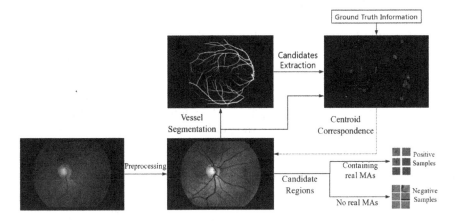

Fig. 4. Sample feature generation for training.

method is used to train the top "thawing" layer of the pre-trained model together with our newly added fully-connected classifier.

In this paper, we use VGG16 fine-tuning model to train the last convolution block of the model with the classifier. According to the extracted feature map, the model classifies the candidate samples of the microaneurysm to determine whether it is a real microaneurysm. Here, we use sigmod-activated single unit at the last level of the classifier (a dense layer with a size of 1), which calculates the probability that the input sample belongs to a microaneurysm. The binary cross-entropy loss is used, which is defined as:

$$loss = -\sum_{i=1}^{n}[y_i \lg \hat{y}_i] + [(1 - y_i)\lg(1 - \hat{y}_i)] \tag{7}$$

Where y_i represents the ground truth value, $\hat{y}_i$ is the predicted value of the trained model and n denotes the number of training samples in a batch.

During the testing process, we perform non-maximal suppression operations on candidate regions according to the probability values of each candidate region. Among the candidate regions with high coincidence rate, we only retain the candidate regions with the largest probability value and remove the other candidate regions.

4   Results

4.1   Data and Settings

In the experiment, a public database e-ophtha [5] is used, which is a color fundus image database designed for the scientific research on diabetic retinopathy (DR). The experiment uses the sub-dataset e-ophtha-MA, which contains 148 images with small aneurysms. The location information of microaneurysms in these images has been identified by ophthalmologists. Before the experiment, the image is scaled according to the original proportion, and the long edge of the scaled image is 1440. The first 74 images of the database are used to form the training set to generate training samples. The last 74 images are used to form the test set to verify the performance of the model.

In the process of training sample generation, we get the mask image of the candidate region, as shown in Fig. 3(d). The white area in the image is a candidate area of microaneurysm, but the area is irregular. Therefore, we take the centroid coordinates of the white area in Fig. 3(d) as the center to intercept the rectangular area with size $(w+L) \times (h+L)$ and then take the rectangular area as the sample of the microaneurysm, where L is a constant, w and h are the width and height of the smallest external rectangle in the white area respectively. In the experiment, the number of positive samples is less than that of negative samples, so we set the L values to $11, 12, \cdots, 17$ to intercept candidate regions with different sizes.

The experiment is carried out in Ubuntu 16.04 operating system. OpenCV is used for image preprocessing, and Keras is used for the realization of convolution neural network and the classifier.

4.2   Evaluation Metrics of Detection Performance

Two examples of the output of our microaneurysm detection model are shown in Fig. 5.

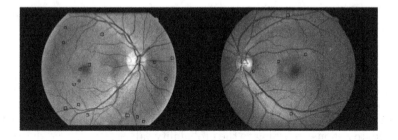

Fig. 5. Examples of microaneurysm detection results.

In the field of medical image, the FROC curve is the most widely used indicator for abnormal point detection, which is similar to the lesion detection in this paper. Therefore, FROC is also used in this paper as the main evaluation metric. In the FROC curve, the abscissa indicates the average number of false positive detections per image (FPI), and the ordinate shows the sensitivity of the model. The Sensitivity formula is as follows:

$$Sensitivity = \frac{TP}{TP + FN} \tag{8}$$

We also calculate the Competition Metric (CPM) as proposed in the Retinopathy Online Challenge [12], which is the average per lesion sensitivity at the average number of FPs per image $\in \{1/8, 1/4, 1/2, 1, 2, 4, 8\}$.

4.3   Comparison Methods

So far, Wu et al. [19] and Orlando et al. [13] have also used e-ophtha database to carry out related research on microaneurysm detection.

The method of Wu et al. consists of four main steps: preprocessing, candidate extraction, feature extraction and classification. A total of 27 feature features, including local features and contour features, are extracted for KNN classifier to distinguish real aneurysms from false lesions.

In Orlando et al.'s method, deep learning is combined with domain knowledge. The learning features of CNN are improved by adding hand-made features. The set vectors of these features are then used to identify real lesion areas using random forest classification. Therefore, our proposed method will be compared with the above two methods.

4.4   Evaluation Result

When selecting training samples, we use different L to intercept multi-scale candidate regions, so we choose different L for testing. The FROC curves of the proposed method at different L are shown and compared in Fig. 6. In the figure, it can be seen that the sensitivity of the test results is better when L takes the value of 13, 14 and 15. Table 1 shows the sensitivity of the proposed method at 7 predefined FPI when L takes 6 different values, and the CPM values are also listed. The CPM value indicates that the performance of the proposed is best when $L = 14$. So we choose $L = 14$ as the parameter setting for the proposed method and compare it with other methods.

Table 1. Sensitivities at predefined FPI for the proposed method at different L value.

L	FPI							
	0.125	0.25	0.5	1.0	2.0	4.0	8.0	CPM
12	0.181	0.192	0.313	0.410	0.518	0.653	0.737	0.429
13	0.184	0.264	0.333	0.480	0.556	0.688	0.795	0.471
14	0.176	0.251	0.342	0.454	0.585	0.725	0.809	0.477
15	0.094	0.171	0.280	0.420	0.551	0.712	0.817	0.435
16	0.085	0.165	0.253	0.398	0.525	0.670	0.799	0.413
17	–	0.093	0.228	0.355	0.495	0.615	0.750	–

Figure 7 shows a comparison of the FROC curves for our method ($L = 14$), Wu's method and Orlando's method. In addition, the sensitivity for the three

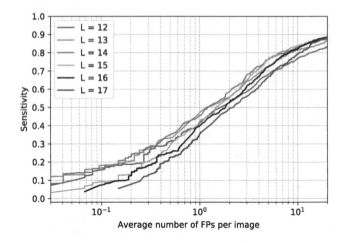

Fig. 6. FROC curves of the proposed method at different L value.

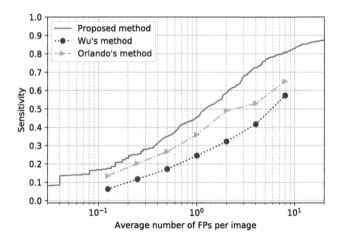

Fig. 7. FROC curves of three methods.

Table 2. Sensitivities at predefined FPI for three methods.

Method	FPI							
	0.125	0.25	0.5	1.0	2.0	4.0	8.0	CPM
Wu's method	0.063	0.12	0.17	0.25	0.32	0.42	0.57	0.273
Orlando's method	0.14	0.20	0.27	0.37	0.45	0.52	0.62	0.367
Proposed method ($L = 14$)	0.176	0.251	0.342	0.454	0.585	0.725	0.809	0.477

methods at 7 predefined FPI are calculated and shown in Table 2. Both the FROC curves in Fig. 7 and CPM in Table 2 show that the proposed method is more sensitive than Orlando's method and Wu's method. It indicates that when the same number of real microaneurysms are detected, the proposed method has fewer false detection than the other two methods.

5 Conclusion

In this paper, object detection algorithm based on deep learning is introduced into the field of medical images, and an microaneurysm detection model based on R-CNN is designed. The proposed method consists of several steps: image preprocessing, candidate region generation, feature extraction, classification and non-maximal suppression. The main contribution of this paper is to propose a preprocessing method for fundus image and a candidate region generation algorithm for microaneurysms. When generating candidate regions, multi-scale amplification is carried out to obtain high quality and large number of training samples in fewer data sets. The trained VGG16 network is then used to extract features of the microaneurysm candidate samples, and a classifier is used to obtain the most likely microaneurysm candidate regions. Finally, the non-maximal suppression operation is used to leave several candidate regions with the highest probability among the overlapping candidate regions. Experimental results on the e-ophtha database show that the average sensitivity of the proposed method is 0.477 for 7 lower average number of FPs per image, which is better than the other two methods.

In the future work, we will use different CNN networks for feature extraction, such as ResNet, Inception, Xception and so on. Furthermore, in order to detect multiple lesions in retinal fundus images, we will cooperate with hospitals to obtain more images containing different lesions.

Acknowledgment. This research was supported by the National Nature Science Foundation of China (No. 61603197 and No. 61772284).

References

1. Abràmoff, M.D., Niemeijer, M.: Mass screening of diabetic retinopathy using automated methods. In: Michelson, G. (ed.) Teleophthalmology in Preventive Medicine, pp. 41–50. Springer, Heidelberg (2015). https://doi.org/10.1007/978-3-662-44975-2_4
2. Antal, B., Hajdu, A.: An ensemble-based system for microaneurysm detection and diabetic retinopathy grading. IEEE Trans. Biomed. Eng. **59**(6), 1720 (2012)
3. Baudoin, C.E., Lay, B.J., Klein, J.C.: Automatic detection of microaneurysms in diabetic fluorescein angiography. Revue D Épidémiologie Et De Santé Publique **32**(3–4), 254–261 (1984)
4. Budak, U., Şengër, A., Guo, Y., Akbulut, Y.: A novel microaneurysms detection approach based on convolutional neural networks with reinforcement sample learning algorithm. Health Inf. Sci. Syst. **5**(1), 14 (2017)

5. Decencière, E., et al.: Teleophta: machine learning and image processing methods for teleophthalmology. IRBM **34**(2), 196–203 (2013). https://doi.org/10.1016/j.irbm.2013.01.010. http://www.sciencedirect.com/science/article/pii/S1959031813000237, special issue: ANR TECSAN: Technologies for Health and Autonomy

6. Frame, A.J., et al.: A comparison of computer based classification methods applied to the detection of microaneurysms in ophthalmic fluorescein angiograms. Comput. Biol. Med. **28**(3), 225 (1998)

7. Girshick, R., Donahue, J., Darrell, T., Malik, J.: Region-based convolutional networks for accurate object detection and segmentation. IEEE Trans. Pattern Anal. Mach. Intell. **38**(1), 142–158 (2015)

8. Gulshan, V., et al.: Development and validation of a deep learning algorithm for detection of diabetic retinopathy in retinal fundus photographs. Jama **316**(22), 2402 (2016)

9. Guo, Y., Budak, Ü.: A novel retinal vessel detection approach based on multiple deep convolution neural networks. Comput. Methods Programs Biomed. **167**, 43–48 (2018)

10. Guo, Y., Budak, Ü., Vespa, L.J., Khorasani, E., Şengür, A.: A retinal vessel detection approach using convolution neural network with reinforcement sample learning strategy. Measurement **125**, 586–591 (2018)

11. Lam, C., Yi, D., Guo, M., Lindsey, T.: Automated detection of diabetic retinopathy using deep learning (2018)

12. Niemeijer, M., Ginneken, B.V., Cree, M.J., Mizutani, A., et al.: Retinopathy online challenge: automatic detection of microaneurysms in digital color fundus photographs. IEEE Trans. Med. Imaging **29**(1), 185–195 (2010)

13. Orlando, J.I., Prokofyeva, E., Fresno, M.D., Blaschko, M.B.: Learning to detect red lesions in fundus photographs: an ensemble approach based on deep learning (2017)

14. Prokofyeva, E., Zrenner, E.: Epidemiology of major eye diseases leading to blindness in Europe: a literature review. Ophthalmic Res. **47**(4), 171–188 (2012)

15. Quellec, G., Lamard, M., Josselin, P.M., Cazuguel, G., Cochener, B., Roux, C.: Optimal wavelet transform for the detection of microaneurysms in retina photographs. IEEE Trans. Med. Imaging **27**(9), 1230–1241 (2008). https://doi.org/10.1109/TMI.2008.920619

16. Reza, A.M.: Realization of the contrast limited adaptive histogram equalization (CLAHE) for real-time image enhancement. J. VLSI Signal Process. Syst. Signal Image Video Technol. **38**, 35–44 (2004)

17. Ronneberger, O., Fischer, P., Brox, T.: U-Net: convolutional networks for biomedical image segmentation. In: Navab, N., Hornegger, J., Wells, W.M., Frangi, A.F. (eds.) MICCAI 2015. LNCS, vol. 9351, pp. 234–241. Springer, Cham (2015). https://doi.org/10.1007/978-3-319-24574-4_28

18. Simonyan, K., Zisserman, A.: Very deep convolutional networks for large-scale image recognition. arXiv e-prints arXiv:1409.1556, September 2014

19. Wu, B., Zhu, W., Shi, F., Zhu, S., Chen, X.: Automatic detection of microaneurysms in retinal fundus images. Comput. Med. Imaging Graph. Off. J. Comput. Med. Imaging Soc. **55**, 106 (2016)

VR Technology-Based Intelligent Cognitive Rehabilitation System for Alzheimer's Disease

Yucheng Hang[1], Wen Ge[1], Hao Jiang[1], HaoJun Li[1],
and Wenjun Tan[1,2,3(✉)] (iD)

[1] School of Computer Science and Engineering,
Northeastern University, Shenyang 110189, China
tanwenjun@cse.neu.edu.cn
[2] Key Laboratory of Intelligent Computing in Medical Image,
Ministry of Education, Northeastern University, Shenyang 110189, China
[3] Cyberspace Institute of Advanced Technology, Guangzhou University,
Guangzhou 510000, China

Abstract. Alzheimer's disease has become a worldwide problem. Cognitive training can effectively slow the progression of Alzheimer's disease and improve the quality of life of patients with Alzheimer's disease. Spatial orientation is an important aspect of cognitive training. Due to the immersive and interactive features of VR (Virtual Reality) technology, VR technology has been gradually applied to cognitive training systems. This paper designs and implements a VR technology-based intelligent cognitive rehabilitation system for Alzheimer's disease for assessing and training the spatial orientation of patients with Alzheimer's disease. First, pre-assess the physiological status and operational ability of patients with Alzheimer's disease. Then, build a realistic environment, guide through endogenous orientation and auditory orientation, and complete orientation training with different difficulty levels. Finally, the system provides relevant data for correlation analysis, combined with computer technology, to help doctors understand the patient's condition to complete further treatment.

Keywords: Spatial orientation · Alzheimer's disease · Virtual reality

1 Introduction

With the increasing number of Alzheimer's patients in low- and middle-income countries, it is predicted that the total number of Alzheimer's patients will reach 75.6 million in 2030 and reach 135.5 million in 2050. Alzheimer's disease is characterized by cognitive decline, accompanied by mental symptoms and behavioral problems, mainly characterized by memory impairment, aphasia, misuse, loss of recognition, visual spatial skills impairment, executive dysfunction, and personality and behavioral changes [1, 2]. In the past few decades, a variety of programs have been proposed for the treatment of Alzheimer's disease, but there has been no substantial breakthrough in drug treatment, and more research has turned to non-pharmaceutical fields with obvious effects [3]. Among the various methods of non-drug intervention in Alzheimer's

© Springer Nature Switzerland AG 2019
H. Wang et al. (Eds.): HIS 2019, LNCS 11837, pp. 213–223, 2019.
https://doi.org/10.1007/978-3-030-32962-4_20

disease, cognitive function training has been shown to be effective in improving cognitive function in patients with Alzheimer's disease [4]. Cognitive function training focuses on the cognitive function of a specific aspect through standardized task setting, which can not only slow the progression of Alzheimer's disease, improve the quality of life of patients with Alzheimer's disease, but also reduce the burden of medical resources and promote the healthy aging of the whole society process. Cognitive function training mainly includes music therapy [5], nostalgic therapy [6], narrative therapy [7], etc., under the guidance of professional guidance, to help patients with brain function remodeling, improve or maintain specific aspects of cognitive function.

The traditional cognitive function training of Alzheimer's disease is mainly led by professional therapists. With the application of computer technology in the medical field, computer-based cognitive function training has a significant effect in healthy elderly, mild cognitive impairment and dementia patients. Studies have shown that cognitive function training based on computer information communication technology can not only reduce the decline of cognitive function in normal elderly population, but also delay the disease progression in patients with Alzheimer's disease [8, 9]. The continuous development of computer technology and equipment has promoted the generation of VR (Virtual Reality) technology. Due to the characteristics of VR immersion and interactivity, VR technology is applied as a new computer-based human-computer interaction form to phobia, depression, nervousness and anxiety. In the clinical medical field [10–14], medical education [15] and clinical skills training [16], the advantages of VR are verified, so researchers will train VR technology and traditional cognitive function. The method was combined to test the patients with Alzheimer's disease, in order to promote VR as a new effective cognitive training tool to the Alzheimer's disease group. However, most of the VR technologies currently used to treat Alzheimer's disease are indoor scenes and cannot interact, which has a negative impact on the treatment effect.

The essence of VR technology applied to cognitive training in Alzheimer's disease is to establish a virtual scene that is similar to reality or does not exist in reality, and incorporates traditional cognitive training tasks, so that people with Alzheimer's disease can immerse and act on the scene to achieve the purpose of cognitive training. Cognitive training focuses on memory, attention, spatial orientation, language skills, ability to judge and solve problems. The training effect was evaluated mainly by the scores of patients' cognitive function, the scores of dementia-related tests, the satisfaction of patients' self-assessment, the changes of mental and psychological conditions, the self-care ability of daily life and the improvement of quality of life.

This paper mainly implements the intelligent cognitive rehabilitation system of Alzheimer's disease based on VR technology. The main task is to simulate outdoor scenes and allow patients to interact in the system to guide patients with Alzheimer's disease to find the path to the target location and to gradually develop the spatial orientation of Alzheimer's disease patients in the process.

2 System Analysis and Design

Because the severity of each Alzheimer's disease is different, it is necessary to set different training methods to meet the needs of different patients, and considering the spatial orientation of Alzheimer's patients is generally poor, so multiple ways should be adopted for guidance. According to this requirement, the system has the following functions:

(1) It has a realistic town scene in the 1990s.

Because the age of Alzheimer's patients is concentrated in the age of 50 and above, the acceptance of new things such as VR is not high. In order to avoid the patient's conflict and aversion, the system built a realistic town scene in the 1990s based on the patient's adaptability, and selected the store and the hospital as the final destination to enhance the practicality and intimacy, so that patients can have a strong sense of reality and immersion in the scene.

(2) Evaluate and train patients' spatial orientation ability.

Spatial orientation is one of the most common and widely used spatial cognitive processes in human life. And the spatial orientation process is a collection of a variety of cognitive processes, involving motion perception, environmental cognition and spatial information acquisition and other related processes, with complexity [17]. The system has three different difficulty paths based on the degree of illness, which can be applied to different Alzheimer's patients. At the same time, guidance is provided through endogenous orientation and auditory orientation, allowing the patient to focus on completing the training to reach the destination. The system provides first-person and third-person perspectives. The first-person perspective is mainly used to move the scene space. The third-person perspective is mainly used for system control and related data collection.

(3) Convenient for the doctor to proceed to the next treatment based on the patient's movement rate and spatial memory.

According to the data obtained by the training, such as the relationship between the correct number of movements and the number of training, whether the destination can be reached again after the instruction is removed, etc., the needs of two evaluations and four treatments as shown in Fig. 1 can be met.

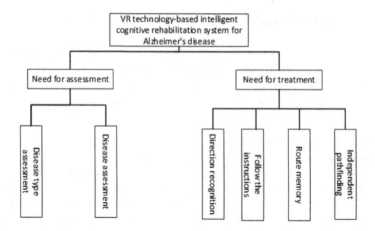

Fig. 1. The system functional requirement

3 Method

3.1 Overview of VR Building

The actual size of the town scene is about 900 square meters. The weather conditions are set to be sunny to facilitate patient adaptation and judgment. It contains more than 80 buildings and 2 destination buildings of different difficulty levels, namely the shop and the hospital. As shown in Fig. 2, there are 6 direction selection points in the scene, namely, A, B, C, D, E, F, and 6 wrong directions, namely, A, B, C, D, E, F, and at least 2 turning points. Choose the route with one of the three difficulties, and the direction selection point and the wrong direction will be reduced or increased appropriately, where A is the starting point, C is the destination store, and F is the destination hospital.

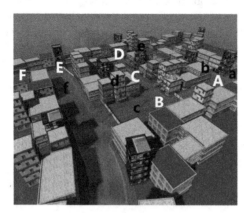

Fig. 2. Scene overview

3.2   Endogenous Orientation and Auditory Orientation

In this system, the central arrow is used to indicate the endogenous orientation in the visual orientation, supplemented by the speech indication as the auditory orientation, to guide the patients with Alzheimer's disease to complete the training.

Attention can be transferred to different spatial positions through two orientations: (1) a top-down approach, also known as "random" or "endogenous" orientations, which are mainly determined by our goals, intentions or task needs; (2) a bottom-up approach, also known as "involuntary" or exogenous orientation, is mainly based on the significance of the stimulus or the potential correlation between the stimuli.

Endogenous orientation usually uses a central symbol clue with a high probability of predicting the target's spatial position, among which the central arrow is the most commonly used. Moreover, studies have found that even though arrow clues have no predictive effect on target position, they can still attract directional attention [18–20]. This shows that, to some extent, the arrow cue can automatically direct attention to the location indicated by the arrow, which is why we chose it as the primary indicator, as shown in Fig. 3.

Give the patient auditory orientation, such as: when the patient selects the right direction at each direction selection point, it will prompt "correct direction"; when the direction is wrong, it will prompt "wrong direction, please re-select" and other instructions.

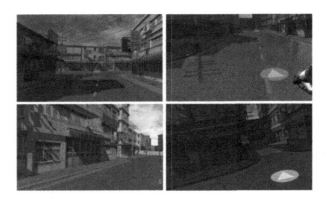

Fig. 3. Directional indication.

3.3   Treatment Protocol

1. *Preliminary work*
(1) Pre-assessment of disease severity, physiological status, and equipment handling capabilities.
    Understand the history of Alzheimer's patients and test their physical features and visual exploration (including linear orientation tests), and perform simple but necessary assessment questionnaires (e.g., Do you use a computer in your life? Have you ever been exposed to virtual reality?

(2) Multiple path selection based on pre-assessment.
According to the pre-assessment results, the optimal difficulty route is determined among the three difficulty levels: simple, moderate and difficult, and the selection operation of the learning handle of the Alzheimer's disease patient is guided (in order to simplify the operation, only the trigger is selected as the selection of the advance button), and the patient is guided to familiarize the route [21–25].

2. *Spatial orientation assessment and training*

(1) Simple route: As shown in Fig. 4, patients start from the starting point A (home) and choose between one correct direction and two wrong directions. If they choose correctly, they will reach the middle point B and then choose between one correct direction and one wrong direction. If they choose correctly, they will reach the target point C (shop).

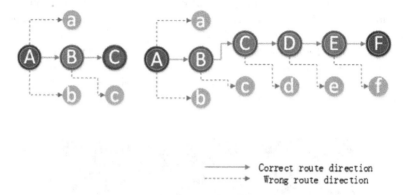

```
──────────▶  Correct route direction
·········▶  Wrong route direction
```

Fig. 4. Simple and moderate route diagram

(2) Moderate route: As shown in Fig. 4, after completing the simple route and reaching the point C (shop), the patient selects in one correct direction and one wrong direction, three times in total, and if the selection is correct, the destination point F (hospital) is reached.

(3) Difficult route: As shown in Fig. 5, after completing the moderate route and reaching the point F (hospital), the patient selects in one correct direction and one wrong direction, four times in total, and if the selection is correct, the destination point A (home) is reached.

3. *Training process*

The flow of each training is shown in Fig. 6.

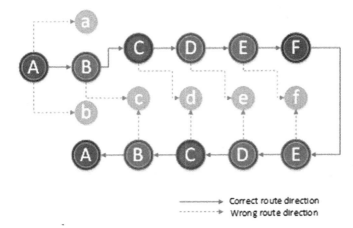

Fig. 5. Difficult route diagram

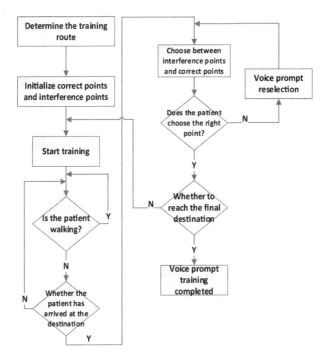

Fig. 6. Training flow chart

4   Experimental Environment

The hardware and software environment of VR technology-based intelligent cognitive rehabilitation system for Alzheimer's disease is as follows:

(1) Hardware environment:
     Processor: Intel(R) Core(TM) i5-4210 M CPU @ 2.60 GHz; Memory: 4 GB; VR device: HTC VIVE
(2) Software Environment:
     Operating system: Windows10 64-bit; Development platform: Unity 3D; Development language: C#; Programming environment and compiler: Visual Studio 2010.

5   Results

5.1   Function Result

The system implements both evaluation and treatment functions. The Montreal Cognitive Assessment (MoCA) is a widely used screening assessment for detecting cognitive impairment. It was created in 1996 by Ziad Nasreddine in Montreal, Quebec. It was validated in the setting of mild cognitive impairment, and has subsequently been adopted in numerous other settings clinically [25–28]. In the assessment phase, we combine MoCA assessment, physiological status assessment and operational capability assessment to conduct a comprehensive and comprehensive assessment of patients and use this as a basis for developing specific treatment plans. During the treatment phase, we conduct spatial orientation training as planned, and at the same time, we conduct an assessment at regular intervals to adjust the treatment plan in time.

5.2   Performance

After conducting experiments on a number of normal people, we estimate that the therapeutic effects as shown in Tables 1 and 2 can be achieved. The patient had more errors in the assessment before treatment and the MoCA score was around 24. After the training, the error will be significantly reduced and the MoCA score will increase, while the treatment effect will remain for more than three weeks, and the regression will occur after the fourth week.

Table 1. Average number of errors in patient's selections in different periods

Point of election	Pre-training (2.5 weeks prior to treatment)	Independent training (Final day)	3 weeks after training	4 weeks after training
A	3	0	0	1
B	1	0	0	0
C	0	0	0	0
D	2	0	0	1
E	1	0	0	0

Table 2. MoCA scores of the patient at different periods

Week	MOCA variant	Overall MOCA score	Visuospatial/executive (/5)	Delayed recall (/5)			All other (/20)
				No cue	Category cue	Multiple choice cue	
2.5-week	7.1 original	24	3	1	1	3	19
Final day	7.1 original	26	5	2	2	1	19
3-week	7.2 variant	25	5	0	3	2	20
5-week	7.1 original	24	3	0	2	2	19

5.3 Stability

The system has strong stability. We tested a number of normal people and found that participants showed some improvement in spatial orientation after training. The specific performance is shortened by the time to complete the route, as shown in Table 3.

Table 3. Time taken by different participants to complete different routes

	Number of selection points	Participant A	Participant B	Participant C	Average time (seconds)
Simple	2	36	38	36	36.66
Moderate	5	84	87	85	85.33
Difficult	10	169	175	173	172.33

6 Conclusion

This paper designs and implements a VR technology-based intelligent cognitive rehabilitation system for Alzheimer's disease for assessing and training the spatial orientation of patients with Alzheimer's disease. First, pre-assess the physiological status and operational ability of patients with Alzheimer's disease. Then, build a realistic environment, guide through endogenous orientation and auditory orientation, and complete orientation training with different difficulty levels. Finally, the system provides relevant data for correlation analysis, combined with computer technology, to help doctors understand the patient's condition to complete further treatment.

Acknowledgments. The authors would like to thank the editor and reviewers for their valuable advices that have helped to improve the paper quality. This work is supported by the Fundamental Research Funds for the Central Universities (N181602014), National Key Research and Development Program of China (2018YFC1314501).

References

1. Janca, A., Hiller, W.: ICD-10 checklists—a tool for clinicians' use of the ICD-10 classification of mental and behavioral disorders. Compr. Psychiatry **37**(3), 180–187 (1996)
2. Small, G.W., Rabins, P.V., Barry, P.P., et al.: Diagnosis and treatment of Alzheimer disease and related disorders. Consensus statement of the American Association for Geriatric Psychiatry, the Alzheimer's Association, and the American Geriatrics Society. JAMA, J. Am. Med. Assoc. **278**(16), 1363–1371 (1997)
3. McLaren, A.N., Lamantia, M.A., Callahan, C.M.: Systematic review of non-pharmacologic interventions to delay functional decline in community-dwelling patients with dementia. Aging Ment. Health **17**(6), 655–666 (2013)
4. Jennifer, R., Caroline, V.H., Martin, B.: Cognitive interventions in healthy older adults and people with mild cognitive impairment: a systematic review. Ageing Res. Rev. **12**(1), 263–275 (2013)
5. Gomez, G.: Effects of a personalized music intervention among older adults with dementia. J. Am. Med. Dir. Assoc. **17**(3), B25–B26 (2016)
6. Van Bogaert, P., Van Grinsven, R., Tolson, D., et al.: Effects of SolCos model-based individual reminiscence on older adults with mild to moderate dementia due to Alzheimer disease: a pilot study. J. Am. Med. Dir. Assoc. **14**(7), 528.e9–528.e13 (2013)
7. McKeown, J., Ryan, T., Ingleton, C, et al.: You have to be mindful of whose story it is': the challenges of undertaking life story work with people with dementia and their family carers. Dement. (Lond. Engl.) **14**, 238–256 (2013)
8. Robert, P.: Recommendations for the use of serious games in people with Alzheimer's disease, related disorders and frailty. Front. Aging Neurosci. **6**, 54 (2014)
9. Manera, V., Petit, P.-D., Derreumaux, A., et al.: Kitchen and cooking', a serious game for mild cognitive impairment and Alzheimer's disease: a pilot study. Front. Aging Neurosci. **7**, 24 (2015)
10. Maskey, M., Lowry, J., Rodgers, J., et al.: Reducing specific phobia/fear in young people with autism spectrum disorders (ASDs) through a virtual reality environment intervention. PLoS ONE **9**(7), e100374 (2014)
11. Hartanto, D., Kampmann, I.L., Morina, N., et al.: Controlling social stress in virtual reality environments. PLoS ONE **9**(3), e92804 (2017)
12. Repetto, C., Gaggioli, A., Pallavicini, F., et al.: Virtual reality and mobile phones in the treatment of generalized anxiety disorders: a phase-2 clinical trial. Pers. Ubiquitous Comput. **17**(2), 253–260 (2013)
13. Standen, P.J., Threapleton, K., Connell, L., et al.: Patients' use of a home-based virtual reality system to provide rehabilitation of the upper limb following stroke. Phys. Ther. **95**(3), 350–359 (2015)

14. Hua, Y., Qiu, R., Yao, W., et al.: The effect of virtual reality distraction on pain relief during dressing changes in children with chronic wounds on lower limbs. Pain Manag. Nurs. **16**(5), 685–691 (2015)
15. Trelease, R.B., Nieder, G.L.: Transforming clinical imaging and 3D data for virtual reality learning objects: HTML5 and mobile devices implementation. Anat. Sci. Educ. **6**(4), 263–270 (2013)
16. Palter, V.N., Grantcharov, T.P.: Individualized deliberate practice on a virtual reality simulator improves technical performance of surgical novices in the operating room: a randomized controlled trial. Ann. Surg. **259**(3), 443–448 (2014)
17. Coluccia, E., Louse, G.: Gender differences in spatial orientation: a review. J. Environ. Psychol. **24**(3), 329–340 (2004)
18. Marotta, A., Lupiáñez, J., Casagrande, M.: Investigating hemispheric lateralization of reflexive attention to gaze and arrow cues. Brain Cogn. **80**(3), 361–366 (2012)
19. Tan, W., Yuan, Y., Chen, A., Mao, L., Ke, Y., Lv, X.: An approach for pulmonary vascular extraction from chest CT images. J. Healthc. Eng. (2019). https://doi.org/10.1155/2019/9712970
20. Tan, W., et al.: an approach to extraction midsagittal plane of skull from brain CT images for oral and maxillofacial surgery. IEEE Access **7**, 118203–118217 (2019)
21. Huang, J., Peng, M., Wang, H., Cao, J., Gao, W., Zhang, X.: A probabilistic method for emerging topic tracking in microblog stream. World Wide Web **20**(2), 325–350 (2017)
22. Zhang, J., Tao, X., Wang, H.: Outlier detection from large distributed databases. World Wide Web **17**(4), 539–568 (2014)
23. Li, H., Wang, Y., Wang, H., Zhou, B.: Multi-window based ensemble learning for classification of imbalanced streaming data. World Wide Web **20**(6), 1507–1525 (2017)
24. Khalil, F., Wang, H., Li, J.: Integrating markov model with clustering for predicting web page accesses. In: Proceeding of the 13th Australasian World Wide Web Conference (AusWeb07), pp. 63–74 (2007)
25. Khalil, F., Li, J., Wang, H.: An integrated model for next page access prediction. Int. J. Knowl. Web Intell. **1**(1), 48–80 (2009)
26. Ma, J., Sun, L., Wang, H., Zhang, Y., Aickelin, U.: Supervised anomaly detection in uncertain pseudoperiodic data streams. ACM Trans. Internet Technol. (TOIT) **16**(1), 4 (2016)
27. Hu, H., Li, J., Wang, H., Daggard, G.: Combined gene selection methods for microarray data analysis. In: Gabrys, B., Howlett, Robert J., Jain, Lakhmi C. (eds.) KES 2006. LNCS (LNAI), vol. 4251, pp. 976–983. Springer, Heidelberg (2006). https://doi.org/10.1007/11892960_117
28. Peng, M., Zeng, G., Sun, Z., Huang, J., Wang, H., Tian, G.: Personalized app recommendation based on app permissions. World Wide Web **21**(1), 89–104 (2018)

Mental Health

Research on the Construction of Autism Knowledge Map Information System in Internet Environment

Wang Zhao[1,2(✉)]

[1] Wuhan University School of Information Management, Wuhan, China
199223263@qq.com
[2] Suzhou Zealikon Healthcare Co., Ltd., Suzhou, China

Abstract. With the development of social economy and the aggravation of environmental pressure, autism has been gradually recognized and its incidence has become higher and higher. At present, the research on autism at home and abroad is still in its infancy, and the research methods and tools are relatively few, especially the research on the acquisition and display of autism-related knowledge is relatively scarce. Doctors and various rehabilitation institutions as well as the vast number of autistic patients have an urgent need to acquire knowledge about treatment and rehabilitation of autism. In the information age, the Internet provides people with convenient access to information and knowledge. The purpose of this study is to use Internet technology to collect information and knowledge about autism. The autism database is designed and the autism information system based on knowledge map is constructed. Autism information system can provide doctors and patients with efficient access to autism information and knowledge, help them to acquire the required knowledge at any time and anywhere, and promote the early diagnosis and treatment of autism.

Keywords: Autism · Knowledge map · Information system

1 Introduction

Autism, also known as autism or autism disorders, is a representative disease of generalized developmental disorders. In recent years, the incidence of autistic children has become higher and higher, experiencing a transition from rare diseases to epidemics, and the number of autistic children has exceeded our imagination. But there are few autism related knowledge websites or information system. It is difficult for people to acquire autism related knowledge. Rehabilitation treatment of autism is generally effective before the age of 6. How to make the knowledge of autism popularized and easily acquired by the public is the focus of current research. Knowledge maps show the relationship between knowledge in a visual form, which makes knowledge easier to understand. With the efficient communication channel of the Internet, the rapid dissemination of autism information and knowledge is possible.

The purpose of this paper is to study the information and knowledge of autism, build the knowledge map of autism, and establish a visual autism query system.

© Springer Nature Switzerland AG 2019
H. Wang et al. (Eds.): HIS 2019, LNCS 11837, pp. 227–237, 2019.
https://doi.org/10.1007/978-3-030-32962-4_21

In order to systematize and standardize the knowledge of autism, promote the diagnosis and treatment of autism, and improve the public's awareness of autism, so as to provide an opportunity for patients with autism to seek medical treatment and treatment as soon as possible.

2   Autism and Its History

Autism (autism disorder) is a neurodevelopmental disorder, also known as autism. The diseases are collectively referred to as autism spectrum disorder (ASD) [1]. Since Kanner, an American child psychiatrist, first reported autism in 1943, the incidence of autism has risen rapidly worldwide. In the 1980s, about 3–5 out of every 10,000 people suffered from the disease, while in 2000, 6.7 out of every 1,000 children suffered from the disease [2]. According to the National Center for Health Statistics, the probability of autism among children aged 3–14 in the United States reached 2.76% in 2016 [3]. The incidence of autism has been increasing steadily for more than 40 years.

There is no statistical survey on autistic children in China. However, according to the data of "Report on the Development of Autism Education and Rehabilitation Industry in China II", the number of autism population in China is estimated to exceed 10 million people, of which 2 million are autistic children. At the same time, it is growing at the rate of nearly 200,000 per year [4].

Autism brings serious financial burden to both society and family. Families with autistic children, on the one hand, spend a lot of time caring for children, working hours are reduced, so that work income is reduced. On the other hand, the cost of family rehabilitation treatment for autistic children is huge, which increases the family's financial burden [5]. According to the survey of family financial burden of pre-school autistic children, 33% of parents of autistic children reported that the care of autistic children seriously affected their career, their annual income was significantly lower than that of ordinary families, with an average annual income loss of 30,957 yuan. Meanwhile, the average annual cost of autistic children's families for children's education and training is significantly higher than that of ordinary families [6]. Society and government also need to invest a lot of money in rehabilitation education for autistic children. At the same time, autism also brings depression to the patients' families, which has a negative impact on their quality of life [7, 8].

It can be seen that the incidence of autism in children is relatively serious, and the harm to society and family is enormous. However, there is no systematic and standardized knowledge system for medical research on autism. Doctors often rely on personal experience to diagnose and treat autism, so it is worthwhile to build a knowledge map of autism. This can provide comprehensive information and knowledge services to autistic children. It plays an important role in alleviating the economic and mental pressure of families with autistic children.

3 Current Situation of Knowledge Map of Autism

3.1 Knowledge Map and Its Application

Knowledge map is an important part of AI. Knowledge maps originate from semantic networks [9]. On May 16, 2012, Google introduced the concept of knowledge map, which aims to improve the accuracy of search engines and make search engines more intelligent [10]. Knowledge map is essentially a semantic network that reveals the relationship between entities and can formally describe the relationship between things in the real world.

In recent years, knowledge map has been applied to search engines, intelligent question answering systems, e-commerce and many other fields. The application of knowledge map makes these software more intelligent. Knowledge map also plays an important role in the process of medical intellectualization. Using knowledge map technology, medical knowledge can be integrated and expressed more accurately and normatively.

3.2 Current Status of Knowledge Map of Autism

Overseas research on knowledge map of autism is relatively early. Before the concept of knowledge map was put forward, many scholars studied the ontology of autism.

The research on the construction and reasoning of children's autism knowledge map is relatively few in China, and most of them are based on literature research hotspots and visual analysis of research status. There are few studies on the construction of autism knowledge map.

Therefore, building an autism information system based on knowledge map has important scientific research and application value.

3.3 The Architecture of Knowledge Map

The main problems studied in this paper are the construction and reasoning of the knowledge map of autism. The key issues involved are knowledge extraction, knowledge fusion and knowledge reasoning of the knowledge map of autism. As shown in Fig. 1, knowledge extraction usually includes named entity recognition, entity relationship extraction and attribute extraction. Knowledge fusion usually includes entity links, entity alignment and so on. In addition, it also involves the storage and application of knowledge maps. Knowledge maps are usually stored in graph-based databases, RDF-based databases and relational databases.

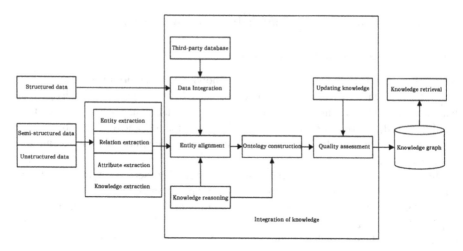

Fig. 1. The architecture of knowledge map

4   Construction of Information System for Autism

Autism information system includes Autism Knowledge Base, Autism Knowledge Map, Data Import, Association Query, User Interface, etc.

4.1   Construction Principles

The construction of information system for autism has several characteristics, such as accuracy, advanced, popular and practical.

- Accuracy: Autism knowledge base is required to be accurate and reliable, in line with hospital and national standards. Current diagnostic criteria for autism include the World Health Organization's International Statistical Classification of Diseased and Related Health Problems (ICD-10) and the American Psychiatric Association's Revised Manual on Diagnosis and Statistics of Mental Abnormalities (DSM-IV-TR, APA, 2000).
- Advanced: The system can collect timely data for the knowledge base, including the latest autism diagnosis, treatment and rehabilitation knowledge. Information system can use the latest technology to meet the knowledge needs of all kinds of users.
- Popularization: The goal of system design is to meet the needs of autism patients to acquire knowledge of autism in any area and at any time through network channels, relying on the Internet and mobile Internet.
- Practicality: The design requirement of information system is to achieve practical purposes, provide comprehensive and necessary autism knowledge, reduce the workload of doctor diagnosis, and reduce the cost of autism diagnosis and treatment.

4.2 Design Idea

Autism information system includes data processing and knowledge visualization display, which includes two main parts: one is the collection of basic data, the other is the analysis and visualization of collected data, including user interface interaction design. The design idea is as follows: The system has the function of automatic data acquisition and processing, and can store and visualize the knowledge data collected before. The principles of user interface design are as follows.

- Beautiful Interface: The interface design meets the requirements of conciseness, professionalism and user-friendliness. Each component of the program interface has independent functions, clear classification and comprehensive information display.
- Visual Knowledge Display: The program can realize the display of knowledge association. For example, after searching for "diagnoses", the information display area can display the knowledge map and specific diagnostic methods of autism diagnosis.
- Structured Presentation of Knowledge: By using knowledge map, the structure and relevance of knowledge can be displayed, and the content of knowledge can be displayed comprehensively and abundantly.

4.3 Overall Structure of the Information System

The information system adopts Browser/Server structure, the server part of the system includes knowledge database, and the client part of the system includes program interface. The overall structure of the system is shown in Fig. 2.

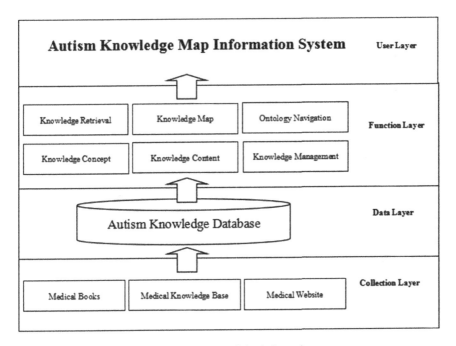

Fig. 2. Overall structure of the information system

The system includes four layers: Collection layer, data layer, function layer and user layer. Each layer depends on each other and gradually forms the whole information system. Collection layer is mainly responsible for collecting various information and knowledge of autism, including medical books, medical knowledge base, medical websites. Data layer is the data center of the information system, which stores information and knowledge about autism. Function layer includes knowledge retrieval, knowledge map, ontology navigation, knowledge concept display, knowledge content editing, knowledge management and other business functions. User layer is the user interface, including the client page and the server page.

4.4   Running Environment Based on B/S/D Three-Tier Architecture

Browser/Server/Database is the most suitable application model for solving public information services and interacting corresponding dynamic services. It realizes the real thin client, and greatly simplifies the distribution, configuration management and version management of the application system. The system adopts a similar structure. The network topology diagram is shown in Fig. 3.

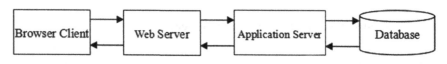

Fig. 3. Network topology diagram

WEB clients are WEB browsers, such as Netscape Navigator or Microsoft Internet Explorer. WEB servers are any HTML-based servers, such as Netscape Enterprise Server or Sybase Application Server. Application server is an extension of WEB server function, responsible for authority, component, transaction, database connection and other management. Users can send requests through WEB browser and communicate with WEB server through HTTP protocol. If it is a data request, the WEB server or application server communicates with the database server and constructs the returned data into a browser page and returns it to the user.

The three-tier architecture is particularly suitable for this information system:

- In the front desk, customers do not need to install a particularly complex and huge application system, just need to use the network browser integrated with the operating system, which makes the front desk system very convenient to promote, suitable for the situation of a very large customer base. The front desk is only responsible for the display of data, and the visualization part is mainly on this layer of display.

- Data processing is entirely in the middle of the application service layer. Customers issue commands through browsers (such as queries, orders, etc.). The application service layer obtains commands, processes them accordingly, and returns user results in the form of HTTP. This is also suitable for decentralized users, centralized processing features.
- Autism-related data is generally stored in a powerful data server, and all users can access the data server through the application server. This can be stored in a data set for easy maintenance and management. This is also the development direction of current data management forms.

From the above description, we can see that this information system has multi-user but needs centralized processing, data needs centralized storage requirements, three-tier structure will be a good software model.

4.5   Design of Knowledge Map of Autism

Autism knowledge map is the key of this study. The key steps of autism knowledge map design include knowledge extraction, knowledge fusion and knowledge reasoning.

Knowledge map are usually stored in graph-based databases, RDF-based databases and relational databases. In this study, relational database is used to complete the storage of knowledge map.

4.5.1   Data Sources

Data is needed to construct the knowledge map of autism. The data sources of the knowledge map of autism include open source medical knowledge map, network resources, scientific research literature and so on. Most of the data such as network resources and scientific research literature are unstructured data, so the construction of knowledge map is mainly based on unstructured data.

4.5.2   Ontology Construction

The ontology construction of knowledge map is the definition of knowledge map structure. The definition of autism knowledge map ontology includes the definition of class and the definition of relationship. Combining various data types and referencing medical knowledge map, this paper defines the following six basic categories: "disease", "symptoms", "drugs", "training and treatment", "examination methods", "pathogenic factors or behavior".

According to the six types of entities, five kinds of semantic relations are created in this paper, which are:

- Symptoms: disease-symptoms, indicating the corresponding relationship between disease and symptoms, namely disease and its corresponding clinical symptoms.
- Pathogenesis: Pathogenic factors or behaviors - diseases, drugs - diseases, used to link pathogenic factors or behaviors with diseases, drugs and diseases, indicating that such pathogenic factors or behaviors and drugs can lead to the disease.
- Examination: Examination mode - disease, used to connect examination mode and disease, indicating that this examination mode can be used to examine and diagnose the disease.

- Treatment: Treatment - disease, treatment - symptoms, used to link treatment and disease, treatment and symptoms, indicating that the treatment is directed at the disease or the treatment is directed at the symptoms.
- Co-occurrence disease: disease-disease, used to connect disease and disease, means that these two diseases can occur in the same patient, that is, the same patient can suffer from both diseases at the same time.

4.5.3   Storage of Knowledge Map

Knowledge map essentially represents entities, their attributes and the relationship between entities and entities in the form of graphs. At present, graph data structure and RDF (Resource Description Framework) structure in Semantic Web framework are widely used to store data in knowledge map.

This paper uses RDF structure database to store data. RDF is a standard data model developed by the World Wide Web Consortium (W3C) to describe real resources on the semantic web, which can be read and understood by computers. In RDF, each resource has its unique URI (Uniform Resource Identifiers). RDF is a set of finite triples (s, p, o). Each triple represents a fact statement sentence, in which s is the subject, P is the predicate and O is the object. Its meaning is that s has the attribute P and its value is o or that there is a relationship p between S and o. For example (autism, symptoms, communication disorder), it means that the symptoms of autism have communication disorder.

4.6   Core Code

The following are the core code to show the relationship between data nodes and the core code to import data.

4.6.1   Core Code of Data Display Function

The following code uses echart to visualize the relationship between data nodes.

```
var myChart = echarts.init(document.getElementById
    ("top_echart"));
var option = {title : { text: 'Autism Information Service
    Platform', x:'right',y:'bottom'},calculable: true,
    tooltip : { trigger: 'item',formatter: '{b}'},
    series : {type:'force',itemStyle: {normal: label: { show:
    true, textStyle: { color: '#333'}}},
    nodeStyle : { brushType : 'both',borderWidth : 0},
myChart.on('mouseup',function(params){var option;}
```

4.6.2   Core Code of Data Import

In order to facilitate the formation of data, the information service platform provides data import function and supports the import of multiple versions of Excel files. The implementation method is as follows.

```
public List<Map<String,String>> importExcelForShow(String
    fileName,   MultipartFile   file)   throws   Exception
    {List<Map<String,String>> listMap=new ArrayList<>();
    boolean isExcel2003 = true;
    if(sheet==null){return listMap;}
  for (int r = 1; r <= sheet.getLastRowNum(); r++)
  { Row row = sheet.getRow(r);
    if (row == null){continue;} String a="";
    if(row.getCell !=null){a= row.getStringCellValue();}
    return listMap;}
```

The program first determines the format of the file, distinguishes the excel version, and imports different versions in different ways. After the file format is correct, the program transforms the file into a stream, starts to read the data line by line, stores each row of data in the Map collection, and stores it in the database.

4.7   System Interface

4.7.1   Main Interface

The main interface of the autism information system is shown in Fig. 4. The following is the description of each display area.

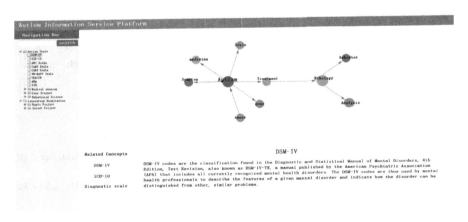

Fig. 4. Main interface

4.7.2   Search and Tree Display

Users can enter keywords in the search bar, search, and display relevant content in the tree structure. See Fig. 5.

4.7.3   Knowledge Map of Autism

Autism knowledge map supports multi-level knowledge display. Nodes at all levels can be dragged, enlarged and narrowed. Clicking on the node can show details of relevant knowledge. See Fig. 6.

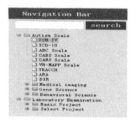
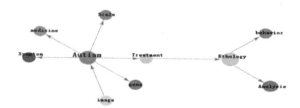

Fig. 5. Search interface   **Fig. 6.** Knowledge map

5   Conclusion

The incidence of autism has become more and more high, which has attracted more and more attention from all aspects of society. Using knowledge map and other tools to build an information system for autism, to meet the public's understanding of autism and the information needs of the treatment and rehabilitation of autistic patients, has become a research hotspot. This paper initially constructs an autism information system based on knowledge map, and achieves the sharing and utilization of autism knowledge. Next, we will study the diagnosis and rehabilitation of autism, expand the business functions of the system, promote the sharing of autism knowledge, and improve public awareness and understanding of autism.

Acknowledgements. This research has been possible thanks to the support of projects: National Natural Science Foundation of China (No. 61772375) and Independent Research Project of School of Information Management Wuhan University (No: 413100032).

References

1. Duan, Y., Wu, X., Jinfeng: Advances in etiology and treatment of autism. Chin. Sci. Life Sci. **09**, 820–844 (2015)
2. Vismara, L.A., Rogers, S.J.: The Early Start Denver Model. J. Early Interv. **31**(1), 91–108 (2008)
3. Zablotsky, B., Black, L.I., Blumberg, S.J.: Estimated prevalence of children with diagnosed developmental disabilities in the United States 2014–2016. NCHS Data Brief **291**, 1–8 (2017)

4. Academy of Autism of Five Coloured Deer: Report on the Development of Autism Education and Rehabilitation Industry in China 2. Huaxia Publishing House (2017)
5. Wu, X., Chen, S., Jinfeng: Research progress on quality of life and its influencing factors of primary caregivers of autistic children. Gen. Nurs. **16**(18), 2206–2208 (2018)
6. Yang, Y., Wang, M.: Employment and financial burdens of families with preschool-aged children with autism. Chin. J. Clin. Psychol. **22**(2), 295–297, 361 (2014)
7. Singh, P., Ghosh, S., Nandi, S.: Subjective burden and depression in mothers of children with autism spectrum disorder in india: moderating effect of social support. J. Autism Dev. Disord. **47**(10), 3097–3111 (2017)
8. Wang, Y., Xiao, L., Chen, R., et al.: Social impairment of children with autism spectrum disorder affects parental quality of life in different ways. Psychiatry Res. **266**, 168–174 (2018)
9. Sireteanu, A.N.: A survey of web ontology languages and semantic web services. Ann. Alexandru Ioan Cuza Univ. Econ. **60**(1), 42–53 (2013)
10. Amit S.: Introducing the Knowledge Graph: things, not strings (2012)

Evidence-Based Analysis
of Neurotransmitter Modulation
by Gut Microbiota

Ting Liu[1] and Zhisheng Huang[1,2(✉)]

[1] Computer Science, Vrije Universiteit Amsterdam, Amsterdam, The Netherlands
ting.liu.vu@hotmail.com, huang@cs.vu.nl
[2] Computer Science, Brain Protection Innovation Center,
Capital Medical University, Beijing, China

Abstract. Gut microbiota that lives in the human gastrointestinal tract impacts on the mental illness through the neurotransmitter-mediated pathway. It's well known that the imbalance of neurotransmitter leads to mental problems. The association between gut microbiota and neurotransmitter needs to be explored in depth. In this paper, we aim at identifying the quality evidence of neurotransmitter modulation by gut microbiota. We use evidence-based medical analysis to characterize the relevant articles to five levels in terms of the strength and reliability of evidence. Thirty-four articles are identified to evaluate their evidence. Gut microbiota not only produces neurotransmitters directly but also modulates neurotransmitters level via metabolism pathways. Also, the growth of some gut microbiota can be counter-regulated by neurotransmitters. This paper provides a comprehensive picture of the association between gut microbiota and neurotransmitter, which give researchers an insight into neurotransmitter modulation by gut microbiota.

Keywords: Gut microbiota · Neurotransmitter · Level of evidence · Evidence-based analysis · Serotonin · Dopamine · Norepinephrine · GABA

1 Introduction

Human gastrointestinal microbiota, also known as gut flora or gut microbiota, are the microorganisms that live in the digestive tracts of humans. The gut microbiota plays a protective role in the host defense against and homeostasis. Researchers have preliminary explored the role of gut microbiota in the development of mood illness. The disorder of gut microbiota plays a causal role in depression [58], anxiety [11], eating disorder [23], and others. This causal relationship involves neurotransmitter imbalance caused by gut microbiota. It's well known that the interruption of neurotransmitter can result in mental disorders

This work was partially supported by the China Scholarship Council.

[36]. The association between gut microbiota and neurotransmitter needs to be explored in depth. In the last few years, many studies on germ-free animals have demonstrated that the absence of microbial colonization altered the expression and turnover of neurotransmitter in both central and enteric nervous systems (CNS and ENS) [6]. Gut microbiota influences the ENS activity by producing local neurotransmitters, such as serotonin, dopamine, norepinephrine, and others [2]. Gut microbiota can modulate the level of neurotransmitter in the host. The current relevant information about neurotransmitter modulation by gut microbiota is fragmented and disorganized because the relevant studies are published by a lot of different researchers in a different time. The information needs to be integrated if we want to insight into the association between gut microbiota and neurotransmitter and identifying the trustworthy evidence.

In this article, we aim to identify the quality evidence of neurotransmitter modulation by gut microbiota. We used the method by extending the meta-data checking that proposed in [18] to automatically identify evidence classes. The evidence is classified to five levels from the strength and reliability of the randomized controlled trials (RCTs) design (Table 1). The classification of the reference evidence levels helpful for determining reliable evidence from the references. This paper provides a comprehensive list of representative gut microbiota which can modulate neurotransmitter produce. By understanding the association, it suggests a possibility for the treatment or prevention of mental illness with microbe-mediate interventions.

Table 1. Hierarchy of evidence based on the strength of RCTs design

Levels	Design of study
1	Evidence obtained from a systematic review or at least one randomized controlled trial
2	Evidence obtained from well designed pseudo-randomized controlled trials of appropriate size
3	Evidence from well-designed trials without randomization, single group pre-post, cohort, interventions or time-series studies
4	Evidence obtained from case series or non-experimental studies from more than one center or research group
5	Opinions of respected authorities, based on clinical experience, descriptive studies or reports of expert committees

2 Related Work

2.1 Gut Microbiota Linked to Mental Illness

Germ-free mice with transplanted fecal microbiota from the depressed patient showed depression-like behaviors and physiological features [63]. Compared to healthy control, the composition of gut microbiota in depressed patients are notable changes in the relative abundance of *Firmicutes, Actinobacteria, Bacteroidetes* [63]. Chronic administration of probiotics, e.g., *L. plantarum*, can reduce the anxiety and depression related behaviors [5,28], also helpful for ameliorating neuropsychiatric disorders [28]. Hyperactive locomotor behavior of germ-free *Drosophila melanogaster* can be rescued by single colonization of *L. brevis* strain [48]. Psychopathology of eating disorders also involves changes in the diversity and composition of gut microbiota [23].

2.2 Neurotransmitter Imbalance Leads to Mental Illness

Clinical evidence of depression suggests that depression inseparable with the disturbance in serotonin, norepinephrine, and dopamine neurotransmission in the CNS [37] and the most common class of anti-depressants target the serotonin network. Decreased gamma-Aminobutyric acid (GABA) levels lead to cases of anxiety disorder [41] and depression [30]. Off-balance of neurotransmitter contribute to one's risk of sleeping disorder [59] and eating disorder [56].

2.3 Gut Microbiota Modulate Neurotransmitter Level

Neurotransmitter often produced in brain and ENS. Roughly 50% dopamine and 95% serotonin of the body synthesized in gastrointestinal tract [13]. Gut microbiota has impacts on the formation of neurotransmitter. Daily intake *L. plantarum* significantly increased the levels of both serotonin and dopamine in mice [28]. The probiotic *L. rhamnosus* encourage the production of GABA in mice [5]. The association of germ-free mice with either *Clostridium* or *E. coli* species result in a drastic elevation of free norepinephrine [2].

3   Evidence-Level Analysis

In medicine, Levels of Evidence (LoE) are arranged in a ranking system used in evidence-based practices to describe the strength of the results measured in a clinical trial or research study [15]. The design of the study and measurement will affect the strength of the evidence of one article. We proposed a rule-based algorithm approach for evidence quality identification that covers the required knowledge for the classification of evidence level [18]. We use the PMID to get the metadata (i.e. Publication Types, Abstract, Title, and MeSH Terms, and others) from PubMed. Then the proposed algorithm checks the metadata and estimates the evidence level. The algorithms for identifying evidence classes are described in detail in that paper [18]. We report several experiments with a detailed evaluation of the proposed methods successfully.

4   Results

Bacteria have been shown to produce and consume a wide range of mammalian neurotransmitters [53], including serotonin, dopamine, norepinephrine, GABA, histamine, and acetylcholine. In this paper, thirty-four articles are identified to evaluate the evidence of neurotransmitter modulation by microbiota and the regulation of neurotransmitter on the growth of microorganisms (Fig. 1 and Table 2). Two of these papers at Level 1, nine papers at Level 2 and the rest papers belong to Level 3.

4.1 Serotonin

As a neurotransmitter in both CNS and ENS, serotonin involves in the regulation of many physiological functions including appetite [56], cognition [20], mood [8] and other aspects. Four level-2 RCTs proved that gut microbiota regulates the serotonin level in the host. Administrate *L. plantarum* to a germ-free mouse model significantly increase the contents of both serotonin and dopamine [28]. The presence of *Cl. ramosum* in gut promote serotonin secretion in germ-free mice [33]. Animal-like gut-brain module detection frequency in human gut-associated microbial genomes identified *B. cereus*, *B. oklahomensis*, *A. baumannii* and *paenibacillus* spp. are act as potential serotonin producers [58].

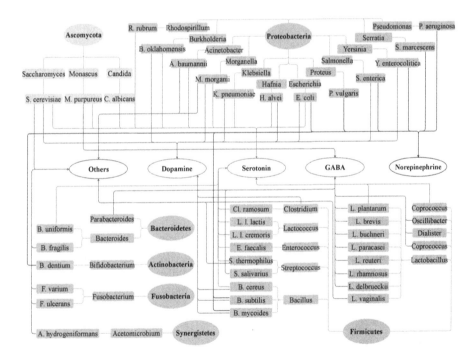

Fig. 1. Neurotransmitter modulation by the gut microbiota. The gut microbiota includes six phyla of bacteria and one phylum of fungi. Light blue backgrounds and lines indicate the species relationship of the bacteria, and light pink represents the fungus. Connection lines with different colors are used to show the link between gut microbiota and neurotransmitters: dopamine (pink), serotonin (green), norepinephrine (blue), GABA (red) and others (grey). Others include histamine and acetylcholine. (Color figure online)

Fecal metabolites analysis show that indigenous spore-forming of *B. uniformis* promote serotonin biosynthesis from Enterochromaffin Cells (ECs) to the mucosa, lumen and circulating platelets [62].

Eight RCTs at Level 3 found that bacteria also produce serotonin *in vitro*. *S. thermophilus* can increase the concentration of serotonin in its growth medium [14]. Serotonin were detected in histidine decarboxylase broth which contain the strains of *H. alvei*, *K. pneumoniae* and *M. morganii*, respectively [43]. Lactic acid bacteria (e.g. *L. plantarum*, *L. l. cremoris* and *L. l. lactis*) can form serotonin in arginine decarboxylase broth [44]. The M-9 or Lysogeny Broth (LB) culture medium of *E. coli* contain nanomolar of serotonin during the late growth phase that is sufficient for animal/human receptors to bind [49]. Bacteria *S. cerevisiae* [32], *R. rubrum* [42], *E. faecalis* [52] and yeast *C. guilliermondii* [52] can be growth-stimulated by serotonin. *C. albicans* is the most common fungal species and member of the human gut microbiota. On one hand, it coats the lining of the intestinal tract and suppresses the ability to produce or secrete serotonin [34]. On the other hand, serotonin has antifungal activity against *Candida* spp. *in vitro* [34].

4.2 Dopamine

The right balance of dopamine is vital for both physical and mental well being. Substantial levels of free dopamine were identified in the gut lumen of both specific pathogen-free mice and germ-free mice with *Clostridium* species [2]. The level of dopamine significantly increased in a germ-free mouse carry with *L. plantarum* strain [28]. *B. oklahomensis* positive correlate with the synthesis of the dopamine metabolite 3,4-dihydroxyphenylacetic acid (DOPAC) [58]. *In vitro* data show that S. thermophilus can increase the concentration of serotonin in the growth medium [14]. The family of *Bacillus* is a potential bacterium that produce dopamine [31,57]. Özoğul et al. certify that *H. alvei*, *K. pneumoniae* and *M. morganii* induce the generate of dopamine in histidine decarboxylase broth [43]. Both the concentrations of serotonin and dopamine increased in *E. coli* growth culture [49,57]. In addition, *P. vulgaris*, *S. aureus* and *S. marcescens* strains have the ability to secrete dopamine [57]. Addition of dopamine in culture medium promote the growth of *Y. enterocolitica*, *E. coli* and *S. enterica* [12]. The proliferation of *S. cerevisiae* EPF cells on solid Maltose-Peptone-Yeast extract medium was stimulated by the addition of monoamine neurotransmitters, such as dopamine, serotonin, and histamine [32].

4.3 Norepinephrine

Norepinephrine plays a determinant role in executive functioning regulating cognition, motivation, and intellect [38]. Several bacteria have been reported to norepinephrine. *Clostridium* increasing the free norepinephrine in the gut lumen of both germ-free and specific pathogen-free mice [2]. In the previous section, we mentioned *E. coli* can produce serotonin and dopamine in both M-9 and LB

Table 2. Representative neurotransmitter-modulating gut microbiota. "+" indicate increased level of neurotransmitters by gut microbiota. "p" present promoted growth of microorganism, whereas "i" present the inhibition.

Neurotransmitters	Levels	Bacterial strain	Effect		Ref.
Serotonin	2	L. plantarum	+		[28]
		Cl. ramosum	+		[33]
		B. oklahomensis, A. baumannii	+		[58]
		B. cereus, Paenibacillus spp.			
		B. uniformis	+		[62]
	3	S. thermophilus	+		[14]
		S. cerevisiae		p	[32]
		C. albicans	+	i	[34]
		R. rubrum		p	[42]
		H. alvei, M. morganii, K. pneumoniae	+		[43]
		L. l. cremoris, L. l. lactis, L. plantarum	+		[44]
		E. coli	+		[49]
		E. faecalis, C. guilliermondii		p	[52]
Dopamine	2	Clostridium spp.	+		[2]
		L. plantarum	+		[28]
		B. oklahomensis	+		[58]
	3	Y. enterocolitica, S. enterica, E. coli		p	[12]
		S. thermophilus	+		[14]
		Bacillus spp.	+		[31]
		S. cerevisiae		p	[32]
		H. alvei, M. morganii, K. pneumoniae	+		[43]
		E. coli	+		[49]
		B. cereus, B. mycoides, B. subtilis, E. coli	+		[57]
		P. vulgaris, S. aureus, S. marcescens			
Norepinephrine	2	Clostridium spp.	+		[2]
	3	Y. enterocolitica, S. enterica, E. coli		p	[12]
		P. aeruginosa		p	[16]
		E. coli	+		[49]
		B. mycoides, B. subtilis	+		[57]
		P. vulgaris, S. marcescens			
GABA	1	Oscillibacter spp.	+		[40]
		Bacteroides, Escherichia, Parabacteroides	+		[54]
	2	B. dentium	+		[9]
		L. reuteri	+		[25]
		B. dentium	+		[46]
		Coprococcus spp., Dialister spp.	+		[58]
	3	L. brevis, B. dentium	+		[4]
		L. rhamnosus	+		[5]
		L. buchneri	+		[7]
		L. paracasei	+		[24]
		L. delbrueckii, L. plantarum, L. rhamnosus	+		[50]
		M. purpureus	+		[55]
		L. brevis	+		[60]
		S. salivarius	+		[61]
Histamine	2	M. morganii	+		[22]
		A. baumannii, F. varium, B. fragilis	+		[58]
	3	L. vaginalis	+		[10]
		S. thermophilus	+		[14]
		S. cerevisiae		p	[32]
		E. coli	+		[47]
Acetylcholine	2	A. hydrogeniformans	+		[58]
	3	L. plantarum	+		[51]

culture medium during the late growth phase. Norepinephrine is another neurotransmitter yield by *E. coli* in its growth medium [49]. *B. mycoides* and *B. subtilis*, both are belong to the genius of *Bacillus*, have the ability to secrete norepinephrine [57]. The authors also found *P. vulgaris* and *S. marcescens* have the same potential [57]. In contract, norepinephrine specific induce the growth of *S. enterica*, *Y. enterocolitica* and *E. coli* [12]. The hormone norepinephrine increasing *P. aeruginosa* growth, virulence factor production, and swimming motility in a concentration-dependent manner [16].

4.4   GABA

Mental disorders such as depression, sleep disorders, stiff-person syndrome, drug and alcohol addiction have been related to the chaos of GABAergic function in the brain. It has been shown that the neurotransmitter GABA can be produced by intestinal bacteria. The *Oscillibacter* type strain has valeric acid as its main metabolic end product, a homolog of neurotransmitter GABA [40]. GABA-producing pathways are actively expressed by *Bacteroides*, *Parabacteroides* and *Escherichia* species are proved by the transcriptome analysis of human stool samples from healthy individuals [54]. Commensal *B. dentium* produces GABA via enzymatic decarboxylation of glutamate by GadB [46]. It can produce GABA in Germ-free mice [9], Sprague-dawly rats [46] and Monosodium Glutamate medium [4]. Gut-brain module analysis of fecal meta-genomes indicated the depletion of *Coprococcus* spp. and *Dialister* spp. have potential roles in microbial GABA production in depression patient [58]. The addition of *L. brevis* to the culturable gut microbiota increased the GABA concentration in the fermented fecal slurry at physiological pH [4]. Wu et al. also found that *L. brevis* is a GABA-producer [60]. Other GABA-producing *Lactobacillus* strain including *L. rhamnosus* [5,50], *L. buchneri* [7], *L. paracasei* [24], *L. delbrueckii* [50], *L. plantarum* [50]. GABA can be formed by *S. salivarius* subsp. *thermophilus* via submerged fermentation [61]. Except for bacteria, the fungus *Monascus* spp. also can produce GABA. Especially *M. purpureus*, the strain with the highest amount of GABA among 16 strains tested in research [55].

4.5   Other Neurotransmitters

Intestinal bacteria can secrete histamine and release histamine from human basophil leukocytes and mast cells which influence on the host immunological processes [3]. Two RCTs at Level 2, prove that *M. morganii*, *A. baumannii*, *F. varium* and *B. fragilis* are four types of histamine secreting bacteria [22,58]. *L. vaginalis* is an another potential histamine-producing strain [10]. *S. thermophilus* isolates had an ability to produce twelve different biogenic amines, including serotonin, dopamine and histamine, in histidine broth and lysine Decarboxylase broth [14]. Bacterial adherence and hemolysin production from *E. coli* induces histamine release from cells [47]. Addition of histamine can stimulate the proliferation of *S. cerevisiae* EPF cells on solid maltose-peptone-yeast extract medium [32]. Acetylcholine serves as primarily excitatory in the CNS. It plays a role in arousal, memory, learning, and neuroplasticity. Stanaszek et al. successfully extracted acetylcholine from the growth medium of *L. plantarum* [51]. *A. hydrogeniformans* promote the synthesis of acetylcholine in host [58]. Increased acetylcholine signaling lead to symptoms of depression and anxiety in both humans and animal models [17].

5   Conclusion

Gut microbiota can stimulate the production of neurotransmitter. *In vitro* and *in vivo* studies showed that gut microbiota has impacts on the level of neurotransmitter. A lot of gut microbes can produce kinds of neurotransmitters in growth medium cultured *in vitro*. By leveraging animal models, accumulating evidence suggests that gut microbiota plays a critical role in regulating host neurotransmitter. A reason is that gut microbiota-generated short-chain fatty acids signal ECs to produce serotonin via expression of tryptophan hydroxylase. The entrance of gut tryptophan into the immune-driven kynurenine pathway plays a major role serotonin dysregulation [1]. Gut microbiota stimulates the production of neurotransmitter by affecting the host metabolism.

Gut microbiota affects mental health by modulating neurotransmitter. Two bacterial genus, *Coprococcus* and *Oscillibacter*, not only involve in the production and metabolism of GABA but also take part in depression [40,58]. *L. rhamnosus* dramatically alters GABA activity in the brain of mice, as well as reduces the anxiety and depression-related behaviors [5,53]. Ingested *L. plantarum* induces the changes of emotional behavior with increasing the level of monoamine neurotransmitters in mouse [28]. These researches implicated a potential role of neurotransmitter in the effects of gut microbiota on mental health.

Gut microbiota is a novel target for the treatment of mental illness. Absence of gut microbiota during early life affects anxiolytic behaviors of mice [45]. Transplant the gut microbiota from depressed patients to germ-free animals produce depressive-like behaviors [21,35,63] and antidepressants use can abolish the impacts [29]. Administration of probiotics contributes to maintaining normal cognitive and emotional management [5,28,48] and reduce anxiety and depression-related behaviors. Modification of gut microbiota through diet and related strategies have significant utility in preventing and treating mental problems.

6   Future Direction

Millions of chemical reactions in the gut-brain work to regulate mood, perceptions, and how we experience life. To be sure, the chemicals are involved in mental illness, but it's not as simple as one chemical being too low or another too high. Gut microbiota not only modulates the neurotransmitters (e.g., serotonin, dopamine, norepinephrine, GABA, etc.) which we mentioned above but also influences other neurotransmitter systems (e.g., peptides, purines, trace amines, etc.). Besides, gut microbiota regulates neurotransmitter by intervention with its receptors. The neurotransmission between brain and gut microbiota depends on the presence of neurotransmitter receptors on the bacteria. Bacteria control the levels of neurotransmitter through neurotransmitter receptors, Such as *L. reuteri* up-regulates GABA receptors in the CNS system [39]. More work is required to insight into the neurochemical changes during the mental illness. In the future, we are interested in building the knowledge graph [19] and neural network [26,27] to model the association between gut microbiota and neurotransmitter.

References

1. Agus, A., Planchais, J., Sokol, H.: Gut microbiota regulation of tryptophan metabolism in health and disease. Cell Host Microbe **23**(6), 716–724 (2018)
2. Asano, Y., et al.: Critical role of gut microbiota in the production of biologically active, free catecholamines in the gut lumen of mice. Am. J. Physiol. Gastrointest. Liver Physiol. **303**(11), G1288–G1295 (2012)
3. Barcik, W., Wawrzyniak, M., Akdis, C.A., O'Mahony, L.: Immune regulation by histamine and histamine-secreting bacteria. Curr. Opin. Immunol. **48**, 108–113 (2017)
4. Barrett, E., Ross, R., O'toole, P., Fitzgerald, G., Stanton, C.: γ-aminobutyric acid production by culturable bacteria from the human intestine. J. Appl. Microbiol. **113**(2), 411–417 (2012)
5. Bravo, J.A., et al.: Ingestion of lactobacillus strain regulates emotional behavior and central gaba receptor expression in a mouse via the vagus nerve. Proc. Natl. Acad. Sci. **108**(38), 16050–16055 (2011)
6. Carabotti, M., Scirocco, A., Maselli, M.A., Severi, C.: The gut-brain axis: interactions between enteric microbiota, central and enteric nervous systems. Ann. Gastroenterol. Q. Publ. Hell. Soc. Gastroenterol. **28**(2), 203 (2015)
7. Cho, Y.R., Chang, J.Y., Chang, H.C.: Production of gamma-aminobutyric acid (GABA) by Lactobacillus buchneri isolated from kimchi and its neuroprotective effect on neuronal cells. J. Microbiol. Biotechnol. **17**(1), 104–109 (2007)
8. Cowen, P.J., Browning, M.: What has serotonin to do with depression? World Psychiatry **14**(2), 158–160 (2015)
9. De Vadder, F., et al.: Gut microbiota regulates maturation of the adult enteric nervous system via enteric serotonin networks. Proc. Natl. Acad. Sci. **115**(25), 6458–6463 (2018)
10. Diaz, M., et al.: Isolation and typification of histamine-producing Lactobacillus vaginalis strains from cheese. Int. J. Food Microbiol. **215**, 117–123 (2015)
11. Foster, J.A., Neufeld, K.A.M.: Gut-brain axis: how the microbiome influences anxiety and depression. Trends Neurosci. **36**(5), 305–312 (2013)
12. Freestone, P.P., Haigh, R.D., Lyte, M.: Specificity of catecholamine-induced growth in Escherichia coli O157: H7, Salmonella enterica and Yersinia enterocolitica. FEMS Microbiol. Lett. **269**(2), 221–228 (2007)
13. Ge, X., Pan, J., Liu, Y., Wang, H., Zhou, W., Wang, X.: Intestinal crosstalk between microbiota and serotonin and its impact on gut motility. Curr. Pharm. Biotechnol. **19**(3), 190–195 (2018)
14. Gezginc, Y., Akyol, I., Kuley, E., Özogul, F.: Biogenic amines formation in Streptococcus thermophilus isolated from home-made natural yogurt. Food Chem. **138**(1), 655–662 (2013)

15. Gross, R.A., Johnston, K.C.: Levels of evidence: taking neurology® to the next level. Neurology **72**(1), 8–10 (2009)
16. Hegde, M., Wood, T.K., Jayaraman, A.: The neuroendocrine hormone norepinephrine increases Pseudomonas aeruginosa PA14 virulence through the las quorum-sensing pathway. Appl. Microbiol. Biotechnol. **84**(4), 763 (2009)
17. Higley, M.J., Picciotto, M.R.: Neuromodulation by acetylcholine: examples from schizophrenia and depression. Curr. Opin. Neurobiol. **29**, 88–95 (2014)
18. Huang, Z., Hu, Q., ten Teije, A., van Harmelen, F.: Identifying evidence quality for updating evidence-based medical guidelines. In: Riaño, D., Lenz, R., Miksch, S., Peleg, M., Reichert, M., ten Teije, A. (eds.) KR4HC 2015. LNCS (LNAI), vol. 9485, pp. 51–64. Springer, Cham (2015). https://doi.org/10.1007/978-3-319-26585-8_4
19. Huang, Z., Yang, J., van Harmelen, F., Hu, Q.: Constructing knowledge graphs of depression. In: Siuly, S., et al. (eds.) HIS 2017. LNCS, vol. 10594, pp. 149–161. Springer, Cham (2017). https://doi.org/10.1007/978-3-319-69182-4_16
20. Jenkins, T., Nguyen, J., Polglaze, K., Bertrand, P.: Influence of tryptophan and serotonin on mood and cognition with a possible role of the gut-brain axis. Nutrients **8**(1), 56 (2016)
21. Jianguo, L., Xueyang, J., Cui, W., Changxin, W., Xuemei, Q.: Altered gut metabolome contributes to depression-like behaviors in rats exposed to chronic unpredictable mild stress. Transl. Psychiatry **9**(1), 40 (2019)
22. Kim, S.H., Ben-Gigirey, B., Barros-Velazquez, J., Price, R.J., An, H.: Histamine and biogenic amine production by Morganella morganii isolated from temperature-abused albacore. J. Food Prot. **63**(2), 244–251 (2000)
23. Kleiman, S.C., et al.: The intestinal microbiota in acute anorexia nervosa and during renourishment: relationship to depression, anxiety, and eating disorder psychopathology. Psychosom. Med. **77**(9), 969 (2015)
24. Komatsuzaki, N., Shima, J., Kawamoto, S., Momose, H., Kimura, T.: Production of γ-aminobutyric acid (GABA) by Lactobacillus paracasei isolated from traditional fermented foods. Food Microbiol. **22**(6), 497–504 (2005)
25. Kunze, W.A., et al.: Lactobacillus reuteri enhances excitability of colonic AH neurons by inhibiting calcium-dependent potassium channel opening. J. Cell. Mol. Med. **13**(8b), 2261–2270 (2009)
26. Lan, G., Benito-Picazo, J., Roijers, D.M., Domínguez, E., Eiben, A.: Real-time robot vision on low-performance computing hardware. In: 2018 15th International Conference on Control, Automation, Robotics and Vision (ICARCV), pp. 1959–1965, November 2018
27. Lan, G., Jelisavcic, M., Roijers, D.M., Haasdijk, E., Eiben, A.E.: Directed locomotion for modular robots with evolvable morphologies. In: Auger, A., Fonseca, C.M., Lourenço, N., Machado, P., Paquete, L., Whitley, D. (eds.) PPSN 2018. LNCS, vol. 11101, pp. 476–487. Springer, Cham (2018). https://doi.org/10.1007/978-3-319-99253-2_38
28. Liu, W.H., et al.: Alteration of behavior and monoamine levels attributable to Lactobacillus plantarum PS128 in germ-free mice. Behav. Brain Res. **298**, 202–209 (2016)
29. Lukić, I., et al.: Antidepressants affect gut microbiota and Ruminococcus flavefaciens is able to abolish their effects on depressive-like behavior. Transl. Psychiatry **9**(1), 133 (2019)
30. Luscher, B., Shen, Q., Sahir, N.: The gabaergic deficit hypothesis of major depressive disorder. Mol. Psychiatry **16**(4), 383 (2011)

31. Lyte, M.: Probiotics function mechanistically as delivery vehicles for neuroactive compounds: microbial endocrinology in the design and use of probiotics. Bioessays **33**(8), 574–581 (2011)
32. Malikina, K., Shishov, V., Chuvelev, D., Kudrin, V., Oleskin, A.: Regulatory role of monoamine neurotransmitters in Saccharomyces cerevisiae cells. Appl. Biochem. Microbiol. **46**(6), 620–625 (2010)
33. Mandić, A.D., et al.: Clostridium ramosum regulates enterochromaffin cell development and serotonin release. Sci. Rep. **9**(1), 1177 (2019)
34. Mayr, A., Hinterberger, G., Dierich, M., Lass-Flörl, C.: Interaction of serotonin with Candida albicans selectively attenuates fungal virulence in vitro. Int. J. Antimicrob. Agents **26**(4), 335–337 (2005)
35. McGaughey, K.D., et al.: Relative abundance of Akkermansia spp. and other bacterial phylotypes correlates with anxiety-and depressive-like behavior following social defeat in mice. Sci. Rep. **9**(1), 3281 (2019)
36. Mittal, R., et al.: Neurotransmitters: the critical modulators regulating gut-brain axis. J. Cell. Physiol. **232**(9), 2359–2372 (2017)
37. Moret, C., Briley, M.: The importance of norepinephrine in depression. Neuropsychiatr. Dis. Treat. **7**(Suppl 1), 9 (2011)
38. Moret, C., Briley, M.: The importance of norepinephrine in depression. Neuropsychiatr. Dis. Treat. **2011**(7), 9–13 (2011)
39. Mu, Q., Tavella, V., Luo, X.M.: Role of Lactobacillus reuteri in human health and diseases. Front. Microbiol. **9**, 757 (2018)
40. Naseribafrouei, A., et al.: Correlation between the human fecal microbiota and depression. Neurogastroenterol. Motil. **26**(8), 1155–1162 (2014)
41. Nuss, P.: Anxiety disorders and GABA neurotransmission: a disturbance of modulation. Neuropsychiatr. Dis. Treat. **11**, 165 (2015)
42. Oleskin, A., Kirovskaia, T., Botvinko, I., Lysak, L.: Effect of serotonin (5-hydroxytryptamine) on the growth and differentiation of microorganisms. Mikrobiologiia **67**(3), 305–312 (1998)
43. Özoğul, F.: Production of biogenic amines by Morganella morganii, Klebsiella pneumoniae and Hafnia alvei using a rapid HPLC method. Eur. Food Res. Technol. **219**(5), 465–469 (2004)
44. Özoğul, F., Kuley, E., Özoğul, Y., Özoğul, İ.: The function of lactic acid bacteria on biogenic amines production by food-borne pathogens in arginine decarboxylase broth. Food Sci. Technol. Res. **18**(6), 795–804 (2012)
45. Pan, J.X., et al.: Absence of gut microbiota during early life affects anxiolytic behaviors and monoamine neurotransmitters system in the hippocampal of mice. J. Neurol. Sci. **400**, 160–168 (2019)
46. Pokusaeva, K., et al.: GABA-producing Bifidobacterium dentium modulates visceral sensitivity in the intestine. Neurogastroenterol. Motil. **29**(1), e12904 (2017)
47. Scheffer, J., König, W., Hacker, J., Goebel, W.: Bacterial adherence and hemolysin production from Escherichia coli induces histamine and leukotriene release from various cells. Infect. Immun. **50**(1), 271–278 (1985)
48. Schretter, C.E., et al.: A gut microbial factor modulates locomotor behaviour in Drosophila. Nature **563**(7731), 402 (2018)
49. Shishov, V., Kirovskaya, T., Kudrin, V., Oleskin, A.: Amine neuromediators, their precursors, and oxidation products in the culture of Escherichia coli K-12. Appl. Biochem. Microbiol. **45**(5), 494–497 (2009)
50. Siragusa, S., De Angelis, M., Di Cagno, R., Rizzello, C., Coda, R., Gobbetti, M.: Synthesis of γ-aminobutyric acid by lactic acid bacteria isolated from a variety of Italian cheeses. Appl. Environ. Microbiol. **73**(22), 7283–7290 (2007)

51. Stanaszek, P.M., Snell, J.F., O'Neill, J.J.: Isolation, extraction, and measurement of acetylcholine from Lactobacillus plantarum. Appl. Environ. Microbiol. **34**(2), 237–239 (1997)
52. Strakhovskaia, M., Ivanova, E., Fraǐnkin, G.: Stimulatory effect of serotonin on the growth of the yeast Candida guilliermondii and the bacterium Streptococcus faecalis. Mikrobiologiia **62**(1), 46–49 (1993)
53. Strandwitz, P.: Neurotransmitter modulation by the gut microbiota. Brain Res. **1693**, 128–133 (2018)
54. Strandwitz, P., et al.: GABA-modulating bacteria of the human gut microbiota. Nat. Microbiol. **4**(3), 396 (2019)
55. Su, Y.C., Wang, J.J., Lin, T.T., Pan, T.M.: Production of the secondary metabolites γ-aminobutyric acid and monacolin K by Monascus. J. Ind. Microbiol. Biotechnol. **30**(1), 41–46 (2003)
56. Treasure, J., Eid, L.: Eating disorder animal model. Curr. Opin. Psychiatr. **32** (2019)
57. Tsavkelova, E., Botvinko, I., Kudrin, V., Oleskin, A.: Detection of neurotransmitter amines in microorganisms with the use of high-performance liquid chromatography. Dokl. Biochem. Proc. Acad. Sci. USSR Biochem. Sect. **372**(1–6), 115 (2000)
58. Valles-Colomer, M., et al.: The neuroactive potential of the human gut microbiota in quality of life and depression. Nat. Microbiol. **4**, 623 (2019)
59. Wirz-Justice, A., Benedetti, F.: Perspectives in affective disorders: clocks and sleep. Eur. J. Neurosci. 1–20 (2019)
60. Wu, C.H., Hsueh, Y.H., Kuo, J.M., Liu, S.J.: Characterization of a potential probiotic Lactobacillus brevis RK03 and efficient production of γ-aminobutyric acid in batch fermentation. Int. J. Mol. Sci. **19**(1), 143 (2018)
61. Yang, S.Y., et al.: Production of γ-aminobutyric acid by Streptococcus salivarius subsp. thermophilus Y2 under submerged fermentation. Amino Acids **34**(3), 473–478 (2008)
62. Yano, J.M., et al.: Indigenous bacteria from the gut microbiota regulate host serotonin biosynthesis. Cell **161**(2), 264–276 (2015)
63. Zheng, P., et al.: Gut microbiome remodeling induces depressive-like behaviors through a pathway mediated by the host's metabolism. Mol. Psychiatry **21**(6), 786 (2016)

Quantifying the Effects of Temperature and Noise on Attention-Level Using EDA and EEG Sensors

Zhengrui Xue[1][(✉)], Luning Yang[2], Prapa Rattadilok[1], Shanshan Li[1], and Longyue Gao[1]

[1] School of Computer Science, University of Nottingham Ningbo China, Ningbo, China
{scyzxl, prapa.rattadilok, zyl8712, zyl8699}@nottingham.edu.cn
[2] School of Mathematical Science, University of Nottingham Ningbo China, Ningbo, China
smylyl@nottingham.edu.cn

Abstract. Most people with Autism Spectrum Disorder (ASD) experience atypical sensory modality and need help to self-regulate their sensory responses. Results of a pilot study are presented here where temperature, noise types and noise levels are used as independent variables. Attention-based tests (ABTs), Electrodermal Activity (EDA) and Electroencephalography (EEG) sensors are used as dependent variables to quantify the effects of temperature and noise. Based on the outcome of the analyses, it is feasible to use off-the-shelf sensors to recognize physiological changes, indicating a possibility to develop sensory management recommendation interventions to support people with ASD.

Keywords: Autism Spectrum Disorder · Sensory management · Sensors · Electrodermal Activity · Electroencephalography

1 Introduction

Autism Spectrum Disorder (ASD) is a neurodevelopment disorder characterized by a range of persistent difficulties in social communication, cognitive and repetitive behavior patterns, as well as differences in perceptual processing [1]. Human senses work by acquiring conscious information that allows them to make classifications in their environment [2]. In the United States, one out of 68 children are diagnosed with ASD [3]. Although there is evidence that sensory deficits can impede the development of the ability to socially interact at an early age [4], the sensory training for children with ASD remains unexplored.

Researchers have categorized the heterogeneity of ASD based on behavioral and physical phenotypes [5]. The Diagnostic and Statistical Manual of Mental Disorders, 4th edition (DSM-IV) applies a multi-categorical system in diagnosing ASD. However, many studies have indicated that the DSM-IV criteria have limited reliability, poor classification of core symptoms and low predicate ability [6, 7]. Instead of a

© Springer Nature Switzerland AG 2019
H. Wang et al. (Eds.): HIS 2019, LNCS 11837, pp. 250–262, 2019.
https://doi.org/10.1007/978-3-030-32962-4_23

multi-categorical system, DSM 5th edition (DSM-5) uses a single diagnostic dimension which removes the clinical subtypes in DSM-IV, and determines that symptoms of ASD are best represented in a two-domain model of social-communication deficits and restricted-repetitive interests/behaviors (RRB) [8]. According to Huerta et al. [9], the specificity of using the new ASD diagnostic criteria is significantly improved. By having any abnormal sensory response to environment or unusual sensory interests within one dimension, researchers can explore the clinical outcomes and treatment response of people with ASD subgroups more efficiently [10].

Some people with ASD have hypersensitive sensory condition and the external stimulus can cause a panic attack or overwhelming sensation [11]. Others could be hyposensitive, with the low perception of temperature and pain. Sensory management plays a critical role in addressing the challenges faced by people with ASD. Sensory technologies are designed to help overcome these restrictions and assist people with ASD to better understand and participate in the social environment [12]. Although the technologies have been shown to support people with ASD effectively [13], no known technological solutions focus on recommending sensory management strategies for people with ASD in real-time. This paper presents a feasibility study of developing a novel sensory management recommendation system, which aims to combine several sensors, working together and providing more comprehensive information.

2   Related Work

2.1   Sound Level Monitors

People with ASD have motor, sound, sensory and visual impairments, but these impairments are not considered in ASD diagnosis [14, 15]. Specifically, children with ASD have delayed neural timing, reduced neural stability, and low sensitivity of pitch changes, when compared with their neuro-typical developing peers, and this may negatively influence their communication capability [16].

A sound level meter is a hand-held device equipped with a display and a microphone on the top, e.g. Casella [17]. It can respond to changes in air pressure caused by sound waves, i.e. automatically convert physical vibration into an electrical signal, and thus measure the sound level that travels through the air [17].

Smartphones have recently become an alternative device for measuring sound level. Although limitations exist, some studies suggest that smartphones can replace the traditional sound level assessment devices in the near future [18]. One study suggests that a mobile application that tracks noise level has a significant difference between measured and true noise levels, indicating the low performance for ambient noise measurement in hardware [19]. The same study also shows that the age of a smartphone will also determine its ability to accurately measure noise, however the relation between accuracy and low volatility requires further research.

NIOSH [20] combines the features of high-accuracy sound level meters and noise dosimeters into a mobile application. The application will record the instantaneous noise level in the laboratory and calculate an average noise level. LENA or Language Environment Analysis has been used in many ASD researches to collect, manage and analyze the audio record. LENA comes with custom-designed clothing with a pocket to insert LENA recorder. LENA provides counts and percentile data on audio measurements. However, its suitability for clinical applications is so far unproven [21].

2.2 Physiological Monitors

2.2.1 Electrodermal Activity (EDA) Sensor

The sweat glands of human are varied and controlled by the sympathetic nervous system. Electrodermal Activity (EDA), also known as Galvanic Skin Response (GSR), refers to changes in sweat gland activity that are reflective of the intensity of our emotional state or arousal. When a person experiences stress or is aroused, moisture collects under the skin, increasing the skin's electrical conductivity which changes the skin temperature and heart rate [22]. Typically, EDA sensors measure the electrical conductance of skin [23] and have been used as an indicator of psychological or physiological arousal.

EDA sensors are widely used for stress assessment and intervention in people with ASD [24, 25]. In addition to an EDA, iCalm [26] also includes a photoplethysmograph (PPG) for the heart rate, 3-axis accelerometer for movements, and an optical infrared thermometer for detecting the skin temperature. One study has tested iCalm for continuous data collection on 7 participants within 48 h, the results shows that iCalm can run continuously for long periods of time and has similar performance to a clinician standard device [28]. In the electronic device market, Empatica E4 uses the cloud to store user's data from four sensors i.e. 3D accelerometer, PPG sensor, EDA sensor and the skin temperature sensor. Samsung Gear watches lack the EDA sensor but are equipped with Gyro and Barometer sensors, and data from Samsung devices were collected directly by Wi-Fi [27].

It should be noted that EDA cannot determine emotion factors and the EDA sensors need physical contact with the body, which may cause danger during aggressive behaviors. In [28], extensive numbers of wearable solutions for physiological and emotional monitoring for ASD is reviewed.

2.2.2 Attention Level Sensor

Attention is the term that has been defined as the behavioral and cognitive process of selectively concentrating on a discrete aspect of information while ignoring other perceivable information and the allocation of limited cognitive process [29].

The Muse Brain sensor is a lightweight headband that uses electroencephalography (EEG) sensors to monitor human brain activity, which corresponds to attention level [30]. MUSE uses seven precisely calibrated EEG sensors, two on the forehead, two behind the ear, and three reference sensors. Signal processing and machine learning techniques are applied to analyze these signals, and visualized as a chart.

The iView X RED eye tracker has been used to detect the attention pattern of people with ASD. In a dark and isolated environment, a small video was provided as a visual stimulus for participants, and an eye tracker was used at a 60 Hz. The subject's gaze pattern is tracked by the device and then analyzed for any atypical patterns in the gaze behavior [31]. However, the device is expensive and requires calibration for every subject. The subject also needs to face the camera, which restricts free movement.

WearCam is a head-mounted eye tracker that measures wide-angle field of view and gaze direction from the perspective of the subject [2]. The video can be analyzed to monitor the subject's focus of attention throughout the session. The mobility of device allows for more natural interactions, but the accuracy is relatively low. Moreover, people who are sensitive to skin contact may not be tolerant the head-mounted devices.

3   Methodology

The aim of the experiment is to measure the attention level of people under different noise levels and temperatures. Attention-level is measured using well-known attention-based tests (ABTs) including Stroop Color and Word Test (SCWT) [32], Dot Cancellation Test (DCT) [33] and mouse tracking task (MTT) [34]. The speed and the accuracy or the correctness in completing these ABTs are used as the quantitative measurements for attention-level. Within-subjects experimental design [35] is used, i.e. each participant participates in all of the experimental conditions. In minimizing the learning effect, i.e. participants became more familiar with the tasks over time, Latin-square design [36, 37] is used to place the order of the tasks for different participants.

The temperature of the experimental room is controlled digitally using an air-conditioner and a heater. A temperature sensor and a sound sensor connected to an Arduino UNO board are used to monitor and record the temperature and the sound level during the experiment. Data from Arduino UNO board is compared with a digital thermostat and the NIOSH app to ensure the accuracy of the measurements. GSR sensor and MUSE headband are used to measure EDA and EEG respectively.

3.1   Stroop Color and Word Test (SCWT)

The SCWT [32] is a test widely used to evaluate the ability of the subject to suppress cognitive interference in neuropsychology. In SCWT, participants are provided colored-words with mismatched colors (Fig. 1). Participants must ignore the meaning of the words and identify the color of the word as soon as possible.

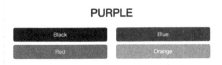

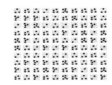

Fig. 1. An example of the SCWT   **Fig. 2.** An example of the DCT

3.2   Dot Cancellation Task (DCT)

The DCT [33] is used to study visual focused attention and sustained attention. Participants are shown a picture containing a large set of black dots groups with a number of black dots including 3 dots, 4 dots and 5 dots on a computer (Fig. 2). They are required to click all the dot groups containing four dots with mouse as quickly as possible.

3.3   Mouse Tracking Task (MTT)

The MTT was designed to replace eye tracking [34]. Participants are required to follow a curve line by using computer mouse (Fig. 3). The tracking matching rate of the cursor on the curve line is used to evaluate the level of attention.

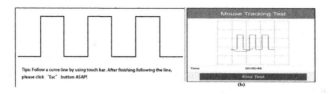

Fig. 3. An example of the MTT and an example of the task result

4   Discussion

4.1   Attention and Noise Level

Three different noise types are used i.e. atmospheric noise, man-made noise and industrial noise, to demonstrate the connection between the noise level and human attention level when participants are asked to complete DCT, and MTT. The atmospheric noise is of rainfall. The man-made noise is of hubbub in a coffee shop. The industrial noise is of large industrial fan blowing at high-speed. The participants listen to each of these noise types whilst completing their ABTs under three different loudness i.e. 40 dB, 60 dB and 80 dB.

4.1.1   Processing Speed of the Dot Cancellation Task (DCT)

Figures 4, 5 and 6 illustrates processing speed of the DCT when participants are listening to different levels of atmosphere noise, industrial noise and man-made noise respectively. The processing speed is calculated by the formula.

$$V = \frac{N}{T} \tag{1}$$

V is the processing speed of the DCT i.e. click per second. The higher the V value, the higher the performance of the participant. N is the number of 4 dot groups the participant processed. T is the total completion time in seconds. The red dots in the figures represent the averages processing speed under different types of noise and levels of noise, which are also summarized in Table 1 and Fig. 7.

Table 1. Average Processing Speed of the DCT under three different noise levels.

	40 dB	60 dB	80 dB
Type 1 atmospheric noise	0.3840	0.5364	0.7324
Type 2 industrial noise	0.8526	0.7560	0.6421
Type 3 man-made noise	0.7030	0.8567	0.8126

As shown in Table 1., average processing speed increases with the increasing levels of noise i.e. from 40 dB to 80 dB when participants are listening to the atmospheric noise and man-made noise whilst completing the ABTs. The average processing speeds under man-made noise are higher for all of the three levels of noise, than the average processing speed under the atmospheric noise. This indicates that the man-made noise may have a positive influence on the performance of participants in the DCT. However, the average processing speed decreases significantly under the industrial noise.

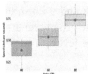 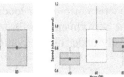 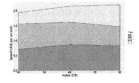

Fig. 4. DCT's processing speed under atmosphere noise. (Color figure online)

Fig. 5. Under industrial noise. (Color figure online)

Fig. 6. Under man-made noise. (Color figure online)

Fig. 7. Avg. of processing speed. (Color figure online)

As shown in Figs. 4, 5 and 6, different noise types significantly affect the performance of the DCT. Figure 7 illustrates the changes in average processing speed when participants are listening to different noise types at different loudness i.e. 40 dB, 60 dB, and 80 dB. Noise type 1, 2 and 3 represents atmosphere noise, industrial noise and man-made noise, and the height of each colour represents the mean of processing speed of each noise type under different levels of noise. As illustrated, the processing speed is at its lowest when the atmosphere noise is used at 40 dB, and the processing speed is at its highest when the man-made noise is used at 60 dB.

4.1.2 Matched Rates of the Mouse Tracking Task (MTT)

$$R_M = \frac{M}{T} \qquad (2)$$

R_M is the matched rate of the testing image. M is the number of black pixels that match the original image. T is the total number of black pixels of the test image.

In the group scenario, 4 participants on 4 computers are sitting in the same room to complete the ABTs. In the individual scenario, the participant is sitting alone in room to the complete the ABTs. Table 2 contains the average match rates under different types of noise and levels of noise.

Table 2. Match Rate – of the group and individual MTT under three different noise levels.

	40 dB	60 dB	80 dB
Group-atmosphere noise	0.6373	0.6583	0.7078
Type 1 atmospheric noise	0.6483	0.6531	0.6380
Type 2 industrial noise	0.6483	0.5967	0.5940
Type 3 man-made noise	0.6483	0.5693	0.6437

From Table 2, there is no significant difference in the average match rate between the group scenario and the individual scenario when participants are completing the ABTs whilst listening to atmospheric noise at any loudness. Figures 8 and 9 illustrate the box whisker plots showing the performance results of MTT from the group scenario and individual scenario respectively under different atmospheric noise levels.

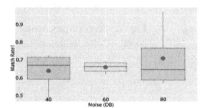
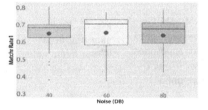

Fig. 8. Results of Matched Rate for group MTT under atmosphere noise.

Fig. 9. For individual.

As shown in Fig. 8, there is a slight increase in the match rate of the group scenario when the level of atmospheric noise increases from 40 dB to 80 dB. However, for the match rate of the individual scenario as shown in Fig. 9, there is only a difference of 0.01 between different levels of noise, which can be deemed negligible. Figures 10 and 11 shows the performance results of the MTT for the individual scenario when participants are listening to different noise levels of industrial noise and man-made noise respectively.

As shown in Figs. 10 and 11, when the individual participants are listening to the industrial noise and man-made noise, the match rates decrease by about 0.2 when the noise level changes from 40 dB to 60 dB. It can be inferred that the effect of the atmosphere noise on the performance of participants in MTT is barely noticeable, but different noise type can affect the performance of the participants in different ways in MTT.

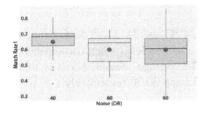

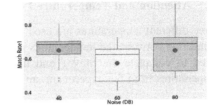

Fig. 10. Matched Rates - individual MTT under industrial noise.

Fig. 11. Under man-made noise.

4.1.3   Calmness Rates of the EEG Device-Muse

Table 3 contains the average calmness rate under different types of noise and levels of noise. Participants were most calm when listening to man-made noise at 60 dB while completing the ABTs. Participants were least calm when listening to industrial noise at 80 dB while completing the ABTs. It should be noted that there is no significant difference in the calmness rate when participants are listening to atmospheric noise at different noise levels.

Table 3. Calmness rate of the participants - individual MTT under three different noise levels.

	40 dB	60 dB	80 dB
Type 1 atmospheric noise	0.5257	0.5055	0.5047
Type 2 industrial noise	0.5257	0.4865	0.4004
Type 3 man-made noise	0.5257	0.6563	0.4313

Figures 12, 13 and 14 show the calmness rates of the participants under different level of atmospheric noise, industrial noise, and man-made noise respectively. The red dots in the figures represent the average calmness rates of the participants under different types of noise and levels of noise.

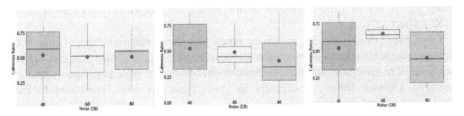

Fig. 12. Calmness rates under atmosphere noise.

Fig. 13. Industrial noise.

Fig. 14. Man-made noise.

4.2   Attention and Temperature Level

Three different temperatures are used i.e. 17 °C, 24 °C and 31 °C, to demonstrate the connection between the temperatures and human attention level when participants are asked to complete the SCWT and the DCT. The average measured values of the temperatures from the experiment are 17.38, 24.13 and 30.50 respectively.

4.2.1   Single-Click Times in the Stroop Color and Word Test (SCWT)

4.2.1.1 The Limitation of no Warm-up Question

Figure 15 shows that the amount of time the participants take to answer each question varies greatly, particularly for the first 9 questions when the participants are completing the ABTs in a room where temperature is set 17 °C i.e. level 1. Following the first nine questions, the average amount of time the participants take to answer each question remains approximately constant. This indicates that the participants require at least 9 questions to warm up for or get used to the SCWT.

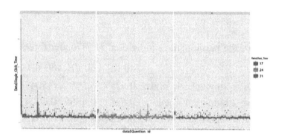

Fig. 15. Single click times for different question ID under three level of temperature

4.2.1.1 The Influence from Gender

Figures 16, 17 and 18 show the average amount of time the participants take to answer each question, splitting by genders i.e. male (1) and female (0), when they are completing the SCWT in a room with the temperature setting equal to 17 °C, 24 °C and 31 °C respectively.

From Figs. 16, 17 and 18, it can be noted that the average amount of time the female participants take to answer each question remains approximate constant under each level of temperature, and the average amount of time the male participants take to answer a question varies significantly in some questions when compared to the female's performance. When investigating the errors made in the SCWT, it is also interesting to note that errors are made by only female participants. This can be inferred that male participants are better at suppressing cognitive interference than females.

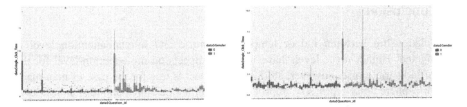

Fig. 16. The boxplot of single click time for different questions for female and male separately under the temperature of 17.

Fig. 17. Under the temperature of 24.

4.2.2 Processing Speed of the Dot Cancellation Task (DCT)

Figures 19 and 20 shows boxplot of processing speed for all participants when completing DCT under three different temperature settings. As shown in Fig. 19, most of the processing speed for all participants are between 0.5 and 0.9 number of 4 dots groups processed per second and the differences under the three temperature settings are barely noticeable. However, as shown in Fig. 20, significant differences exist as the temperature changes for some participants, and the tendency cannot be predicted.

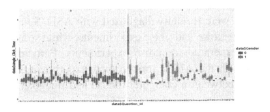

Fig. 18. The boxplot of single click time for different questions for female and male separately under the temperature of 31.

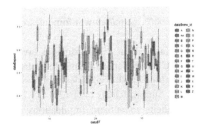

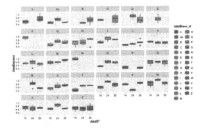

Fig. 19. The boxplot of data processing speed for each participant when they are tested under three different temperature

Fig. 20. The boxplot of data processing speed for each participant when they are tested under three different temperature

5 Conclusion

The relationship between indoor temperature, noise and human attention level is investigated. Higher noise levels have negative impacts on the attention-level for the case of industrial noise, however, an opposite impact is true for the case of man-made and atmosphere noise types. The impact of different temperatures on the attention-level of the female participants are lower than the male participants. However, it is interesting to note that the ability to suppress cognitive interference are lower in females as indicated by the errors made during the SCWT.

According to DSM-5, restricted and repetitive patterns of behavior, interests or activities is a part of the condition. This manifests in four varieties including sensory aspects of the environment. Further investigations are required to evidence the feasibility of using off-the-shelf devices to develop a sensory management recommendation system for people with ASD. However, the preliminary assumption here is that the impact from temperature and noise will be even more noticeable than in the case of neuro-typical people.

6 Limitations

There are 40 participants in total, including males and female with age range between 18 and 40. None of them were formally diagnosed with ASD. Some of the participants participated in both temperature and noise experiments, while some of the participants participated in either temperature or noise experiments. Participants were asked to familiarize themselves with the ABTs prior to their experiment. Participants of MTT were allowed to choose between a computer mouse and trackpad.

References

1. Cashin, A., Barker, P.: The triad of impairment in autism revisited. J. Child Adolesc. Psychiatr. Nurs. **22**, 189–193 (2009)
2. Introduction to Sensorial: Montessori Primary Guide (2006). http://www.infomontessori. com/sensorial/introduction.htm. Accessed 13 July 2018
3. Developmental Disabilities Monitoring Network Surveillance Year 2010 Principal Investigators; Centers for Disease Control and Prevention (CDC): Prevalence of autism spectrum disorder among children aged 8 years - autism and developmental disabilities monitoring network, 11 sites, United States, 2010. MMWR Surveill. Summ. **63**(2), 1–21 (2014)
4. Caminha, R.C., Lampreia, C.: Findings on sensory deficits in autism: implications for understanding the disorder. Psychol. Neurosci. **5**(2), 231–237 (2012)
5. Ingram, D., Takahashi, N., Miles, J.: Defining autism subgroups: a taxometric solution. J. Autism Dev. Disord. **38**, 950–960 (2008). https://doi.org/10.1007/s10803-007-0469-y
6. Walker, D., Thompson, A., Zwaigenbaum, L., Goldberg, J., Bryson, S., Mahoney, W.: Specifying PDD-NOS: a comparison of PDD-NOS, asperger syndrome, and autism. J. Am. Acad. Child Adolesc. Psychiatry **43**, 172–180 (2004). https://doi.org/10.1097/00004583-200402000-00012

7. Macintosh, K., Dissanayake, C.: Annotation: the similarities and differences between autistic disorder and asperger's disorder: a review of the empirical evidence. J. Child Psychol. Psychiatry **45**, 421–434 (2004). https://doi.org/10.1111/j.1469-7610.2004.00234.x

8. Frazier, T., Youngstrom, E., Speer, L., Embacher, R., Law, P., Constantino, J.: Validation of proposed DSM-5 criteria for autism spectrum disorder. J. Am. Acad. Child Adolesc. Psychiatry **51**, 28–40 (2012). https://doi.org/10.1016/j.jaac.2011.09.021

9. Huerta, M., Bishop, S., Duncan, A., Hus, V., Lord, C.: Application of DSM-5 criteria for autism spectrum disorder to three samples of children with DSM-IV diagnoses of pervasive developmental disorders. Am. J. Psychiatry **169**, 1056–1064 (2012)

10. Grzadzinski, R., Huerta, M., Lord, C.: DSM-5 and autism spectrum disorders (ASDs): an opportunity for identifying ASD subtypes. Mol. Autism. **4**(1), 12 (2013). Accessed 15 May 2013

11. Gillingham, G.: Autism: Handle with Care: Understanding and Managing Behaviour of Children and Adults with Autism. Future Education Inc., Arlington (1995)

12. El Kaliouby, R.: Affective computing and autism. Ann. N. Y. Acad. Sci. **1093**, 228–248 (2006)

13. Aresti-Bartolome, N., Garcia-Zapirain, B.: Technologies as support tools for persons with autistic spectrum disorder: a systematic review. Int. J. Env. Res. Public Health **11**, 7767–7802 (2014)

14. Simmons, D.R., Robertson, A.E., McKay, L.S., Toal, E., McAleer, P., Pollick, F.E.: Vision in autism spectrum disorders. Vis. Res. **49**(22), 2705–2739 (2009)

15. Gowen, E., Hamilton, A.: Motor abilities in autism: a review using a computational context. J. Autism Dev. Disord. **43**(2), 323–344 (2013)

16. Otto-Meyer, S., Krizman, J., White-Schwoch, T., et al.: Exp. Brain Res. **236**, 733 (2018). https://doi-org.ezproxy.nottingham.edu.cn/10.1007/s00221-017-5164-4

17. Sound Meter Source LLC (2018). https://soundmetersource.com/index.html

18. Murphy, E., King, E.A.: Testing the accuracy of smartphones and sound level meter applications for measuring environmental noise. Appl. Acoust. **106**, 16–22 (2015)

19. Murphy, E., King, E.A.: Testing the accuracy of smartphones and sound level meter applications for measuring environmental noise. Appl. Acoust. **106**, 16–22 (2016)

20. App Store: NIOSH Sound Level Meter, EA LAB (2019)

21. Warren, S.F., et al.: Whatautomatedvocal analysis reveals about the vocal production and language learning environment of young children with autism. J. Autism Dev. Disord. **40**, 555–569 (2010)

22. Critchley, H.D.: Electrodermal responses: what happens in the brain. Neuroscientist **8**, 132–142 (2002)

23. Chen, W., Cesar, P.: Physiological Measurement on Students' Engagement in a Distributed Learning Environment (2015)

24. Ruiz-Robledillo, N., Moya-Albiol, L.: Lower electrodermal activity to acute stress in caregivers of people with autism spectrum disorder: an adaptive habituation to stress. J. Autism Dev. Disord. **45**(2), 576–588 (2015)

25. Fenning, R.M., Baker, J.K., Baucom, B.R., et al.: Electrodermal variability and symptom severity in children with autism spectrum disorder. J. Autism Dev. Disord. **47**(4), 1–11 (2017)

26. McCarthy, C., Pradhan, N., Redpath, C., Adler, A.: Validation of the Empatica E4 wristband. In: Proceedings of the 2016 IEEE EMBS International Student Conference (ISC), Ottawa, ON, Canada, 29–31 May 2016, pp. 1–4 (2016)

27. Yekta, S.C., Niaz, C., Deniz, E., Cem, E.: Continuous stress detection using wearable sensors in real life: algorithmic programming contest case study. Sensors **19**(8), 1849 (2019)

28. Taj-Eldin, M., Ryan, C., O'Flynn, B., et al.: A review of wearable solutions for physiological and emotional monitoring for use by people with autism spectrum disorder and their caregivers. Sensors **18**(12), 4271 (2018)

29. Anderson, J.R.: Cognitive Psychology and Its Implications, 6th edn, p. 519. Worth Publishers, New York (2004)

30. Hayden, S.: Can this brain-sensing headband give you serenity, CNN (2014). http://edition.cnn.com/2014/08/18/tech/can-this-brain-sensing-headband/

31. Chawarska, K., Macari, S., Shic, F.: Decreased spontaneous attention to social scenes in 6-month-old infants later diagnosed with autism spectrum disorders. Biol. Psychiatry **74**, 195–203 (2013)

32. Stroop, J.R.: Studies of interference in serial verbal reactions. Exp. Psychol. **18**, 643 (1935)

33. Crawford, J.R., Parker, D.M., McKinlay, W.W.: A Handbook of Neuropsychological Assessment. Psychology Press, London (1992)

34. Buscher, G., et al.: Eye tracking analysis of preferred reading regions on the screen. In: CHI 2010 Extended Abstracts on Human Factors in Computing Systems (2010)

35. Budiu, R.: Between-Subjects vs. Within-Subjects Study Design (2018). https://www.nngroup.com/articles/between-within-subjects/

36. Gao, L.: Latin Squares in Experimental Design (2005). http://compneurosci.com/wiki/images/9/98/Latin_square_Method.pdf

37. The Latin Square Design. https://newonlinecourses.science.psu.edu/stat503/node/21/

Semantic Processing of Personality Description for Depression Patients

Zhisheng Huang[1,2,3], Qing Hu[1,2,3], Haiyuan Wang[1], Yahan Zhang[1],
Jie Yang[1,4], and Gang Wang[1,4(✉)]

[1] Advanced Innovation Center for Human Brain Protection,
Capital Medical University, Beijing, China
gangwangdoc@163.vip.com
[2] Department of Computer Science, VU University Amsterdam,
Amsterdam, The Netherlands
[3] College of Computer Science and Technology,
Wuhan Univesity of Science and Technology, Wuhan, China
[4] Beijing Anding Hospital, Capital Medical University, Beijing, China

Abstract. The personality description has been considered to be an important part of the electronic medical records (Emrs) for depression in-patients. However, the personality description of a patient is usually provided by a family member of the patient when he or she is admitted to the hospital. Because of non-professional background of those family members, personality descriptions in EMRS have various problems such as non-standard description, confusion between personality and behavior, and others. In this paper, we propose an approach to dealing with non-standard description of personality for depression patients by introducing a semantic relevance measure of personality. Furthermore, we make a mapping of those personality description items into the personality items in the well-known personality model of the Sixteen Personality Factor Questionnaire (16PF). We find some interesting observations on the connection between existing personality description in EMRs and the personality items in the 16PF model, and suggest possible improvement of the personality description in EMRs for depression patients.

Keywords: Depression · Personality · Semantic processing · Semantic relevance measure · 16 Personality Factor (16PF)

1 Introduction

Major depressive disorder (MDD), also known simply as depression, is a serious mental problem for the people in the modern society. Major depression disorder significantly affects the personal life of the patient, also has deep impact on the patient's family and personal relationships. The impact of MDD on functioning and well-being has been compared to that of other chronic medical diseases such as hypertension and diabetes. Major depressive disorder affects approximately

© Springer Nature Switzerland AG 2019
H. Wang et al. (Eds.): HIS 2019, LNCS 11837, pp. 263–275, 2019.
https://doi.org/10.1007/978-3-030-32962-4_24

216 million people in 2015, which is about the three percent of the population all over the world.

Personality description has been considered to be an important part in their electronic medical records (EMRs) for depression in-patients. The personality description of a patient is usually provided by a family member of the patient when the patient is admitted to the hospital. Because of non-professional background of those family members, personality descriptions in EMRS have various problems, such as non-standard description, confusion between personality and behavior, and others. It is very hard to use a statistical tool to explore the relationship between personality and diagnosis.

The research questions in this paper are: (i) Is it possible to obtain a meaningful list of personality items which can serve as the optional item list in EMRs for the personality description? (ii) Is it meaningful to use a standard glossary which is based on a theory of personality as the optional list in EMRs for depression patients.

In this paper, we propose an approach to dealing with non-standard description of personality for depression patients. The main idea is to introduce a semantic relevance measure to detect similar personality description, by which we can significantly reduce arbitrary description of personality and provide a standard way for the representation of personality description in EMRs. Compared it with well-known approach in machine learning such as Word2Vec approach, we can show that semantic relevance measure approach has a significant advantage over the traditional machine learning approach. We use the 2792 patient data of depression in Beijing Anding Hospital, which consists of 8954 personality descriptions. By *personality item*, we mean a primitive description of personality. A personality description consists of a set of personality items. We obtain 439 personality items from the 8954 personality descriptions over 2792 EMRs. By using the semantic relevance measure approach and others, 439 personality description items can be reduced into 172 items (61% reduced). That reduced list can serve as the optional list for the personality items in EMRs. That improvement also provides the possibility to use a statistical tool to make the analysis on the relationship between personality and diagnosis.

The Sixteen Personality Factor Questionnaire (16PF)[1] is a well-known modeling for the personality theory which is developed by Raymond B. Cattell, Maurice Tatsuoka and Herbert Eber [2]. The 16PF provides a measure of normal personality and can also be used by psychologists, and other mental health professionals as a clinical instrument to help diagnose psychiatric disorder [9,12]. In this paper, we explore the relationship between the reduced list of the personality items and the personality elements in 16PF. We have several interesting observations on that relations. Our observations are (i) the list of personality items in 16PF does not cover all of the personality items which are needed for depression patients, and (ii) the list of personality items in 16PF is too large to serve as a candidate list for depression patients. That answers our second research question.

---

[1] https://en.wikipedia.org/wiki/16PF_Questionnaire.

The contributions of this paper are: (i) we propose a semantic relevance measure to deal with arbitrary description of personality for depression patient, (ii) we show how this semantic relevance measure can be used for the standardization of personality description, (iii) we show the proposed approach has better performance that which is used on traditional machine learning approach, (iv) we report several observations on the relationship between the reduced list of personality item and the personality items in 16PF.

This paper is organized as follows: Sect. 2 presents the basic structure of personality description in EMRs and their problems. Section 3 presents the framework of semantic processing on personality description, and proposes an approach based on semantic relevance measure over the descriptions. Section 4 reports our experiments. Section 5 explores the relation between the reduced list of personality description and those in 16PF. Section 6 discusses related work, future work, and make the conclusions.

2   Personality Description in Depression Patient Data

The personality description usually appears in the front page of EMRs, like this:

- Patient ID: 61152
- Gender Female
- Age: 40
- Diagnosis: Recurrent depressive disorder, currently severe depressive episode without psychotic symptoms
- ICD10 Code: F32.2
- Main complaint: Low mood, insomnia for 9 years, aggravated for 2 weeks
- Current medical history: In 2008, after half a year of laparotomy, the patient did not like to go out, lazy, insomnia, lack of energy, did not like to talk, did not contact family and outsiders, and was diagnosed as "postpartum depression" at a local hospital. One month, after giving the drug treatment, she was discharged from the hospital. Five years ago, after leaving the company due to unsatisfactory work, the above symptoms appeared. She was diagnosed as "anxious and depressed state". .... Three months ago, the company began to lay off employees, patients lost their jobs, worried about mortgage after losing their jobs, worried about the future, to adjust their mood, took their son and parents to travel to Lijiang two weeks ago, worked hard, and returned to Beijing, the mood was depressed, not willing to go out and don't want to see people. Lie in bed all day, repeatedly go online to find disease-related information, occasionally have a concept of suicide, no self-injury, no suicide plan, poor eating, insomnia, and night sleep for about 3 h....
- Pre-disease personality: Timid, sensitive and suspicious, temperament, guilty, inferior.

Namely, the personality description is provided as one of the most important items at the front page of EMRs. The personality is described for that of the patient before she or he suffers from the disease. Those personality descriptions are usually provided by a family member when the patient is admitted into the hospital. However, because of unprofessional background of the family member, personality descriptions in EMRs have various problems:

Here are some typical problems at the personality description:

- Unnecessary Additional Description: Some unnecessary additional words are used to describe the personality. For example, "active" is described as "personality is active when she was young".
- Inappropriate Description: Use some inappropriate words to describe the personality. For example, "lively" is described as "somehow lively".
- Composition: Combing several personality items into a single one. For example, "inferior" and "does not like to talk" is described as "does not like to talk because of personality".
- Confusion between personality and result: Use the words about the result to describe the personality. For example, use the word "study grades are good at the school" to describe the personality.

Arbitrary and non-professional description of personality in depression patient data would make it very hard to use a statistical tool to explore the relationship between personality and diagnosis. Ideally, EMR systems should provide a standard list for the personality description, so that it can be selected by the family member when the patient data is made. The work of this paper is an attempt to obtain a meaningful list of personality list from existing EMRs for depression patients, The selected list for the personality items would be able to provide all the necessary items for the description and would not contain too many non-relevant items for the selection, In the following we will discuss how the goal can be achieved.

3   Framework

In this section, we will propose a framework to obtain a meaningful list of personality items, which can be used for EMRs for depression patients. Figure 1 presents the main workflow for the processing.

- *Extract Personality Description:* It is rather easy to extract personality description from EMRs. As shown in the previous section, personality description is usually provided as a separated items at the front page of EMRs. It is easy to detect and extract the personality description from the XML-formatted file.
- *Extract Personality Item:* We can extract personality items from extracted personality descriptions. Those personality items are usually separated by the comma.
- *Pre-processing Personality Items:* We need the pre-processing on the personality items to remove the items contain those typical errors which are discussed in the previous section, It is quite easy to detect those errors, either by using a NLP tool or by manual.

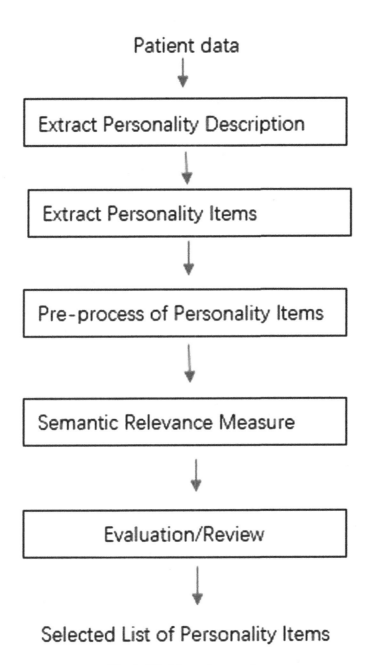

Fig. 1. Workflow of processing

- *Semantic Relevance Measure:* After the pre-processing, we can obtain a candidate list of personality items, we use a semantic relevance measure to detect similar items which are semantically equivalent, then we can merge those detected items.
- *Evaluation and Review:* In the procedure of review, we examine the ranking result of the semantic relevance measure. That examination would start from the top items in the ranking, and decide which item would be merged with their semantically closest items and which items would not be merged.

There are various methods for the semantic relevance measure. It can be based on a machine learning approach like word2vec. It can be based on a domain ontology/terminology approach in which the semantic distance can be calculated based on the connected edge numbers in the ontology. In this paper, we will propose a semantic relevance measure to detect synonym of those personality description items, so that they can be merged and reduced with respect to their semantic meaning, based on Search engine. The advantage of using semantic relevance measure with a search engine is that the relevance measure can be calculated simply via the co-occurrence of terms in a search engine such as Google. The semantic relevance measure is based on the assumption that the more frequently two terms co-occur in the same paper, the more semantically related they are. This assumption is inspired by the Normalized Google Distance from [3,4]. The equation for our Normalized Google Distance (NGD) is as follows:

$$NGD(x,y) = \frac{max\{\log f(x), \log f(y)\} - \log f(x,y)}{\log M - min\{\log f(x), \log f(y)\}}$$

or Where $f(x)$ is the number of Google hits for the search term x; $f(y)$ is the number of Google hits for the search term y; $f(x,y)$ is the number of Google hits for the search terms x and y; M is the number of webpages indexed in Google. $NGD(x,y)$ can be understood intuitively as the symmetric conditional probability of co-occurrence of x and y.

The relation between the semantic relevance and the semantic distance is that the less the semantic distances of two items are, the more the semantic relevance of two items are. We have used this semantic relevance measure approach for medical guideline update [5–7]. We have shown that Google-based semantic distance measure has much better performance, compared with that by using other methods [5–7].

4   Experiment and Results

We have developed a system which can do the processing based on the framework which is proposed in the previous section. We have conducted the experiments for the processing. We use the 2792 patients data of depression in Beijing Anding Hospital, which consists of 8954 primitive personality descriptions. 8954 primitive personality description consist of 433 personality items. In the stage of pre-processing, we remove the items which suffer from the typical problems above by manually checking and merge those duplicated description. That procedure results in 233 personality items.

We implement a tool for a semantic relevance measure by using Google distance calculation. For those 233 personality items, semantic distance values are obtained. In the stage of evaluation/review, we examine the two personality items in which the semantic distance is almost zero (<0.0013). The semantic distance with zero means that those two items may be semantically equivalent. Thus, we detect 42 meaningful pairs out of 64 combinations (65.6%). That process results in 172 primitive (i.e., non-compositive) personality items. Those selected 172 personality items can serve as the candidate list which can be used in EMRs for depression patients.

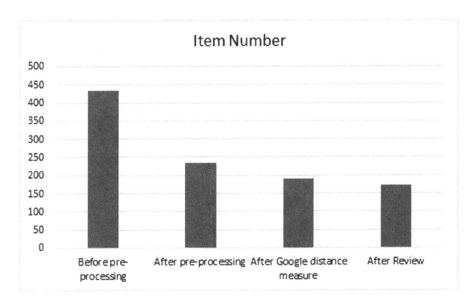

Fig. 2. Item numbers in the workflow

The change of the item numbers in the workflow is shown in Fig. 2. The change of the reduction rate in the workflow is shown in Fig. 3.

We also make a comparison work with that by using the approach word2vec, a well-known method in machine learning, for similar word processing. Word2vec can effectively represent a word into a vector through the optimized training model, according to the given corpus. Word2vec contains two models, skip-gram and Continuous Bag of Word (CBOW) [11, 13]. The direct purpose of skip-gram and CBOW models is to obtain high-quality word vectors, and simplify the training steps to optimize the model, which directly reduces the computational complexity. In this way, the relationship among words can be measured quantitatively, and the distance of two words can be calculated by Word2vec.

We get and train some Chinese text such as news, Baidu encyclopedia and novels from the Web as the Chinese corpus to train on the computer and form

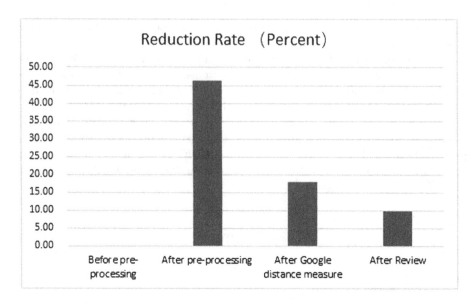

Fig. 3. Reduction rate in the workflow

a vector file about 1.5G. Based on this corpus, the following testing steps are designed:

1. Segment the personality items by the word segmentation model Jieba.
2. Check the segmentation effect, and extract the central word from the multiple segmentations.
3. Retrieve whether the central word is in the corpus.
4. Calculate the distance between each two words.

The model Jieba may cause some segmentation errors in some oral descriptions, so step 2 is indispensable. After step 3, 185 of the 233 personality items are available (79%), as the central word cannot be extracted from the items or the item is not in the corpus. The calculation results show that there are only 3 pairs of these items with a distance of less than 0.05 and 30 pairs with a distance of less than 0.1. In the calculation of lexical distance based on Word2Vec, the corpus has a great influence on the results and can directly determine whether the results are available or not. This corpus is based on news or encyclopedias, with few descriptions of mental illness and people's feelings.

5   Exploring Relations with 16PF

Personality has been well studied in Psychology. The Sixteen Personality Factor Questionnaire (16PF) is a widely used tool for the personality test, as we have discussed above. Raymond Cattell's 16 Personality Factors cover the primary factor such as Warmth, which corresponds with the personality items such as

Personality Factor	Factor Abbr	High/Low Range	Element Number
Warmth	A	+	9
Warmth	A	-	4
Reasoning	B	+	6
Reasoning	B	-	5
Emotional Stability	C	+	4
Emotional Stability	C	-	5
Dominance	E	+	11
Dominance	E	-	4
Liveliness	F	+	7
Liveliness	F	-	7
Rule-Consciousness	G	+	9
Rule-Consciousness	G	-	3
Social Boldness	H	+	8
Social Boldness	H	-	5
Sensitivity	I	+	2
Sensitivity	I	-	2
Vigilance	L	+	4
Vigilance	L	-	0
Abstractedness	M	+	6
Abstractedness	M	-	0
Privateness	N	+	0
Privateness	N	-	7
Apprehension	O	+	10
Apprehension	O	-	4
Openness to Change	Q1	+	5
Openness to Change	Q1	-	1
Self-Reliance	Q2	+	5
Self-Reliance	Q2	-	5
Perfectionism	Q3	+	13
Perfectionism	Q3	-	5
Tension	Q4	+	4
Tension	Q4	-	4
Unknown	UK	N/A	9
		Total	173

Fig. 4. Mapping Personality Elements into 16PF. "+" means the high range, and "-" means the low range. Factor Abbr means the abbreviation of the personality factor.

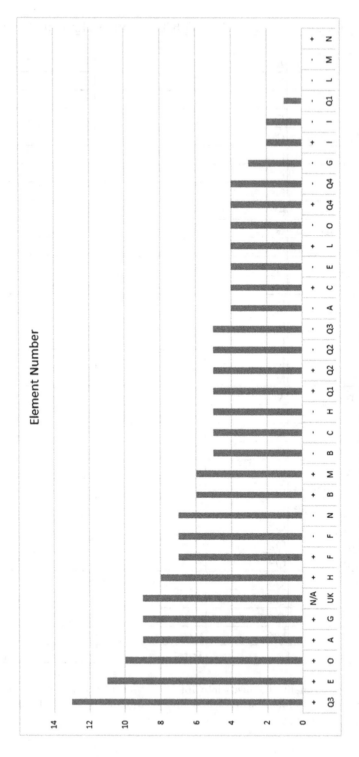

Fig. 5. Ranked distribution of personality elements in the 16PF.

Impersonal, distant, cool, reserved, detached, formal, aloof at the Descriptors of low range, and the personality items such as Warm, outgoing, attentive to others, kindly, easy-going, participating, likes people at the Descriptors of high range. The primary factor Reasoning corresponds with the items such as concrete thinking, lower general mental capacity, less intelligent, unable to handle abstract problems at the Descriptors of low range, and the personality items such as Abstract-thinking, more intelligent, bright, higher general mental capacity, fast learner at the Descriptors of high range. The other primary factors are Emotional Stability (e.g. easily upset or mature), Dominance (e.g. obedient or competitive), Liveliness (e.g. taciturn or lively), Rule-Consciousness (e.g. disregards rules or rule bound), Social Boldness (e.g, shy or venturesome), Sensitivity (e.g. tough minded or tender minded), Vigilance (e.g., easy or skeptical), Abstractedness (e.g., practical, or impractical), Privateness (e.g., open, or discreet), Apprehension (e.g., self-satisfied or self blaming), Openness to Change (e.g., traditional, or free thinking), Self-Reliance (e.g., group-oriented or solitary), Perfectionism (e.g. flexible or organized), and Tension (e.g. relaxed, or impatient).

We have made a mapping from the 173 personality elements which are obtained by the semantic processing above into the elements in the 16 PF. Figure 4 shows that how many personality elements can be mapped into their personality factor with respect to high range or low range in the 16PF. From the mapping, we have the following interesting observation:

– The most frequent personality elements for depression patients appear in the high range of the personality factor Perfectionism Q3 (13 elements). The second most frequent personality elements appear in the high range of the personality factor Dominance E (11 elements), and the third one the rank is in the high range of the personality factor Apprehension O (10 elements). The ranked factors are shown in Fig. 5.
– There are no personality elements for depression patients which occur in the low range of the personality factor Vigilance, and in the low range of the personality factor Abstractedness, and in the high range of the personality factor Privateness.
– There are nine personality elements (such as generous and humorous, etc.) which cannot be found their corresponding elements in the 16PF.

The frequent appearance of personality elements at the high range of the personality factor Perfectionism supports for the claim that maladaptive, unhealthy, or neurotic perfectionism, where anything less than perfect is unacceptable, can leave individuals vulnerable to depression [1, 10]. We can also find some similar evidence to explain the reason why the high range of the factor Dominance is the second top one [8]. There are three ranges which have no any personality elements. Furthermore, there exist significant amount of personality elements which can classified into ones in the ranges of any personality factor. Those justify that the 16PF model cannot be simply used in EMRs for depression patients.

6   Discussion and Conclusion

In this paper, we have presented a semantic-distance-based approach for processing personality elements in EMRs for depression patients. Our experiment shows that we can obtaining a meaningful selected list of the personality elements. That selected list can serve as a standard list for the personality description when a family member states the personality traits of the patients. We also make the comparison work with those obtained by using the machine learning approach word2vec.

We have also made the mapping of those selected list of personality elements into the elements in well-known model 16PF. We have several interesting observation on the connection between selected personality elements and those in 16PF. That mapping provides an easy way to obtain the 16PF result from EMRs which use the selected list of personality elements. That also justifies that we cannot simply use 16PF model in the EMR system for depression patients. The work done in this paper provides the possibility for further exploration on the connection between personality and diagnosis for various types of depression. That would be one of our future work.

References

1. Blatt, S.J.: The destructiveness of perfectionism. Implications for the treatment of depression. Am. Psychol. **50**(12), 1003–1020 (1995)
2. Cattell, R.B.: The description of personality: basic traits resolved into clusters. J. Abnorm. Soc. Psychol. **38**(4), 476–506 (1943)
3. Cilibrasi, R., Vitanyi, P.M.B.: The google similarity distance. IEEE Trans. Knowl. Data Eng. **19**, 370–383 (2007)
4. Cilibrasi, R., Vitanyi, P.: Automatic meaning discovery using Google. Technical report, Centre for Mathematics and Computer Science, CWI (2004)
5. Hu, Q., Huang, Z., ten Teije, A., van Harmelen, F.: Detecting new evidence for evidence-based guidelines using a semantic distance method. In: Holmes, J.H., Bellazzi, R., Sacchi, L., Peek, N. (eds.) AIME 2015. LNCS (LNAI), vol. 9105, pp. 307–316. Springer, Cham (2015). https://doi.org/10.1007/978-3-319-19551-3_39
6. Hu, Q., Huang, Z., van Harmelen, F., ten Teije, A., Gu, J.: Evidence-based clinical guidelines in semanticCT. In: Zhao, D., Du, J., Wang, H., Wang, P., Ji, D., Pan, J.Z. (eds.) CSWS 2014. CCIS, vol. 480, pp. 198–212. Springer, Heidelberg (2014). https://doi.org/10.1007/978-3-662-45495-4_18
7. Huang, Z., ten Teije, A., van Harmelen, F., Aït-Mokhtar, S.: Semantic representation of evidence-based clinical guidelines. In: Miksch, S., Riaño, D., ten Teije, A. (eds.) KR4HC 2014. LNCS (LNAI), vol. 8903, pp. 78–94. Springer, Cham (2014). https://doi.org/10.1007/978-3-319-13281-5_6
8. Johnson, S.L., Leedom, L.J., Muhtadie, L.: The dominance behavioral system and psychopathology: evidence from self-report, observational, and biological studies. Psychol Bull. **138**(4), 692–743 (2012)
9. Karson, W., O'Dell, J.W.: A Guide to the Clinical Use of the 16PF. University of Michigan Press, Ann Arbor (1976)
10. Melrose, S.: Perfectionism and depression: vulnerabilities nurses need to understand. Nurs. Res. Pract. **2011**, 858497 (2011)

11. Mikolov, T., Chen, K., Corrado, G., Dean, J., et al.: Efficient estimation of word representations in vector space. Computer Science (2013)
12. Schuerger, J.M.: Career assessment and the sixteen personality factor questionnaire. J. Career Assess. **3**(2), 157–175 (1995)
13. Mikolov, T., Sutskever, I., Chen, K., Corrado, G.S., Dean, J.: Distributed representations of words and phrases and their compositionality. Adv. Neural Inf. Process. Syst. **26**, 3111–3119 (2013)

Healthcare

Genetically Tailored Sports and Nutrition Actions to Improve Health

Jitao Yang[(⊠)]

School of Information Science, Beijing Language and Culture University,
Beijing 100083, China
yangjitao@blcu.edu.cn

Abstract. With the development of molecular biology techniques, genomics is broadly introduced to expound the individual difference and molecular mechanism. Effects of genetic diversity on sports performance have been more and more found by scientists. For instance, studies on association of gene polymorphisms and training response mainly intend to discover the effects of different genotypes on the effectiveness of aerobic exercise training to increase aerobic physical fitness. Genes related to training response primarily include PPARD, PPARGC1A, ACTN3, ACE, HBB, TFAM, NFR2, AR and etc. Gene polymorphisms of PPARD and PPARGC1A are shown to be associated with post-training individual anaerobic threshold. ACE is one of the earliest and most studied gene in genes related to endurance performance that ACE is a carboxypeptidase, the key enzyme in Renin-angiotensin system, it was found in many tissues in the body including skeletal muscle, associated to functions of degrading bradykinin and transferring angiotensin I to angiotensin II. Therefore, genetic testing can help people to know the precise information on how body uniquely responds to exercise. Based on the deeper understanding of a person's genetics and physiology information, in this paper, we provide a platform with sports and nutrition actions that are tailored specifically for different people to optimize their sports performance and effects as well as improve their health.

Keywords: Genomics · Genetics · Sports · Nutrition · Healthcare

1 Introduction

Due to the fast development of molecular biology techniques, genomics is broadly introduced to expound the individual difference in sports performance, sport-related injuries, sports nutrition, and sports effects. Sports genomics [2,3] is used to build individualized training plans and personalized nutrition to improve health.

The physical capacity of individual is a complex phenotype that affected by human genome and environmental contexts. Sports abilities and competences are associated with many genes, variations in our genes influences the components of muscles, effect of training to improve endurance capacity, effect of physical

© Springer Nature Switzerland AG 2019
H. Wang et al. (Eds.): HIS 2019, LNCS 11837, pp. 279–286, 2019.
https://doi.org/10.1007/978-3-030-32962-4_25

activities on improving blood glucose, exercise fatigue degree, anterior cruciate ligaments protection ability, exercise time choice, etc.

To receive a good sports effect, we should know that people's sports capacity and sports nutrition requirements are different from each other. However, these differences in our personal sports and nutrition actions are ignored by most of the current sports guidance.

Genomics technologies and polygenic model [1] are closely connected to the development of personalized health, sports genomics has a great influence in establishing sports and nutrition advice for individuals.

In this paper, we demonstrate our sports genomics algorithm platform, based on which, we can analyze people's DNA and provide genetically tailored sports and nutrition actions for people to improve their sports effects and health.

2   Sports and Nutrition Genomics

The sports capacity of a person is affected by a variety of factors, including environment and genes. Based on the scientific evidences [4,5], it looks promising that genes influence the sports and nutrition effects. For instance, hundreds of scientific articles [16] provide solid evidence that the genes of ACE I/D and ACTN3 R577X have associations with endurance and power-related performance [5]; PPARD and PPARGC1A both have effects on the effectiveness of aerobic exercise training [22]. COL12A1 gene encodes the alpha chain of type XII collagen, a member of the FACIT (fibril-associated collagens with interrupted triple helices) collagen family, COL12A1 has a connection with the risk of having ACL (Anterior Cruciate Ligaments) injury [25]. COL3A1 [26] and COL1A1 [27] are also genetic risk factors for ACL injury. Therefore, DNA test in sport and nutrition is available to identify personal capacity for better respond to training and nutrition, while lesser suffer from injuries.

3   Sports and Nutrition Actions

3.1   DNA Test

To have a DNA test, a saliva collection kit will be sent to the user, after splitting saliva to a special saliva collection tube, the user should register the sample number, user name, age, gender, and the other personal information through the online WeChat or mobile App system, then the saliva tube should be mailed to the genomics lab to extract the DNA. The DNA will be sequenced by sequencing equipment, such as next generation sequencing NovaSeq [8], or iScan [7] with Infinium Global Screening Array-24 Kit [6]. Then the sequenced DNA data will be analyzed and interpreted by our genomics and genetics algorithm platform.

3.2   DNA Genetic Interpretation

We have designed and developed an algorithm platform for analyzing personal genetic data to recommend individually tailored sports and nutrition actions.

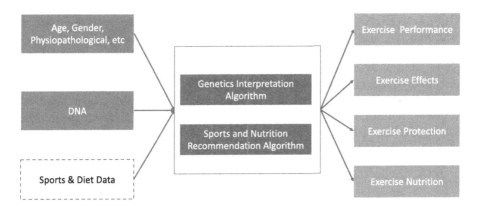

Fig. 1. The sports genomics and tailored actions working mechanism.

The platform models how SNPs (Single nucleotide polymorphisms) impact the Exercise Performance, Exercise Effects, Exercise Protection, and Exercise Nutrition, with the following genetic testing items:

- Exercise Performance: Inborn Endurance VS. Power, Endurance, Power, Effect of Training to Improve Endurance Capacity.
- Exercise Effects: Core Temperature Increasing Speed while Exercising, Exercise Fatigue Degree, Effect of Physical Activities on Losing Weight, Effect of Physical Activities on Improving Blood Glucose, Effect of Physical Activities on Improving Blood Pressure, Effect of Physical Activities on Improving Blood Lipid.
- Exercise Protection: Achilles Tendon Protection Ability, Anterior Cruciate Ligaments Protection Ability, Lumbar Inter-vertebral Disc Protection Ability, Rotator Cuff Protection Ability.
- Exercise Nutrition: Carbohydrate Choice while Exercising, Protein Choice while Exercising, Vitamin D Requirement while Exercising, Omega-3 Requirement while Exercising, Folate Requirement while Exercising, Effect of Caffeine on Exercise, Exercise Time Choice.

Figure 1 demonstrates the working mechanism from sports genomics to individually tailored actions. We now give a few examples to explain the relationships between genes and sports.

(1) Genes related to endurance performance:
A lot of extensive and in-depth researches have disclosed the association between genes and endurance performance. The genes: Angiotensin Converting Enzyme (ACE), Mitochondrial DNA (mtDNA), Peroxisome Proliferator Activated Receptors (PPARs), Adrenaline Receptors (ADR), Guanine Nucleotide Binding Protein β Polypeptide 3 (GNB3), and Nuclear Respiratory Factor 2 (NRF2) have been studied to have close connections with endurance performance. The genes including CKMM, BDKRB2, GH1, NOS3, COL5A1 [9],

COL6A1, VEGF, and VEGFR2 also have associations with endurance performance.

ACE is a carboxypeptidase, which is the key enzyme in Renin-angiotensin system. It was found in many tissues in the body including skeletal muscle, associated to functions of degrading bradykinin and transferring angiotensin I to angiotensin II [10]. ACE is the earliest and most studied gene related to endurance performance [11]. The first study concerning ACE was appeared in 1998 [12], followed by many researches finding ACE II genotype is probably a genetic marker for better endurance performance compared with DD genotype. The researches were conducted with marathoner [13,14], rower and ice skater.

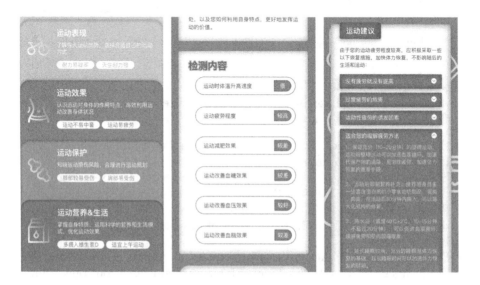

Fig. 2. The Home Screen (left), DNA Test Results (middle), and Sports Actions (right)

(2) Genes related to power performance:

Power in exercise is an ability to produce force with high speed, playing a major role in short-distance and high-speed sports. Compared with the researches of gene polymorphisms in endurance performance, studies of genes related to power are carried out fairly late [15]. The genes [16] involved include α-Actinin 3 (ACTN3), Angiotensin Converting Enzyme (ACE), Growth Differential Factor-8 (GDF-8), Interleukin-6 (IL-6), hypoxia-inducible factor-1 (HIF-1), etc.

ACTN3 encodes a member of alpha-actin binding protein family, as a structural component of sarcomeric Z line, primarily expressed in skeletal muscle and functions. There are four members in alpha-actin binding protein gene family: α-Actinin 1 & 4 were found in unstriated muscle, α-Actinin 2 was found in all skeletal muscle fibers, while α-Actinin 3 (ACTN3) was found in fast muscle fiber only [17]. Scientists mainly focus on gene variation of ACTN3 R577X (rs1815739), on which C-T variation can cause termination of the coding. Once the coding is

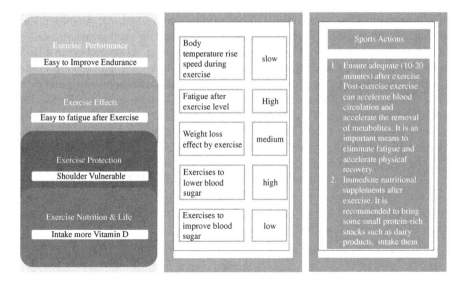

Fig. 3. The Home Screen (left), DNA Test Results (middle), and Sports Actions (right), Fig. 2 was partially translated in English

terminated, deletion of α-Actinin 3 will occur [18]. In 2003, Australian Institute of Sport and University of Sydney found that ACTN3 RR genotype has significantly higher percentage in power athletes and power Olympians compared to endurance athletes and other power athletes, especially in female athletes. The research was conducted with participants from track athletes (<800 m), swimmers competing in events <200 m, judo athletes, short-distance track cyclists and speed skaters [19].

(3) Genes related to training response:
Studies on association of gene polymorphisms and training response mainly intend to discover the effects of different genotypes on the effectiveness of aerobic exercise training to increase aerobic physical fitness [20,21]. Genes related to training response primarily include PPARD, PPARGC1A, ACTN3, ACE, HBB, TFAM, NFR2, AR, and so on [23]. Gene polymorphisms of PPARD and PPARGC1A were shown to be associated with post-training individual anaerobic threshold [22]. In addition, a person's ACTN3 (R577X) with genotype XX demonstrated a greater 1-repetition maximum (60% increase) after resistance training compared with the person whose ACTN3's genotype is RR (30% increase) [24].

3.3 Actions

Figure 2 demonstrates the user interface (in Chinese) of our delivered online mobile smartphone application, Fig. 3 partially translates the contents of Fig. 2 into English. The homepage (Fig. 3, left) summarizes the DNA test results categorized in 4 panels: sports performance, sports effect, sports protection, and sports nutrition. The emphasized DNA testing results (such as: Shoulder Vulnerable, Easy to Improve Endurance) were highlighted in each panel.

Click each panel, more sub test items will be shown, as described in Fig. 3, middle. Each item is listed through a bar frame that the left side is item name, the right side is the genetic testing result with a colored background button.

For more information concerning the testing item, user can click on the bar frame, then as shown in Fig. 3, right, the detail testing information about the item, the suggested sports actions, the scientific background about the testing item, and the reference scientific publications are displayed in separate blocks.

Based on different individual's genetic testing result, our platform can give suggested actions from different aspects. For example, ACL is located in front of the knee joint, behind the patella, it plays a very important role in physical activities, based on the testing result of ACL related genes, the platform will consider the following aspects:

- Risk-related Sports: it is important for users to know what kind of sports are related to ACL injury, in order to be more caution when doing these sports.
- Risk factors: the platform will tell users the specific movements in different sports could possibly cause ACL injury.
- Symptoms: users will know the sign of ACL injury and do self-check easily at home.
- Prevention solution: this part provides important and specific advice and solution in daily life and exercise that can prevent from incidence of ACL injury.
- Nutrition and supplements: suitable nutritional supplement is will be provided for sport performance and recovery.

The actions will include unique warm up, performance, recovery, nutrition, and supplementation suggestions for each person. These actions are designed to empower individuals and encourage the development of new habits and training strategies to help individuals optimize their sports performance and health.

4   Conclusions

Sport and nutrition are very important part of our daily life, general population are currently more and more interested in finding solutions to find the sports activities that are personalized for them, people are also trying to find solutions to optimize their sports performance and sports effects, the fast recovery after sports will be helpful for people to get back quickly to their jobs and daily life, most importantly, people do not want to get injured in sports. The physical capacity of individual is a complex phenotype that affected by environmental contexts as well as human genome. Although it is important to know that the environment impacts many aspects of sports, genes are very critical factors that influence the sports abilities and effects of different people.

In this paper, based on DNA sequencing data, we demonstrate our sports and nutrition genomics data analysis platform, which is available to create more precise and tailored sports and nutrition actions to individuals, so that to help people to optimize sport performance and effects. Please note that, the platform also supports to consider the dynamic sports (from sports bracelet) and diet data to give personalized daily sports and nutrition advice, the research will be published in the near future.

Acknowledgment. This work was partially supported by the Science Foundation of Beijing Language and Culture University (supported by "the Fundamental Research Funds for the Central Universities") (19YJ040010, 17YJ0302, 15YJ030001, 18YJ030006)

References

1. Khera, A.V., et al.: Genome-wide polygenic scores for common diseases identify individuals with risk equivalent to monogenic mutations. Nat. Genet. **50**(9), 1219–1224 (2018)
2. Eynon, N., et al.: The FTO A/T polymorphism and elite athletic performance: a study involving three groups of European athletes. PLoS ONE **8**(4), e60570 (2013). https://doi.org/10.1371/journal.pone.0060570
3. Ahmetov, I.I., Fedotovskaya, O.N.: Sports genomics: current state of knowledge and future directions. Cell. Mol. Exerc. Physiol. **1**, e1 (2012)
4. Lippi, G., Longo, U.G., Maffulli, N.: Genetics and sports. Br. Med. Bull. **93**(1), 27–47 (2010)
5. Guth, L.M., Roth, S.M.: Genetic influence on athletic performance. Curr. Opin. Pediatr. **25**(6), 653–658 (2013)
6. Infinium Global Screening Array-24 Kit. https://www.illumina.com/products/by-type/microarray-kits/infinium-global-screening.html. Accessed 11 June 2019
7. iScan System. https://www.illumina.com/systems/array-scanners/iscan.html. Accessed 11 June 2019
8. NovaSeq 6000 Sequencing System. https://www.illumina.com/systems/sequencing-platforms/novaseq.html. Accessed 11 June 2019
9. Raleigh, S.M., van der Merwe, L., Ribbans, W.J., Smith, R.K., Schwellnus, M.P., Collins, M.: Variants within the MMP3 gene are associated with Achilles tendinopathy: possible interaction with the COL5A1 gene. Br. J. Sport Med. **43**(7), 514–520 (2009)
10. Jones, A., Woods, D.R.: Skeletal muscle RAS and exercise performance. Int. J. Biochem. Cell Biol. **35**(6), 855–866 (2003)
11. Sawczuka, M., Maciejewska, A., Cieszczyk, P., Eider, J.: The role of genetic research in sport. Sci. Sports **26**(5), 251–258 (2011)
12. Gayagay, G., et al.: Elite endurance athletes and the ACE I allele-the role of genes in athletic performance. Hum Genet. **103**(1), 48–50 (1998)
13. Hruskovicova, H., Dzurenkova, D., Selingerova, M., Bohus, B., Timkanicova, B., Kovacs, L.: The angiotensin converting enzyme I/D polymorphism in long distance runners. J. Sports Med. Phys. Fitness **46**(3), 509–513 (2006)
14. Tobina, T., et al.: Association between the angiotensin I-converting enzyme gene insertion/deletion polymorphism and endurance running speed in Japanese runners. J. Physiol. Sci. **60**(5), 325–330 (2010)
15. Eynon, N., et al.: Genes for elite power and sprint performance: ACTN3 leads the way. Sports Med. **43**(9), 803–817 (2013)

16. Ma, F., et al.: The association of sport performance with ACE and ACTN3 genetic polymorphisms: a systematic review and meta-analysis. PLoS ONE **8**(1), e54685 (2013)

17. Grealy, R., Smith, C.L., Chen, T., Hiller, D., Haseler, L.J., Griffiths, L.R.: The genetics of endurance: frequency of the ACTN3 R577X variant in Ironman World Championship athletes. J. Sci. Med. Sport **16**(4), 365–371 (2013)

18. Cieszczyk, P., Sawczuk, M., et al.: ACTN3 R577X polymorphism in top-level Polish rowers. J. Exerc. Sci. Fit. **10**(1), 12–15 (2012)

19. Yang, N., et al.: ACTN3 genotype is associated with human elite athletic performance. Am. J. Hum. Genet. **73**(3), 627–631 (2003)

20. Karavirta, L., et al.: Individual responses to combined endurance and strength training in older adults. Med. Sci. Sports Exerc. **43**(3), 484–490 (2011)

21. Perusse, L., et al.: Advances in exercise, fitness, and performance genomics in 2012. Med. Sci. Sports Exerc. **45**(5), 824–831 (2013)

22. Stefan, N., et al.: Genetic variations in PPARD and PPARGC1A determine mitochondrial function and change in aerobic physical fitness and insulin sensitivity during lifestyle intervention. J. Clin. Endocrinol. Metab. **92**(5), 1827–1833 (2007)

23. Bae, J.S., Kang, B.Y., Lee, K.O., Lee, S.T.: Genetic variation in the renin-angiotensin system and response to endurance training. Med. Princ. Pract. **16**(2), 142–146 (2007)

24. Clarkson, P.M., Devaney, J.M., et al.: ACTN3 genotype is associated with increases in muscle strength in response to resistance training in women. J. Appl. Physiol. **99**(1), 154–163 (2005)

25. Posthumus, M., September, A.V., O'Cuinneagain, D., van der Merwe, W., Schwellnus, M.P., Collins, M.: The association between the COL12A1 gene and anterior cruciate ligament ruptures. Br. J. Sports Med. **44**(16), 1160–1165 (2010)

26. Stepien-Slodkowska, M., et al.: Overrepresentation of the COL3A1 AA genotype in Polish skiers with anterior cruciate ligament injury. Biol. Sport **32**(2), 143–147 (2015)

27. Posthumus, M., et al.: Genetic risk factors for anterior cruciate ligament ruptures: COL1A1 gene variant. Br. J. Sports Med. **43**(5), 352–356 (2009)

Research on Evaluation Method of TCM Intervention Technology for Obesity Based on Literature

Feng Lin[1], Shusong Mao[2], and Dan Xie[1(✉)] iD

[1] Hubei University of Chinese Medicine, Wuhan 430065, China
dinaxie@hbtcm.edu.cn
[2] Hubei Provincial Hospital of Traditional Chinese Medicine,
Wuhan 430062, China

Abstract. Traditional Chinese Medicine (TCM) for weight loss is a personalized medical treatment which is widely used and effective at present. The evaluation of TCM intervention technology for different obesity grades can provide a basis for optimizing treatment schedule. This study retrieved and selected 640 literatures about the treatment of simple obesity with Body Mass Index (BMI) information from 1980 to 2016. Through literature research, expert consultation, mathematical statistics, and machine learning, from the perspective of single intervention technology and intervention technology combination, the evaluation index system of single intervention technology based on literature and the evaluation method of intervention technology combination were established. Empirical study takes overweight patients (BMI 25–26) in obesity grade as an example. Single intervention technology evaluation found that the comprehensive top-ranking TCM intervention technology is "acupuncture, catgut embedding, electro-acupuncture and ear acupoint". Intervention technology combination evaluation found that the most commonly used TCM intervention techniques were "electro-acupuncture and acupuncture", "ear acupoint and acupuncture", "ear acupoint and electro-acupuncture", "ear acupoint, electro-acupuncture and ear acupuncture", and "acupuncture and catgut embedding". The conclusion was in line with clinical practice, thus confirming the rationality of the method. The establishment of this method provides a powerful reference for the clinical selection of appropriate TCM intervention technologies for obesity.

Keywords: Evaluation method · Intervention technology · Obesity

1 Introduction

Traditional Chinese medicine for weight loss is a medical means to help obese patients reduce excessive fat and weight through acupuncture, massage, TCM intervention technology under the guidance of TCM theory, and ultimately improve the health level of obese patients. In recent years, TCM for weight loss has achieved gratifying clinical results as a medical method with definite curative effect. In clinic, there are many kinds of TCM intervention techniques for obesity, and different levels of obesity patients

H. Wang et al. (Eds.): HIS 2019, LNCS 11837, pp. 287–297, 2019.
https://doi.org/10.1007/978-3-030-32962-4_26

have different intervention techniques. Therefore, it is necessary to find out different TCM intervention techniques for different obesity levels. Establishing a scientific and reasonable evaluation index system of obesity grading intervention technology is of great significance to the selection of appropriate intervention technology [1]. This study intends to analyze the clinical research results of obesity TCM intervention technology from the perspective of literature, and construct the evaluation system of obesity TCM intervention technology, in order to determine the intervention technology suitable for different obesity grades from many intervention technologies. In the course of treatment, many kinds of intervention techniques are often used, so machine learning method is used to find the combination laws of intervention techniques in order to make a powerful supplement to the evaluation of intervention techniques.

2   Intervention Technology Evaluation Method

2.1   Establishment Process

Through literature research and expert consultation, the project team analyzed the intervention techniques in the existing literature. Considering whether intervention technology has its own characteristics or combination characteristics, intervention technology evaluation is divided into two categories: intervention technology evaluation and combination evaluation of intervention technology. The former refers to a single intervention technology, which is evaluated by establishing an evaluation indicator system, while the latter explores the relationship among the intervention techniques through a variety of machine learning techniques. Firstly, the relevant literature is searched according to keywords and conditions, and the scope of research is defined. Then the evaluation methods are determined from two dimensions. Finally, the evaluation results are summarized and refined to form an effective scheme. The specific construction process is shown in Fig. 1.

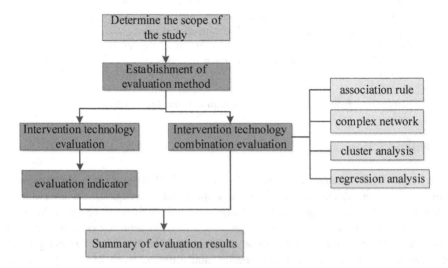

Fig. 1. Construction process of intervention technology evaluation method.

2.2   Research Methods

Different study objects adopt different research methods. For single intervention technology, its effectiveness can be assessed through the evaluation indicator system, while for combination evaluation of intervention techniques, machine learning technology is used to explore the combination law.

Construction Method of Intervention Technology Evaluation Indicator. Literature research and expert consultation are usually used to construct evaluation indicator. The operation steps are as follows:

- Draw up the framework of evaluation system through literature research and conference discussion.
- Optimize the evaluation indicators according to the expert consultation method.
- Validate and revise the evaluation indicator system in practice [2].

Methods of Combination Evaluation of Intervention Technology. In order to explore the relationship between various intervention techniques, there are many machine learning techniques that can be used. Through these methods, we can analyze and obtain frequently combined intervention techniques. In this paper, four methods which are widely used at present are adopted [3]:

- *Association Rule* is an important technique of machine learning, which reflects the interdependence and correlation between things. It is used to find the correlation between valuable data items from large-scale data sets.
- *Complex Network* refers to networks with small world, scale-free, self-organization, self-similarity and some or all attractors. They mainly describe the relationship between individuals and the collective behavior of the system.
- *Clustering Analysis* refers to the process of grouping the set of physical or abstract objects into multiple classes consisting of similar objects.
- *Regression Analysis* is a statistical analysis method to determine the quantitative relationship between variables.

2.3   Establishment of Evaluation Indicator

Through expert consultation, literature research and other methods, the project team initially established an evaluation system of intervention technology [4, 5]. The details are as follows (Table 1):

Table 1. Evaluation indicator of intervention technology.

Primary indicator	Secondary indicator	Description
Scientificity	Evidence classification	The scientific nature of the technical implementation scheme (see Table 2 for details)
Practicability	Total number of cases	Number of patients participating in clinical treatment in the literature
Medical technology level	Effectiveness	Average Effectiveness = Number of Effective Cases/Total Number of Cases
	Recommendation	Assessment by clinical experts is divided into complete recommendation, selective recommendation and non-recommendation
Social recognition	Number of literatures	Number of papers using this intervention technology
	Number of authoritative authors	Author (First Author) with outstanding performance in this field
	Classification of first author units	Unit level is divided into provincial, municipal and county levels
	Project classification	The projects are divided into national, provincial, ministerial, bureau, municipal and below levels

According to the research quality and reliability of the literature, the project team counted the evidence classification. The evidence classification basis is shown in Table 2 [6].

Table 2. The evidence classification basis.

Evidence classification	Description
Ia	Evidence body consisting of at least two different types of studies in four types of studies: randomized controlled trials, cohort studies, case-control studies and case series, and the effects of different research results are consistent
Ib	A single randomized controlled trial with sufficient certainty
IIa	Semi-randomized controlled trials or cohort studies
IIb	Case-control study
IIIa	Historically controlled case series
IIIb	Self-controlled case series
IV	Long-term widely used clinical case reports and historical records of treatment
V	Expert opinions and clinical experience that have not been systematically validated, and therapies that have not been widely used in clinical practice for a long time and documented in historical data

3 Case Study

This study used the above evaluation methods to conduct empirical research on TCM intervention technology for obesity. Firstly, we retrieve the relevant literatures of TCM treatment of obesity, extract and standardize the TCM intervention technology used in the literature, and determine the research object of intervention technology. The intervention technology was evaluated to determine whether the evaluation results were in accordance with the clinical practice, so as to verify the rationality of the evaluation method.

3.1 Data Sources

CNKI, Wanfang and VIP were used as data sources. The key words of retrieval literature were combined with "simple obesity" and "obesity" with "traditional Chinese medicine" respectively. The papers on the treatment of simple obesity by traditional Chinese medicine from 1980 to 2016 were searched.

Inclusion criteria: diagnosis is simple obesity; clinical research literature on the treatment of simple obesity with traditional Chinese medicine.

Exclusion criteria: literature containing secondary obesity; republished literature is taken only once; summary literature, popular science articles, animal experiment literature [7, 8].

According to the inclusion criteria and exclusion criteria, 1477 papers were obtained. The title, age, source of literature, first author, first author unit, intervention technology, evidence classification, recommendation, total number of cases, efficiency, BMI information were entered into Excel.

3.2 Data Preprocessing

Intervention techniques are classified to obtain uniformly described technical names.

- The names of multiple intervention techniques with the same meanings are grouped into one, for example, "acupuncture" and " acupuncture and moxibustion" are unified into "acupuncture".
- A variety of intervention techniques fall into one category, such as "aerobic exercise" and "running" are classified as "exercise".
- The same type of intervention technology can be classified into one category: all traditional Chinese medicine prescriptions are unified as "Chinese medicine herb"; all Chinese patent medicine are unified as " Chinese patent medicine"; all electronic instruments and equipment are unified as "instrument".

Through the classification principle, 21 types of intervention techniques were classified: acupuncture, exercise, diet, ear acupoint, catgut embedding, electro-acupuncture, Chinese medicine herb, western medicine, massage, cupping, instrument psychological intervention, health education, moxibustion, Chinese patent medicine, tea-based drink, acupoint application, medical supervision, scraping, sweat steaming, needle knife.

From the results of literature research, under the guidance of TCM experts and from the actual clinical situation, 10 commonly used TCM intervention techniques for obesity were screened out, which were divided into external treatment and internal treatment, including seven external treatment intervention techniques: acupuncture, catgut embedding, electro-acupuncture, ear acupoints, moxibustion, cupping, acupoint application, and three internal treatment intervention techniques: Chinese medicine herb, Chinese patent medicine, tea-based drink.

The diagnostic and therapeutic criteria for simple obesity, revised by the 5th National Academic Conference on Obesity in 1997, were adopted. According to Body Mass Index (BMI), obesity was classified into five grades: less than 25 as normal, 25–26 as overweight, 26–30 as mild obesity and 30–40 as moderate obesity and more than 40 as severe obesity. A total of 640 articles including BMI and 10 kinds of TCM intervention techniques were screened out, of which 369 were involved in the treatment of overweight patients.

3.3   Experiment and Analysis

Intervention Technology Evaluation. The intervention technology used in 369 literatures for overweight patients was comprehensively analyzed. The evaluation indicators of intervention technology were shown in Tables 3 and 4.

Table 3. "Scientificity, practicability and medical technology level" secondary evaluation indicators of TCM intervention techniques for overweight patients.

Intervention technique	Evidence classification					Total number of cases	Effectiveness (%)	Recommendation	
	Ib	IIa	IIb	IIIa	IIIb			Complete	Selective
Acupuncture	122	24	7	0	61	9486	90.48	125	89
Catgut embedding	58	9	0	0	25	3511	90.26	57	35
Electro-acupuncture	57	8	6	0	26	3781	88.76	59	38
Ear acupoint	33	4	5	1	39	3696	88.91	33	49
Moxibustion	6	2	0	0	4	492	88.62	6	6
Cupping	12	5	0	0	2	822	90.88	12	7
Acupoint application	7	0	0	0	1	80	97.5	7	1
Chinese medicine herb	31	1	0	1	13	1599	85.93	31	15
Chinese patent medicine	4	0	0	0	4	156	89.1	4	4
Tea-based drink	3	0	0	0	2	301	88.37	3	2

Table 4. "Social recognition" secondary evaluation indicators of TCM intervention techniques for overweight patients.

Intervention technique	Number of literatures	Number of authoritative authors	Classification of first author units			Project classification			
			Provincial level	Municipal level	County level	National level	Provincial and ministerial level	Bureau level	Municipal level and below
Acupuncture	214	9	129	83	2	9	6	17	9
Catgut embedding	92	1	52	38	2	2	5	9	4
Electro-acupuncture	97	5	63	33	1	5	5	5	2
Ear acupoint	82	2	42	37	3	5	2	4	2
Moxibustion	12	1	10	2	0	2	0	1	1
Cupping	19	1	7	12	0	0	0	3	4
Acupoint application	8	0	3	5	0	0	0	1	0
Chinese medicine herb	46	1	19	21	6	2	4	5	0
Chinese patent medicine	8	0	4	4	0	1	0	1	0
Tea-based drink	5	0	1	3	1	0	1	1	1

According to Table 3, it was found that in the scientific aspect of technical implementation, the evidence classification was mainly concentrated in Ib, mostly single randomized controlled trials, followed by IIIb, mostly self-control experiments. The top 5 intervention techniques with the number of cases are "acupuncture, electro-acupuncture, ear acupoint, catgut embedding and Chinese medicine herb". In the level of medical technology, the top 5 intervention techniques in terms of efficiency are "acupoint application, cupping, catgut embedding, Chinese patent medicine and acupuncture"; Most of the recommendations are "recommendation" opinions more than "selective recommendation" opinions, and there is no "non-recommendation".

It was found from Table 4 that the top five social recognition of intervention technology are "acupuncture, electro-acupuncture, catgut embedding, ear acupoint and Chinese medicine herb".

Combination Evaluation Method of Intervention Technology

Association Rule Analysis. We use the Apriori algorithm of Weka software to analyze the association rules. After many experiments, the minimum support(min_sup) is 1% and the minimum confidence(min_conf) is 60%. The frequent itemsets are shown in Table 5. The association rules are shown in Table 6.

From Table 5, the combinations of intervention techniques often used in overweight patients are frequent 2-item set: "electroacupuncture and acupuncture", "ear acupuncture and acupuncture", etc., and frequent 3-item set: "ears, electricity Needle and acupuncture, "electroacupuncture, acupuncture and embedding".

The greater the confidence of the association rule, the greater the probability that the latter appears when the former appears. The combinations of intervention techniques found in Table 6 includes "electroacupuncture, diet and acupuncture", "ear acupoints, instruments and acupuncture", "cupping, electroacupuncture and acupuncture".

Table 5. Frequent itemsets of intervention techniques for overweight patients. (min_sup = 1%, min_conf = 60%)

Frequent n-item sets	Intervention techniques name	Support (%)
n = 1	Acupuncture	57.99
	Electro-acupuncture	26.29
	Catgut embedding	24.93
	Ear acupoint	22.22
	Chinese medicine herb	12.47
	Catgut embedding	5.15
n = 2	Electro-acupuncture, acupuncture	21.68
	Ear acupoint, acupuncture	15.45
	Ear acupoint, electro-acupuncture	8.4
	Acupuncture, catgut embedding	4.61
	Electro-acupuncture, catgut embedding	4.07
	Cupping, acupuncture	3.25
n = 3	Ear acupoint, electro-acupuncture, acupuncture	6.78
	Electro-acupuncture, acupuncture, catgut embedding	2.71
	Ear acupoint, cupping, acupuncture	1.08
	Cupping, electro-acupuncture, acupuncture	1.08

Table 6. Association rules of intervention techniques for overweight patients. (min_sup = 1%, min_conf = 60%)

Association rules	Support (%)	Confidence (%)	Lift (%)
Electro-acupuncture, diet ==> acupuncture	1.9	100	1.72
Ear acupoint, instrument ==> acupuncture	1.08	100	1.72
Cupping, electro-acupuncture ==> acupuncture	1.08	100	1.72
Electro-acupuncture, exercise ==> acupuncture	1.63	85.71	1.48
Electro-acupuncture ==> acupuncture	21.68	82.47	1.42
Ear acupoint, electro-acupuncture ==> acupuncture	6.78	80.65	1.39

Complex Network Analysis. In order to show the correlation between intervention techniques, the number of times that two intervention techniques appear at the same time is taken as the weight. Gephi software is used to show the relationship between intervention technologies in a graphical way, as shown in Fig. 2. The thickness of the line represents the number of connections of the two nodes. The thickness of the connection between nodes represents the distance of their relationship. The color depth of the node represents the connection degree between nodes. The color of the node indicates how many nodes are associated with this node.

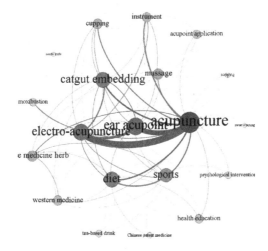

Fig. 2. Complex network diagram of intervention technique for overweight patients.

As can be seen from Fig. 2, the core intervention techniques for overweight patients are acupuncture, electro-acupuncture, ear acupoints, catgut embedding, diet, sports, and Chinese medicine herb.

Cluster Analysis. The k means algorithm provided by the Spss software is used to partition and cluster analysis, and different K values (K = 2, 3,..., 6) are set to obtain different classifications. The results are shown in Table 7.

Table 7. K means cluster analysis result of intervention techniques for overweight patients

K value	Cluster result
K = 2	Acupuncture; diet and exercise
K = 3	Acupuncture; catgut embedding; acupuncture, diet and exercise
K = 4	Electro-acupuncture, acupuncture; Chinese medicine herb; catgut embedding; acupuncture
K = 5	Acupuncture, instrument; catgut embedding; diet, exercise; acupuncture; electro-acupuncture, acupuncture
K = 6	Diet, catgut embedding, moxibustion; Chinese medicine herb, medicine; health education, diet, Chinese patent medicine, exercise; instrument, massage; ear acupoint, psychological intervention, exercise; cupping, electro-acupuncture, acupuncture, catgut embedding

From Table 7, we can see that the results of clustering with K = 5 are most satisfied with clinical experience. The clustering results of intervention techniques for overweight patients are "acupuncture and instrumentation", "catgut embedding", "diet and exercise", "acupuncture", "electro-acupuncture and acupuncture".

Regression Analysis. We use logistic regression analysis to obtain the combinatorial relationship between various intervention techniques and their weights, reflecting the therapeutic effect of each intervention technique. Intervention technology is an independent variable, while efficiency is a dependent variable. Then we set efficiency of less than 90% to 1 and efficiency of more than 90% to 2, which can be divided into two categories, and used the logistic regression algorithm provided by SPSS software to carry on the regression analysis, and found that the positively correlated TCM intervention techniques were "cupping, massage, catgut embedding, instrument and acupuncture".

4 Conclusion

In this study, an evaluation system of TCM intervention technology for obesity was constructed, including four first-level indicators and eight second-level indicators. So the case study about overweight patients were evaluated from four aspects: scientificity, practicability, medical technology level and social recognition. It was found that the top 4 TCM intervention techniques were "acupuncture, catgut embedding, electro-acupuncture and ear acupoint". The common machine learning methods (association rules, complex networks, clustering and regression analysis) were used to find the combination laws of intervention technologies. It was found that the top 5 combination laws were "electro-acupuncture and acupuncture", "ear acupoint and acupuncture", "ear acupoint and electro-acupuncture", "ear acupoint, electro-acupuncture and acupuncture", and "acupuncture and catgut embedding". The evaluation method proposed in this study can guide clinical doctors and nurses to choose appropriate intervention technology. However, there are still some short-comings in this study, mainly as follows: firstly, the English literature databases such as PubMed should be included in the search scope because of the small amount of literature; secondly, the evaluation indicators of intervention technology has some limitations and needs to be further expanded; thirdly, the more suitable machine learning methods should be selected for the intervention technology combination.

Acknowledgements. This study was supported by the Key Scientific Research Project of Hubei Province Department of Education. (No. D20172003)

References

1. Liu, R., Qin, Y., Zhou, L., Li, Q.: Study on the evaluation method of suitability of earthquake emergency medical technology. Med. J. of Chin. People's Lib. Army **36**(06), 669–670 (2011)
2. Chen, L., Liu, G., Luo, C., Zhao, X.: Establishment and application of evaluation index system for new clinical technique. Chin. Hosp. Manage. **30**(09), 12–13 (2010)
3. Wu, D., Zhang, X., Gan, Y., Yu, S.: Application of data mining algorithms in traditional Chinese medicine research. China Pharm. **29**(19), 2717–2722 (2018)
4. Zhou, Y., Ma, W., Zhou, Z.: Establishment of comprehensive evaluation index system for special medical technique. Hosp. Adm. J. Chin. People's Lib. Army **2008**(09), 871–873 (2008)

5. Huang, X., Zhong, W., Li, L., Lu, H., Huang, W.: Evaluation and application management mode for new clinical technologies. Mod. Hosp. **17**(11), 1590–1593 (2017)
6. Chen, W., Fang, S., Liu, J., Chen, K.: The introduction of evidence-based medicine classification system in China and the challenges it faces in the field of traditional Chinese medicine. Chin. J. Integr. Tradit. W. Med. **37**(11), 1285–1288 (2017)
7. Chen, X., Huang, W., Hu, F., Jin, Y., Hong, Z., Zhou, Z.: Regularity of acupoint selection for simple obesity treated by acupoint catgut embedding based on complex network technology. Acupunct. Res. **43**(09), 585–590 (2018)
8. Chen, X., et al.: Prescription analysis of electroacupuncture for simple obesity based on complex network technique. Chin. Acupunct. Moxib. **38**(03), 331–336 (2018)

Bibliometrics Analysis of TCM Intervention Technology for Simple Obesity Patients

Ziqin Fei, Feng Lin, and Dan Xie$^{(\boxtimes)}$ (iD)

Hubei University of Chinese Medicine, Wuhan 430065, China
dinaxie@hbtcm.edu.cn

Abstract. The bibliometrics method is used to analyze the literature related to the treatment of simple obesity with Traditional Chinese Medicine (TCM), to understand the current situation and the development tendency of obesity intervention technology. From a variety of literature databases, the papers on the treatment of simple obesity by TCM from 1980 to 2016 are selected, and 640 papers are finally included. The papers are analyzed from six dimensions: time distribution, type of publication, distribution of authors and units, fund projects, titles and key words. According to the study, since 2001, the number of articles published has been steadily increasing; Beijing, Guangzhou and other first-tier cities have paid more attention to obesity, and some core research teams have formed; high-frequency keywords of intervention technology mainly include "acupuncture", "electro-acupuncture", "acupoint catgut embedding", "ear acupoint" and "cupping". The results show that the research of TCM intervention technology for obesity is in the rapid development stage with broad application prospects. This paper can provide reference for clinical practice of TCM treatment of obesity.

Keywords: Bibliometrics · TCM intervention technology · Simple obesity

1 Introduction

In recent years, with the continuous improvement of people's living standards and the change of diet structure, as well as the formation of various bad habits and environmental factors, the overweight and obesity rates in China have been rising. From 1992 to 2015, the overweight rate has risen from 13% to 30%, and the obesity rate has risen from 3% to 12%. Simple obesity [1] is the most common type of obesity, accounting for about 95% of the obese population. Bibliometrics is a cross-science that uses statistical methods to quantitatively analyze knowledge carriers. It is often used in current situation investigations and the development tendency research. In this study, the literature of traditional Chinese medicine in the treatment of simple obesity is analyzed by Bibliometrics, hoping to explore the current situation and development tendency of TCM intervention technology in the treatment of simple obesity, and provide reference for future research.

© Springer Nature Switzerland AG 2019
H. Wang et al. (Eds.): HIS 2019, LNCS 11837, pp. 298–305, 2019.
https://doi.org/10.1007/978-3-030-32962-4_27

2   Materials and Methods

2.1   Literature Search

Based on the data sources of CNKI, Wanfang and VIP, the keywords of Chinese retrieval literature combine "Traditional Chinese Medicine" with "simple obesity" and "obesity" respectively, and the papers on the treatment of simple obesity by TCM from 1987 to 2016 are searched [2].

2.2   Data Acquisition

Criteria for Inclusion and Exclusion of Literature. The diagnostic and therapeutic criteria for simple obesity, revised by the 5th National Academic Conference on Obesity in 1997, were adopted. According to Body Mass Index (BMI), obesity was classified into five grades: less than 25 as normal, 25–26 as overweight, 26–30 as mild obesity and 30–40 as moderate obesity and more than 40 as severe obesity. This criterion is used to select documents.

Inclusion criteria: simple obesity is diagnosed clearly; treatment methods include literature on ten kinds of TCM intervention techniques: acupuncture, catgut embedding, electro-acupuncture, ear acupoint, moxibustion, cupping, acupoint application, Chinese medicine Herb, Chinese patent medicine and tea drinking; The BMI (Body Mass Index) index [3] is clearly given in the literature.

Exclusion criteria: repeated literature is selected only once; literature on secondary obesity is included [4]; review literature, popular science literature, and animal experimental research literature are selected.

Literature Screening. According to the criteria of inclusion and exclusion, 640 literatures are obtained. The title, source, publication time, author, author unit, key words and fund items of each document are extracted.

2.3   Data Analysis Method

This paper uses Excel conventional statistical analysis technology to analyze the time distribution, Journal distribution, author and unit distribution, fund distribution, etc. CiteSpace [5] software is used for collaborative network analysis and keyword co-occurrence analysis. In order to discover the research hotspot of weight loss in traditional Chinese medicine, the word cloud map technology was used to construct the word cloud map of literature title.

3   Results

3.1   Time Distribution

The amount of publications is an important index to measure a scientific research activity, and the time distribution of literature reflects the development process of this research. From the number of literatures, when the subjects start, reach their peak and mature can be seen. The statistics of this paper are from 1987 to 2016. The time distribution of the literature is shown in Fig. 1.

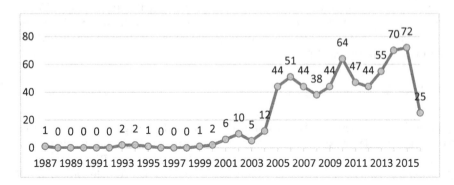

Fig. 1. Trends in literature publication from 1987 to 2016.

Figure 1 shows that the period from 1987 to 2000 is the initial stage in this field, and only 9 papers have been published in 13 years. The period from 2001 to 2016 is the development stage in this field, especially after 2004, there has been an explosive growth, which has been in a stable growth state. It can be seen that the growth of national economic level has triggered great concern about obesity, and the TCM intervention technology for obesity patients has gradually attracted the attention of researchers.

3.2   Type Distribution of Publications

Literatures obtained in this study are strictly screened by doctors according to inclusion and exclusion criteria. There are three types of journals retrieved: journals, dissertations and conference papers. Among 640 papers, 544 papers are published in journals, accounting for 85% of the total literature; 89 dissertations, accounting for 14% of the total literature; and 7 conference papers, accounting for 1% of the total literature. Most of the literature selected in this research comes from journals, which shows that journals have asserted great influence on the research and development of this field. In the course of the research, it is found that many research results of dissertations have been published in journals.

3.3   Author and Unit Distribution

First Author. According to the distribution of the first authors and their units, 592 authors published papers by the first authors. Most of them only published one paper, totaling 553, 32 authors published two papers, 5 authors published three papers, and 2 authors published four papers. Authors and organizations who have published three or more papers are listed in Table 1.

Table 1. High-yielding first author and its unit

ID	Author	Unit	Number of papers
1	Kong Yueqing	Third Affiliated Hospital of Henan Luohe Medical College	4
2	Zhang Zhongcheng	Second Clinical Medical College of Guangzhou University of Traditional Chinese Medicine	4
3	Guan Zhenmin	People's Hospital of Baoan District, Shenzhen City, Guangdong Province	3
4	Lei Yue	Shenzhen Fourth People's Hospital	3
5	Liu Peng	Xiyuan Hospital, Shiyan City, Hubei Province	3
6	Tan Guangxing	People's Hospital of Gaoming District, Foshan City, Guangdong Province	3
7	Wang Lili	Xinjiang Medical University	3

Authoritative Author. Authoritative authors refer to groups with strong influence in a certain field. According to statistics, there are 21 authoritative authors in these literatures. The most representative ones are Li Yuehua, director of the National Medical Center for Middle-aged and Elderly Diseases, Lu Yonghui, director of the Acupuncture and Moxibustion Society of Traditional Chinese Medicine, and Li Chunsheng, deputy director of the Society of Geriatrics, Beijing Branch of the Chinese Medical Association. They have great influence in this field, making the research results of this subject more authoritative and persuasive.

Research Team. In order to study the scale of development of existing research teams in intervention technology, CiteSpace is used to analyze the cooperative network of the first author. The results are shown in Fig. 2.

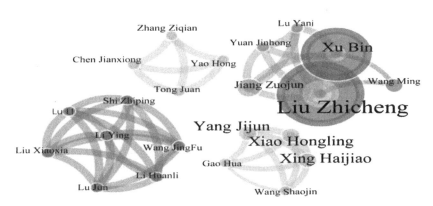

Fig. 2. Analysis of the first author's cooperative network.

Using CiteSpace to analyze the author's collaborative network can show the author's relationship more intuitively. The size and chromatogram of the nodes represent the frequency and duration of the author's writing, respectively. The warmer the nodes are, the later the author's publication time is, and the thicker the connection is, the higher the degree of cooperation of the author is. According to the graph, several large-scale research groups have been formed in this field, the largest of which is represented by Liu Zhicheng. He has published 15 articles and worked in the laboratory of Nanjing University of Traditional Chinese Medicine. Related project funding numbers are 30873307, 39970923, 30873307, 39970929. This research team has played a great role in promoting the development of TCM intervention technology for obesity patients. The result about the research team shows that TCM intervention technology for obesity patients has received some attention, which will play an extremely significant role in the in-depth study of the TCM intervention technology for obesity patients.

3.4   Fund Project Distribution

The number of fund papers in a certain field is an important criterion for evaluating the scientific research ability and level of research groups. To a certain extent, the number of fund papers can reflect the attention and development tendency of this field. According to the statistics of fund distribution in this part of the literature, a total of 123 fund projects are involved, including 14 national funds, 31 provincial and ministerial funds, 32 department and bureau-level funds, 46 municipal funds. Among them, there are three state-level fund projects, four provincial and ministerial fund projects, and eight department-level fund projects which have published two or more papers, as shown in Table 2.

Table 2. Number of articles issued by fund projects.

Fund projects level	Fund projects name	Number of papers
National level	National Natural Science Foundation (30873307)	16
	National Science Fund subsidized project (39970923)	2
	National Natural Science Foundation funded project (39770929)	2
Provincial level	Guangdong Science and Technology Plan Funding Project (2010B030700033)	3
	Hebei Provincial Science and Technology Department Support Project (08276101D-95)	2
	Guangdong Province Social Development and Science and Technology Research Project (2006B35601014)	2
	Guangdong Natural Science Fund Project (020782)	2

(*continued*)

Table 2. (*continued*)

Fund projects level	Fund projects name	Number of papers
Bureau level	Hebei Provincial Administration of Traditional Chinese Medicine Science and Technology Research Project Funded Project (2007028)	4
	Funded Project of Outstanding Science and Technology Innovation Team of Blue and Blue Engineering of Colleges and Universities in Jiangsu Province	3
	Jiangsu Province Featured Advantages Funding Project	3
	Guangdong Provincial Bureau of Traditional Chinese Medicine (2009184)	2
	Henan Provincial Department of Education 2012 Henan Province Higher Education Youth Key Teachers Funding Project (2012GGJS-270)	2
	Jiangsu Provincial Traditional Chinese Medicine Bureau Science and Technology Project (LZ11111)	2
	Shanghai Key Discipline Construction Funding Project (T0302)	2
	Capital Chinese Medicine Research Project (14ZY13)	2

From Table 2, we can see that there are more articles published in national projects, followed by provincial, ministerial and bureau levels, which shows that the state pays more attention to the research of the TCM intervention technology for obesity patients. The main funds come from developed areas such as Guangdong and Jiangsu. It can be seen that the fund support for this study in underdeveloped areas is slightly inadequate.

3.5   Analysis of Literature Title with Word Cloud

"Word cloud" is to visually highlight the "keywords" which appear frequently in the text, to form a "keyword cloud" or "keyword rendering", to extract a large amount of text information, and to quickly grasp the theme of the text [6]. The project team construct word clouds for 640 titles of literatures in order to discover the research hotspots of weight loss in traditional Chinese medicine. In order to show the intervention technology more clearly, the dictionary of intervention technology and the dictionary of stop words are constructed, and the cloud is used as the background to draw the word clouds, as shown in Fig. 3.

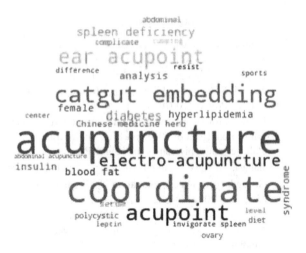

Fig. 3. Word cloud map of literature title

From Fig. 3, we can find that "acupuncture", "catgut embedding" and "electro-acupuncture" is the dominant intervention technology in the literature.

3.6   Analysis of Key Words in Literature

Using CiteSpace for keyword co-occurrence network analysis can show the relationship between keywords more intuitively. The results of keyword analysis are shown in Fig. 4.

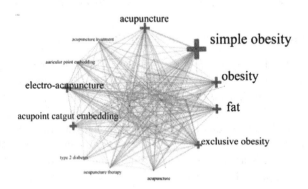

Fig. 4. Keyword clustering analysis diagram (Color figure online)

In Fig. 4, the size and chromatogram of nodes represent the frequency and duration of keyword occurrence, respectively. The warmer the color (e.g. red) is, the later the time occurs, and the thicker the connection is, the higher the degree of co-occurrence between keywords is. From Fig. 4, as the intervention technology is concerned, the color of "acupoint catgut embedding" is orange, the color of "acupuncture", "auricular point embedding" and "electro-acupuncture" is light green. It can be seen that "acupoint catgut embedding" is used earlier, and "acupuncture", "auricular point embedding" and "electro-acupuncture" are used later.

4 Discussion

In this paper, Bibliometrics is used to visualize the TCM intervention techniques for obesity patients in recent 30 years. The results show that from the perspective of the time distribution, the publication volume of literatures in this field has been growing steadily in recent years, and now it is at the development stage. The author predicts that the research of TCM intervention technology for obesity patients will start a research upsurge with the development of the economy. At present, most of the literature in this field comes from journals, which shows that journals play an important role in the development of this field. Researchers mainly come from universities and hospitals. There are fewer basic-level researchers and fewer authoritative authors, but some considerable research teams have been formed. The support degree of the national fund is high, but the input of the local fund is biased towards the developed areas, so the amount of publications in the developed areas is high. According to the key words, the ten intervention techniques such as "catgut embedding", "acupuncture", "ear acupoint" and "electro-acupuncture" are widely used. The conditions for the screening of literature are stringent, including not only TCM intervention technology, but also the BMI level. The number of documents that meeting the inclusion criteria is limited. At present, there is no literature research on the TCM intervention technology of obesity, so this paper has a high reference value for the research group concerned about the TCM intervention technology of obesity patients.

Acknowledgements. This study was supported by the Health Commission of Hubei Province Guiding Project (#WJ2019F185).

References

1. Luo, C., Sun, Y.: Advances in research of traditional Chinese medicine in treating simple obesity. Mod. J. Integr. Tradit. Chin. West. Med. **19**(31), 3482–3484 (2010)
2. Chen, X., et al.: Prescription analysis of electroacupuncture for simple obesity based on complex network technique. Chin. Acupunct. Moxib. **38**(03), 331–336 (2018)
3. Wen, X., Chen, Y., Lan, G., et al.: Consistency between self-evaluation of body weight and BMI category among senior high school students in Nanchang city. Chinese public health, pp. 1–5
4. Guo, L., Zhang, C.: Advances in studies on the effects of galanin receptor 1 and endurance exercise on secondary obesity in patients with metabolic syndrome. J. Gannan Med. Coll. **38**(08), 839–842 (2018)
5. Shi, L., Zhou, J., Mao, Z., et al.: Global health hotspots and frontier analysis based on CiteSpace. Mod. Prev. Med. **46**(10), 1801–1805 + 1810 (2019)
6. Li, X.: Research status of infant sports literature in core periodicals in recent five years based on word cloud analysis. Sports **2014**(05), 79–81 (2014)

Ways for Enhancing the Substance in Consumer-Targeted eHealth

Marjo Rissanen[✉]

Aalto University School of Science, Espoo, Finland
mkrissan@gmail.com

Abstract. The purpose of health consumer–targeted digital information chan-nels is to enhance the knowledge levels of consumers and patients, and thus, increase the intensity of care. Medical information content as a knowledge entity forms the essence, the substance of these systems, and all the other development work should be constructed around the content. Despite broad efforts, recent evidence shows that refinement is needed in the design of information systems in this core area, as well as in its assessment. In addition to tools for evaluating the quality of information, there is a continuing need for design strategies that produce better information quality. Values and their constant evaluation also have an important role in producing high-quality information.

Keywords: Medical knowledge content · Translational design · Consumer targeted e-Health

1 Introduction

In the eHealth sector, consumer-targeted information systems still contain many problems regarding the quality of the medical information content. Information content is the substance layer of such digital services. The accuracy and reliability levels of medical and health-related information, thus, describe the essential quality value of systems. Health care organizations, companies, and national institutions are constantly developing more customized tools for offering medically oriented information to their consumers, as well as aids for evaluating webpages. The purpose is to enhance the intensity of care with the aid of these tools and systems. Enhancing the knowledge level of health consumers can improve service users' abilities to evaluate the quality of their care episodes, and also courage consumers to seek "second opinions" in uncer-tain situations. This brings more balance for communication, and thus, transparency for the health care system. Understanding the meaning of such aims and values affect designers' motivations, and can encourage consumers to use these services. In addition to quality tools for information evaluation, there is a need for practical guidelines and strategies for offering medical information to consumers, with enhanced clarity in problem areas observed in design practice.

© Springer Nature Switzerland AG 2019
H. Wang et al. (Eds.): HIS 2019, LNCS 11837, pp. 306–317, 2019.
https://doi.org/10.1007/978-3-030-32962-4_28

2 Methods

The design scheme in IT typically contains the following key cycles [1]: relevance (requirements, testing), design (processes in design and evaluation), and rigor (knowledge base, theories, and additional sources). The rigor cycle connects the design science activities with the knowledge base, experience, expertise, and creative insights [1]. Accurate medical information content, supporting guidelines and strategies for its enhancement, form part of the knowledge base in contextual design. Medical knowledge content as a large theoretical layer also regulates artifact design. In the design-based research agenda, researchers and designers together analyze problems in practice, make proposals and recommendations for solving the problem, and validate models with tests and iterative cycles for principles in design practice [2]. Thus, a Design-Based Research-framed solution phase contains such principles that can guide the design.

This research considers common problems in the medical core area and available evaluative instruments which represent a partial solution today for the prevailing problems. In this research, examples of guidelines for such interventions which can help control problems observed in this area are presented. The information quality dilemma is also considered more broadly, which helps designers internalize that a quality tools check means assessing the basics, which should be in order. This study highlights that evaluation of information quality (IQ) means, in addition to quality instruments, strategies, creative insights, and value re-framing. This study illuminates this quality dilemma with the following research questions: (1) What kinds of critical problems in medical knowledge content do we face in current consumer-targeted eHealth? (2) What kinds of practical interventions could enhance the situation in the critical problem areas in design practice? (3) What role do values and creative insights have in the scheme for evaluating the quality of the information?

3 Substance as a Translational Design Challenge

Translational design in eHealth targets production strategies which take into account interaction, interoperability, and service synergy requirements [3]. The design of IT artifacts brings together ethical, economic, social, and organizational issues [4], and this also concerns quality thinking in eHealth design. The purpose of patient-targeted medical information is enhanced interaction, and thus, better outcomes. Knowledge translation represents processes ranging from learning to actually using such knowledge in different circumstances [5]. Socially responsible design refers to designers' influence on product and service design [6] as part of "design argumentation" [7]. Content design in eHealth means an area where ethical aspects and social responsibility have a profound role. If medical knowledge content is somehow unclear, too limited, or non-satisfactory in its knowledge intensity, then the usability of the information channel is questionable. However, this does not mean that "aspects of design as indirect indicators of quality" [8, 9] are less important. Less successful design can also mean users lose interest, even if the core knowledge is good quality [10].

4 Quality of Digital Medical Information

4.1 Information Quality and Evaluation Instruments in eHealth

In eHealth, there are several concepts, frameworks, and tools for assessing the quality of the information. In the absence of a general standard for online information quality in eHealth, existing quality tools are utilized as the basis for criteria development [11]. Some evaluative instruments focus on information content, and some on content and aspects of design. These tools differ in aims while concentrating on a specific disease, clinical practice guidelines, health research reports, or online medical information in general, and they serve health professionals, researchers, providers, designers, and health service consumers.

As the core indicators for evaluating information quality are considered aspects like accuracy, completeness, currency, and lack of bias [8]. Indirect proxy indicators for information quality include aspects as readability, design, and disclosures [8, 9]. A model for high-quality data of electronic health records has three categories (information, communication, and security), and sub-categories [12]. Subcategories for information are aspects of accuracy, completeness, consistency, relevance, timeliness, usability, communication contains provenance and interpretability, and security focuses on aspects of privacy and confidentiality [12]. A tool for assessing the quality of mobile apps [13] contains the main areas of engagement, functionality, aesthetics, information, and subjective quality. In this tool, the information category includes the following aspects: accuracy of the app description, goals, quality of the information, quantity of information, visual information, credibility, and evidence base [13]. Robillard et al. [11] developed the Quality Evaluation Scoring Tool (QUEST) for assessing online health information which integrates the strengths of existing popular tools, and contains items such as attribution, currency, authorship, tone (appearance of limitations and contrasting findings), complementarity, and conflicts of interests. In the comparison [11], the authors used widely used criteria-based tools, such as the Health Website Evaluation Tool (HONcode), Sandvik criteria, and the DISCERN instrument, which focuses on the quality of the treatment information. QUEST tool serves especially health consumers, researchers, clinicians, and providers [11]. Health Literacy INDEX [14] is a tool that can be used as a checklist for developers in assessment of health information materials. It contains [14] the areas of plain language, clear purpose, supporting graphics, user involvement, skill-based learning, audience appropriateness, user instruction, development details, evaluation methods, and strength of evidence. It is remarked [11] that quality evaluation tools for online health information will not always work as standalone artifacts, and thus, additional work is required to determine how these tools can best be used to complement health communication strategies. In comparisons it is noticed [15] fair agreement among most instruments even if quality instruments differ in the range of items assessed. Robillard et al. [11] also remarked that the quality criteria across available tools often overlap.

4.2   Realizing the Current Quality Problems of Medical Information

Incorrect, incomplete, or superficial content of health-related websites cause harm for users [16]. Diagnosis level consideration shows problems in many areas. In the heart disease area, producing independent and reliable content, providing regular content updates, and generating patient-tailored content for self-care and adherence present challenges [17]. A sample of ten mobile apps targeted for cancer education were evaluated using 22 criteria, and six of the ten selected apps were rated poor or insufficient [18]. The information connected to cancer-related physical activity, and sedentary behavior on leading cancer websites is of variable quality and accuracy [19]. The majority of patient information on the Internet regarding shoulder arthritis is of mixed quality, without comprehensive sources [20]. Web-based information on stoma disorders has varying content, and the quality of the authorship and information sources remains often unclear [21]. Most websites targeted for self-management support for people with persistent pain, lack cultural tailoring, or have limited or no evidence of clinical efficacy [22], and apps providing information on pain management strategies lack evidence of results for people with persistent pain [23]. In research that covered 36 pain management apps, problems such as a lack of clinician and end-user involvement in app development were demonstrated [24]. Available online patient education materials related to opioid management are written above the recommended reading level [25]. Online information on breast biopsy lesions requiring surgery is too complex for the general public [26]. The results highlight great variability in the quality in health information specifically for tinnitus on the Internet [27]. Popular websites on overactive bladder are low quality, giving potentially biased information on the topic [28].

In social media, an analysis showed that data from 18 publically available Facebook pages hosted by parents of children with leukemia showed that 19% of all cancer information exchanged was not medically accurate, and 14% described unproven treatment modalities [29]. Studies on the use and implications of YouTube for healthcare communication are in the preliminary phase and there is a need for design interventions that enable consumers to assimilate the posted information [30]. The views of elderly end users are often overlooked in design of health-related tools and websites. [31]. Current knowledge on creating interfaces for elderly people is not well applied within mobile health application designs and thus suitable usability assessment methods are needed in this area [32]. Partnering with consumers seems to be challenging, in particular, at the strategic level [33]. Understandability and usability tools have been developed for health-related material, but they have limitations, and have often been tested on a narrow number of health issues [34].

In summary, in the eHealth evaluation literature the problems regarding the delivery of quality medical information are related to problems involving information accuracy, readability, problems in the knowledge intensity offered (too complicated vs. too superficial content), poor testing (and thus, missing evidence of clinical efficacy), lack of clinician and end-user involvement in development, missing design guidelines in interface design for older people, and missing transparency of the information sources.

4.3   Noticing Target Groups in Danger of Too Low Care Intensity Levels

Non-justified low-level care intensity represents always non-professional care intensity [35], and may increase the rate of complications, referrals, and mortality. In design, attention should be paid to target groups that have problems in reaching the professional intensity level of care. Elderly patients, in particular, face possibilities of underdiagnosis or undertreatment. Asthma [36, 37], osteoporosis [38], pelvic insufficiency fractures [39], chronic obstructive pulmonary disease [40], obstructive sleep apnea [41], neuro-muscular diseases, such as myasthenia gravis [42], and hyperparathyroidism [43] are only a few examples of such phenomena. "Elderly patients do not always receive standard surgery for solid tumors, because they are considered unfit for treatments as a consequence of inaccurate estimation of the operative risk" [e.g., 44]. In aortic valve replacements (AVRs), risk-benefit ratios should be better evaluated, and guidelines should be refined among elderly patients with severe aortic stenosis [45]. Patient refusal has seldom been mentioned for denial of AVR, and this is likely to be influence by the responsible doctor [45]. A cooperative evaluation with the patient is needed to assess whether patients' physical condition or advanced age is a real obstacle for intense and efficient care procedures. In interface design, cognition skills, physical activity, and possible motivational barriers for older adults must be taken into account [32].

5   Ways to Support the Substance

5.1   Focus on the Essence (the Medical Core)

What substance knowledge in the medical and health-related context is important for health service users? Knowledge needs can be many, and typically, information systems for consumers as a whole cover a wide area of different components reaching out to many kinds of home services, differently organized other service concepts, etc. Medical records may be connected to certain service concepts, and therefore, can also form one part of the information entity. Core medical knowledge areas, and those general supporting areas that are deeply connected to medical and health-related information, cover the following areas, which are presented in Fig. 1:

- Information connected to a disease or medical problem, e.g., diabetes, or blood pressure, or heart diseases, their care options and prevention.
- Information connected to a treatment: operations, anesthesia, and demanding investigations in different specialty areas and their care options.
- Information connected to complication risks of treatments but also to possible disadvantages of conservative care options, including statistics and patient case examples.
- Information connected to use of services, accessibility, continuity of care, or pre- and post-operative procedures.
- Links to pharmaceutical core knowledge.
- Glossary for all medical terms and a channel for frequently asked questions (FAQ).

Support areas for the medical core can be seen as the following key areas: information connected to laboratory, radiology, scanning, or other investigations and connected analysis, paramedical services (such as physiotherapy, psychology, nutrition, other therapists, connected social services or patient representative services), or other support agencies, tools for self-health management, educational and supportive parts, such as guidelines, feedback, questions, and contact forums, etc. (The role of medication is linked to the subject but it needs a separate analysis).

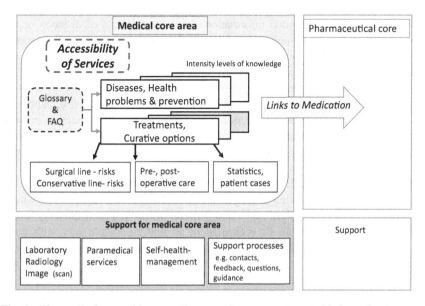

Fig. 1. The medical core with supportive areas in customer-targeted information systems.

5.2   More Clarity with Knowledge Intensity Levels

Users' frustrations are typically connected to such issues as the information is too superficial and incomplete or too detailed, difficult or complicated information content, or missing clarity or logic in presentation. A possibility to select a suitable knowledge intensity level, thus, may mean better customer and product quality in this area. At least two optional levels are recommendable: a basic information level (the compact option) and a specific level with wider specifications. In some sub-areas, a wider professional, demanding level might be included. Connecting advisory text can help users in selecting the right knowledge intensity level. Optional intensity levels are recommendable in the parts of information systems that form the hard medical core (basic knowledge of diseases, treatments, and their care options) (see Fig. 1, medical core area). Textbooks for students often present key facts in a separate box before the detailed presentation. In principle, the same idea streamlined could work in this context.

Compact level of information; low knowledge intensity level. The compact approach could contain most of the basic knowledge of the selected topic. Typically, all users start from this level, including more knowledgeable and professional users, because learning is more convenient if the basics are mastered first. This means the "be aware" point. For the designer, the compact level requires the ability to filter the knowledge amount efficiently in such a way that the essence remains. Producing this level means the most challenging information level in view of design. Minimalism in content design means "more skilled developers with greater development efforts" [46]. All necessary information (the so-called "key facts") must be compressed in a way that is understandable for all kinds of users.

The specific level of information (the deep knowledge intensity level) includes the basic picture, but contains all such key details that might come into question. This level typically contains more detailed information about mechanisms of diseases or treatments, treatment options, complication risks, medicines, and statistical information for different age groups. This knowledge intensity level is specific enough for most users. However, a deeper professional type of intensity level might be useful in very knowledge-intensive sub-areas.

Professional information (the sophisticated knowledge intensity level), in principle, contains nearly the same basic information that doctors need in their practice, presented in understandable, plain language. Doctors have background information and understanding according to their specialty areas, and naturally, the purpose is not to gather all this information to be presented. Producing sophisticated information for patients' use is not problematic, if specific medical language and difficult terms are clarified. This level is needed by those who already know much about the area, those who are professionals, or those who want know and learn all details at a deep intensity level. In addition, versatile entities can be presented in an understandable way with needed specifications, if enough resources are used for these design processes. In practice, the task of producing advanced medical text without using medical terms is demanding. An attached medical glossary expands the subject in certain cases, and therefore, is a recommendable aid for readers. However, a sophisticated presentation includes aspects that are less understandable. It is recommendable that language experts evaluate the final version, and its readability.

These systems are often very self-directive, and therefore, advisory parts (guidelines for use) are often seen as unnecessary. Despite the functional self-directness of systems, guidelines can decrease frustrations. FAQ sections are standard in information channels, and are recommendable in medically oriented phases.

5.3   More Accuracy with Enhanced Self-evaluation

Attribution and accuracy tasks refer to the evidence base and reliability of the information [47], and the connected medical expertise. In eHealth design projects, medical expertise is needed typically from the core medical areas, but possibly also from the assisting medical sub-areas. In many situations, medical treatments are performed in an area of expertise, but additional information about connective medical sub-areas would support understanding. In addition, care in the recovery section, complications or post-operative care may contain information from other areas of specialty, e.g., infection medicine, nutrition, physiotherapy etc. Case-based evaluation is needed in assessing the needed width of the offered presentation. Often, projects represent only a certain medical specialty area, and team members typically evaluate their work contribution in many ways. However, in addition to a chosen project team of health professionals, it is recommendable that the project has auditive medical experts, or sub-specialists who should evaluate substance and its transparency in the final iteration rounds. The second opinion assessment round helps regardless in maturation purposes. In any case, applications are evaluated by several experts when tools are used, but possible observations do not always reach designers.

5.4 Transparency with Enhanced Balance and More Versatile Information

Accuracy is also connected to balanced information. Treatments, for example, surgical operations or demanding investigations, typically have their own specifications which should be fulfilled, if certain treatments can be recommended for a patient, and patients, typically, are commonly and openly informed about these risks. However, even conservative care options may have risks, such as possible shorter life expectancy, sometimes even lower quality of life, etc. Inaccurate estimations of operative risks and careless turning to conservative care options may also mean a non-professional care intensity level. Health care consumers should also be informed of the risks and problems of conservative care options, especially in care for the elderly. Balanced information for care choices encourages patients to take a more active role in their care and decision making when it comes to preferable cure options. Available data on patient outcomes for different treatments, as well as patient experiences of optional care alternatives, should be openly available (hospital-based and general information about treatments, complications, etc., in different age groups). The concept of best practices must be clarified not only for health professionals but also for consumers.

5.5 More Equity with Observation of Groups with Intensity Risks

In design policy, more attention is needed for patients who are in danger of receiving care that has too low intensity levels, such as elderly individuals. Knowledge intensity levels should be selectable, but likewise, presentation modes should, in certain cases, be selectable because of individual differences. For the elderly, information should also be available in audio and video formats. Such options would lower the motivational barriers to utilization of information systems. Thoughtfully designed minimalism in eHealth [48], especially, is a theme that is valuable for interface design for the elderly.

5.6 Space for Innovations with Creative Insights

The knowledge base in the DBR cycle contains different theories, methods, expertise, experience, and meta-artifacts [1]. However, creative insights as inspirational sources are also needed [1, 49]. Creative insights are also necessary in producing high-quality products. This kind of touch is also needed in quality evaluation. Such consideration contains questions such as the following: What can be done more efficiently? What kinds of new approaches could more efficiently help end-users? How could different types of users be supported more precisely? This type of attitude and questioning is needed so that applications and tools can advance more efficiently.

5.7   Toward Sophistication with an Awareness of Values

Prevailing values dictate what is worth presenting, and what knowledge is useful and needed by consumers. The mission refers to the target grouping, audience, and clarity of the meaning and goals of a tool, but the mission also describes values. For example, how are groups in danger of care that has too low intensity observed and taken into account in design, and how are their abilities observed in the media selections? Health care consumers' understanding of medical information in enough specificity makes the interaction more flexible, and increases the equity and transparency in patient–doctor interaction. Internalization of this fact and values is certainly a motivational factor for designers.

6   Discussion and Conclusions

Today, there are many information quality instruments which aid end-users, healthcare professionals, researchers, and designers in evaluating quality aspects, and there is also continuing development in this area. These tools help designers check that the basics are in order. However, in addition to these evaluation aids for information quality, there is a constant need for strategies and design practices that help designers produce more trustable and functional medical core content. This research presented selected examples of ideas that could enhance the current situation by improving the accuracy, readability, and transparency in customer-targeted medical information.

Discovering useful innovations means that the connected value basis needs constant re-evaluation. Trusting only evaluation toolkits may easily lead to too mechanistic assessment procedures; profound self-evaluation may suffer, and very new views are easily forgotten, which makes evaluation work less useful. Designers' skills in constructing and evaluating the artifact mean more rigorous design [1]. Designers need versatile understanding of all the aspects that helps produce high-quality information systems. In translational design aspirations, the question is also about thinking, attitudes, and their re-evaluation. If designers recognize this critical development area in their work, it aids in executing and integrating new function and thinking models to their work. It is emphasized [7] that designers should be "prepared for action" instead of being "guided in action" by a set of detailed prescriptive procedures. When the essential meaning of the medical core, and the connected design challenges, as a multifaceted theoretical knowledge and value frame area is internalized by designers, it can make them more prepared for action.

References

1. Hevner, A.R.: A three cycle view of design science research. Scand. J. Inf. Syst. **19**, 4 (2007)
2. Amiel, T., Reeves, T.C.: Design-based research and educational technology: rethinking technology and the research agenda. J. Educ. Technol. Soc. **11**, 29–40 (2008)
3. Machado, C.M., Rebholz-Schuhmann, D., Freitas, A.T., Couto, F.M.: The semantic web in translational medicine: current applications and future directions. Brief. Bioinform. **16**, 89–103 (2013)

4. Goes, P.B.: Design science research in top information systems journals. MIS Q.: Manage. Inf. Syst. **38**(1), iii–viii (2014)
5. Zidarov, D., Thomas, A., Poissant, L.: Knowledge translation in physical therapy: from theory to practice. Disabil. Rehabil. **35**, 1571–1577 (2013)
6. Koo, Y.: The role of designers in integrating societal value in the product and service development processes. Int. J. Des. **10**(2), 49–65 (2016)
7. Stolterman, E.: The nature of design practice and implications for interaction design research. Int. J. Des. **2**(1), 55–65 (2008)
8. Burkell, J.: Health information seals of approval: what do they signify? Inf. Commun. Soc. **7**, 491–509 (2004). https://doi.org/10.1080/1369118042000305610
9. Fahy, E., Hardikar, R., Fox, A., Mackay, S.: Quality of patient health information on the internet: reviewing a complete and evolving landscape. Australas. Med. J. **7**, 24–28 (2014)
10. Robins, D., Holmes, J.: Aesthetics and credibility in web site design. Inf. Process. Manage. **44**, 386–399 (2008). https://doi.org/10.1016/j.ipm.2007.02.003
11. Robillard, J.M., Jun, J.H., Lai, J.-A., Feng, T.L.: The QUEST for quality online health information: validation of a short quantitative tool. BMC Med. Inform. Decis. Making **18**, 87 (2018). https://doi.org/10.1186/s12911-018-0668-9
12. Almutiry, O., Wills, G., Alwabel, A., Crowder, R., Walters, R.: Toward a framework for data quality in cloud-based health information system. In: International Conference on Information Society (i-Society 2013), pp. 153–157. IEEE (2013)
13. Stoyanov, S.R., Hides, L., Kavanagh, D.J., Zelenko, O., Tjondronegoro, D., Mani, M.: Mobile app rating scale: a new tool for assessing the quality of health mobile apps. JMIR mHealth uHealth **3**, e27 (2015). https://doi.org/10.2196/mhealth.3422
14. Kaphingst, K.A., Kreuter, M.W., Casey, C., et al.: Health literacy INDEX: development, reliability, and validity of a new tool for evaluating the health literacy demands of health information materials. J. Health Commun. **17**, 203–221 (2012). https://doi.org/10.1080/10810730.2012.712612
15. Breckons, M., Jones, R., Morris, J., Richardson, J.: What do evaluation instruments tell us about the quality of complementary medicine information on the internet? J. Med. Internet Res. **10**, e3 (2008). https://doi.org/10.2196/jmir.9
16. Zhang, Y., Sun, Y., Xie, B.: Quality of health information for consumers on the web: a systematic review of indicators, criteria, tools, and evaluation results. J. Assoc. Inf. Sci. Technol. **66**, 2071–2084 (2015)
17. Rosselló, X., Stanbury, M., Beeri, R., Kirchhof, P., Casadei, B., Kotecha, D.: Digital Learning and the Future Cardiologist. Oxford University Press, Oxford (2019)
18. Böhme, C., von Osthoff, M.B., Frey, K., Hübner, J.: Development of a rating tool for mobile cancer apps: information analysis and formal and content-related evaluation of selected cancer apps. J. Cancer Educ. **34**, 105–110 (2019)
19. Buote, R.D., Collins, R.H., Shepherd, J.H., McGowan, E.L.: Evaluation of the accuracy and availability of cancer-related physical activity and sedentary behaviour information on English-language websites. J. Psychosoc. Oncol. **36**, 754–767 (2018)
20. Somerson, J.S., Bois, A.J., Jeng, J., Bohsali, K.I., Hinchey, J.W., Wirth, M.A.: Quality of internet-based decision aids for shoulder arthritis: what are patients reading? BMC Musculoskelet. Disord. **19**, 112 (2018). https://doi.org/10.1186/s12891-018-2018-6
21. Connelly, T.M., Khan, M.S., Alzamzami, M., Cooke, F.: An evaluation of the quality and content of web-based stoma information. Colorectal. Dis. **21**, 349–356 (2019)
22. Devan, H., et al.: Do pain management websites foster self-management support for people with persistent pain? a scoping review. Patient Educ. Couns. (2019). https://doi.org/10.1016/j.pec.2019.04.009

23. Devan, H., Farmery, D., Peebles, L., Grainger, R.: Evaluation of self-management support functions in apps for people with persistent pain: systematic review. JMIR mHealth uHealth. **7**, e13080 (2019)

24. Zhao, P., Yoo, I., Lancey, R., Varghese, E.: Mobile applications for pain management: an app analysis for clinical usage. BMC Med. Inform. Decis. Making **19**, 106 (2019)

25. Kumar, G., Jaremko, K.M., Kou, A., Howard, S.K., Harrison, T.K., Mariano, E.R.: Quality of patient education materials on safe opioid management in the acute perioperative period: what do patients find online? Pain Med. (2019). https://doi.org/10.1093/pm/pny296

26. Miles, R.C., Baird, G.L., Choi, P., Falomo, E., Dibble, E.H., Garg, M.: Readability of online patient educational materials related to breast lesions requiring surgery. Radiology **291**(1), 112–118 (2019)

27. Manchaiah, V., Dockens, A.L., Flagge, A., et al.: Quality and readability of English-language internet information for tinnitus. J. Am. Acad. Audiol. **30**(1), 31–40 (2019)

28. Clancy, A.A., et al.: Patient-targeted websites on overactive bladder: what are our patients reading? Neurourol. Urodyn. **37**, 832–841 (2018)

29. Gage-Bouchard, E.A., LaValley, S., Warunek, M., Beaupin, L.K., Mollica, M.: Is cancer information exchanged on social media scientifically accurate? J. Cancer Educ. **33**, 1328–1332 (2018)

30. Madathil, K.C., Rivera-Rodriguez, A.J., Greenstein, J.S., Gramopadhye, A.K.: Healthcare information on youtube: a systematic review. Health Inform. J. **21**, 173–194 (2015)

31. Nguyen, M.H., et al.: Optimising eHealth tools for older patients: collaborative redesign of a hospital website. Eur. J. Cancer care **28**, e12882 (2019)

32. Wildenbos, G.A., Jaspers, M.W.M., Schijven, M.P., Dusseljee-Peute, L.W.: Mobile health for older adult patients: using an aging barriers framework to classify usability problems. Int. J. Med. Inform. **124**, 68–77 (2019)

33. Farmer, J., Bigby, C., Davis, H., Carlisle, K., Kenny, A., Huysmans, R.: The state of health services partnering with consumers: evidence from an online survey of Australian health services. BMC Health Serv. Res. **18**, 628 (2018)

34. Beaunoyer, E., Arsenault, M., Lomanowska, A.M., Guitton, M.J.: Understanding online health information: evaluation, tools, and strategies. Patient Educ. Couns. **100**, 183–189 (2017)

35. Rissanen, M.: Intensity thinking as a shared challenge in consumer-targeted eHealth. In: Siuly, S., Lee, I., Huang, Z., Zhou, R., Wang, H., Xiang, W. (eds.) HIS 2018. LNCS, vol. 11148, pp. 183–192. Springer, Cham (2018). https://doi.org/10.1007/978-3-030-01078-2_17

36. Hwang, E.-K., et al.: The predictors of poorly controlled asthma in elderly. Allergy, Asthma Immunol. Res. **4**, 270–276 (2012)

37. Dunn, R.M., Busse, P.J., Wechsler, M.E.: Asthma in the elderly and late-onset adult asthma. Allergy **73**, 284–294 (2018)

38. Ostergaard, P.J., Hall, M.J., Rozental, T.D.: Considerations in the treatment of osteoporotic distal radius fractures in elderly patients. Curr. Rev. Musculoskelet. Med. **12**, 50–56 (2019)

39. García, F.J.S., Estrada, J.A.D.H., Johnson, H.M.D.: Pelvic insufficiency: underdiagnosed condition, therapeutic diagnostic review. Coluna/Columna **17**, 151–154 (2018)

40. Stellefson, M.L., et al.: Web-based health information seeking and eHealth literacy among patients living with chronic obstructive pulmonary disease (COPD). Health Commun. **33**, 1410–1424 (2018)

41. Zeineddine, S., Chowdhuri, S.: Apnea in elderly. Curr. Sleep Med. Rep. **5**, 13–22 (2019)

42. Aragonès, J.M., Altimiras, J., Molist, N., Roura, P., Amblàs-Novellas, J.: Under-diagnosis of neuromuscular diseases in patients of 80 years and older. Revista espanola de geriatria y gerontologia (2018)

43. Dombrowsky, A., Borg, B., Xie, R., Kirklin, J.K., Chen, H., Balentine, C.J.: Why is hyperparathyroidism underdiagnosed and undertreated in older adults? Clin. Med. Insights: Endocrinol. Diabetes **11**, 1179551418815916 (2018)

44. Audisio, R.A.: Shall we operate? preoperative assessment in elderly cancer patients (PACE) can help a SIOG surgical task force prospective study. Crit. Rev. Oncol. Hematol. **65**(2), 156–163 (2008)

45. Iung, B., Cachier, A., Baron, G., et al.: Decision-making in elderly patients with severe aortic stenosis: why are so many denied surgery? Eur. Heart J. **26**, 2714–2720 (2005)

46. Carroll, J.M., Van Der Meij, H.: Ten misconceptions about minimalism. IEEE Trans. Prof. Commun. **39**, 72–86 (1996)

47. El Sherif, R., Pluye, P., Thoër, C., Rodriguez, C.: Reducing negative outcomes of online consumer health information: qualitative interpretive study with clinicians, librarians, and consumers. J. Med. Internet Res. **20**, e169 (2018). https://doi.org/10.2196/jmir.9326

48. Rissanen, M.: "Machine Beauty" – should it inspire eHealth designers? In: Zhang, Y., et al. (eds.) HIS 2014. LNCS, vol. 8423, pp. 1–11. Springer, Cham (2014). https://doi.org/10.1007/978-3-319-06269-3_1

49. Csikszentmihalyi, M.: Flow and the Psychology of Discovery and Invention, vol. 39. Harper Perennial, New York (1997)

Author Index

Printed in the United States
By Bookmasters